AF316791

Oral Modified Release Drug Delivery Systems

Oral Modified Release Drug Delivery Systems

Piush Khare

Mohini Chaurasia

Sarvesh K. Paliwal

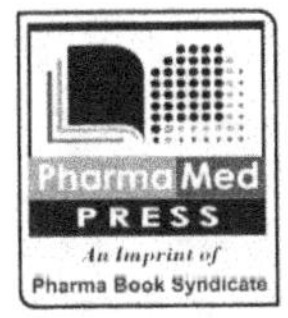

PharmaMed Press

An imprint of Pharma Book Syndicate

A unit of BSP Books Pvt. Ltd.

4-4-309/316, Giriraj Lane,

Sultan Bazar, Hyderabad - 500 095.

Oral Modified Release Drug Delivery Systems
by *Piush Khare, Mohini Chaurasia and Sarvesh K. Paliwal*

© 2018, *by Publisher,* All rights reserved.

No part of this book or parts thereof may be reproduced, stored in a retrieval system or transmitted in any language or by any means, electronic, mechanical, photocopying, recording or otherwise without the prior written permission of the publishers.

Published by

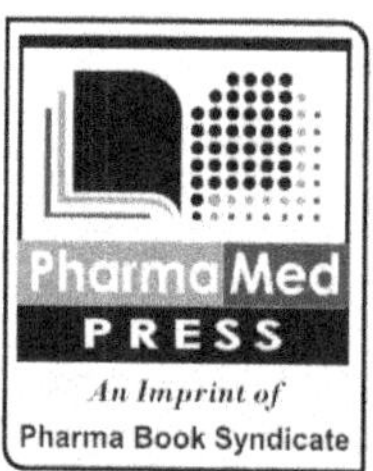

PharmaMed Press
An imprint of Pharma Book Syndicate
A unit of BSP Books Pvt. Ltd.
4-4-309/316, Giriraj Lane, Sultan Bazar, Hyderabad - 500 095.
Phone: 040-23445600, 23445688; Fax: 91+40-23445611
E-mail: info@pharmamedpress.com
www.pharmamedpress.com/pharmamedpress.net

ISBN: 978-93-87593-14-5 (Hardbound)

Preface

In the era of the advancement and technology when majority of the tributaries of science are being marked by developments. The present book was conceptualized in order to bridge the gap between the conventional and the novel frontier of the pharmaceutical science specifically the formulation science. It is well known that the ideology has been shifted towards the development of the novel carriers however since most of the developed novel systems are finding place in the market on yet mass scale, the present priorities of the pharmaceutical niche also seems to be on development modified release delivery systems which may either be amalgam of novel and conventional system or may be full-fledged novel. These are leap ahead from the conventional dosage forms. Needless to say that oral delivery has been most lucrative and still finds the most palatable and convenient mode for the administration of the drug. For decades scientists have played with the drug properties and modified the conventional systems in order to achieve oral delivery for therapeutic cause. The most fascinating fact about the oral delivery is that all forms of the dosage forms and delivery systems are amenable for oral delivery ranging from the conventional to novel systems. Although there has been availability of wide range of the dosage forms which even today lead the market and many have been designed to cater for specific need along with the enormous amount of research put into, there still remain unexplored facets of the oral delivery. This specifically was the thought process which instigated our minds to conceptualize the book.

We are well aware of the fact that there are numerous articles and literature available for one to refer but we feel that all the material especially related to the oral modified release systems and related advancements in oral delivery is scattered and the book in present form is an effort to bring maximum available information in form of different topics under one roof for the convenience of the reader. Sections have been drafted in order that they cover maximum facts spanning from the basic principles to high end advancement introduced till now. This in turn make the book suitable not only for the students at graduate and post graduate level to read in order to accomplish basic learning as per syllabus but also to the research students who can refer the compilation in order to have better insight for their research.

The chapters have been carefully drafted in order to provide the basic understanding of the facts in very precise and simplified manner.

Contributors have tried their level best to design the chapters to deliver the content directly to the mind-set of the reader in a very meek language. Chapters have been designed based on discrete topics which cover almost all the vistas of the oral delivery. Efforts have been levied to provide each chapter with exhaustive learning with possible examples for better understanding. Flow charts, tables, self-explanatory diagrams and schemes, wherever possible have been embedded in the chapters for quick reference. Moreover stress has been laid to interlink the theoretical principles to the practical examples in order to bridge the gap which generally exists.

Finally we believe that the book will cater to the needs of the students, formulation scientists and research scholars and will serve as comprehensive database as well quick reference for their study and research.

Piush Khare
Mohini Chaurasia
Sarvesh K. Paliwal

Acknowledgement

The book as you find in its present shape is a product of many reactions which took place between the ideas and thoughts of different people. On the occasion of the release of book we would like to extend our sincere thanks to all those who have made this project a reality. To begin with we would like to express our deepest sense of gratitude to the authors whose dedicated and diligent efforts with quality input in form of informative chapters paved the path for completion of the present compilation. They really worked hard and supported us at any moment from the conception to end. Constant encouragement and constructive criticism received from our mentors played a significant role in bringing the book in its final form. Thanks are due to the team which assisted in designing, proof reading, preparation of content and constant support in many miscellaneous works. In no ways their efforts can be undermined.

We are highly indebted to the family members who sacrificed their quality time and at the same moment encouraged us in this venture.

Thanks to BSP Books Pvt. Ltd. and their team for introducing the book and transforming it into readable format.

Piush Khare
Mohini Chaurasia
Sarvesh K. Paliwal

List of Contributors

Ankit Jain, Sri Aurobindo Institute of Pharmacy SAIMS Campus, Indore-Ujjain Highway, Indore-453 111, India.

Arvind Gulbake, Centre for Interdisciplinary Research, D.Y. Patil University, Kolhapur-416 003, Maharashtra, India.

Ashish Parashar, School of Pharmacy & Technology Management, NMIMS, SHIRPUR Campus, Dhule-425 405 Maharashtra, India.

Giriraj T. Kulkarni, School of Pharmacy, ITM University, Gwalior-474 001, India.

Jaya Gopal Meher, Pharmaceutics Division, CSIR-Central Drug Research Institute, Lucknow-226 031, India.

Kamlendra Bhadoriya, School of Pharmacy, ITM University, AH-43, Bypass, Jhansi Road, Gwalior-475 001, India.

Kanika Dhote, Truba Institute of Pharmacy, Karond - Gandhi Nagar Bypass Road, Bhopal-462 038, India.

M.S. Sudheesh, Faculty of Pharmacy, VNS Group of Institutions, Neelbud, Bhopal-462 044, India.

Manish K. Chourasia, Pharmaceutics Division, CSIR-Central Drug Research Institute, Lucknow-226 031, India.

Mohini Chaurasia, Amity Institute of Pharmacy, Amity University, Lucknow-226 028, India.

Nitin K. Jain, Department of Biotechnology, Ministry of Science & Technology, New Delhi-400 003, India.

Pankaj K. Singh, Pharmaceutics Division, CSIR-Central Drug Research Institute, Lucknow-226 031, India.

Piush Khare, Eiman Pharma Pvt Limited, 1/1 Palm Road, Shipra Sun City (Gaziabad), National Capital Region, 201 014, India.

Pramod Kumar, School of Life Sciences, The University of Nottingham, Nottingham, U.K. NG7 2RD.

Prashant Khare, Baylor Institute for Immunology Research, Dallas, TX-75204, USA.

Priya Singh Kushwaha, Babasaheb Bhimrao Ambedkar University, Lucknow-226 025, India.

Punit Bhatnagar, Rishiraj College of Pharmacy, Behind SAIMS Campus, Indore-Ujjain Highway, Indore-453 331, India.

Rajendra Awasthi, Department of Pharmaceutics, Laureate Institute of Pharmacy, Kathog, Kangra-177 101, India.

S. K. Paliwal, Department of Pharmaceutical Sciences, Banasthali University, Banasthali-304 022, India.

Sharad P. Pandey, Truba Institute of Pharmacy, Karond - Gandhi Nagar Bypass Road, Bhopal-462 038, India.

Tripti Shukla, School of Pharmacy, Peoples University, Bhanpur Bypass Road, Bhopal- 462 037, India.

Vandana Soni, Department of Pharmaceutical Sciences, Dr. H.S Gour Central University, Sagar-470 003, India.

Vinod Dhote, Truba Institute of Pharmacy, Karond - Gandhi Nagar Bypass Road, Bhopal-462 038, India.

Vivek K. Pawar, Pharmaceutics Division, CSIR-Central Drug Research Institute, Lucknow-226 031, India.

About the Editors

Piush Khare is B.Pharm (2002), M.Pharm (2004) and Ph.D (2011) from Department of Pharmaceutical Sciences, Dr H.S. Gour University-Sagar. He has to his credit 19 publicationsand 02 book chapters in journals and books of repute. He is recipient of outstanding oral presentation award at International Conference of Biomedical Engineering-Singapore in the year 2008. He has more than 10 years of research and teaching experience and has guided more than 14 students for their research/dissertation work at postgraduate (M.Pharm) level. His research interests include controlled and targeted drug delivery including approaches for oral drug delivery.

Mohini Chaurasia (M. Pharm, PhD) is working as Assistant Professor in Amity Institute of Pharmacy, Amity University, Lucknow. She has been involved in the drug delivery research since last one decade and published her research work in various reputed scientific journals. As an academician she has more than 12 years of experience in teaching pharmaceutical sciences to graduate and post graduate students. In her teaching carrier she has guided more than 30 post graduate students for research work. Her experience is well reflected in this book in fulfilling the actual need for students pursuing pharmaceutical education in India.

Prof. Sarvesh K. Paliwal obtained his Bachelor's degree in Pharmacy from JSS, College of Pharmacy, Ooty, Master's degree in Medicinal & Pharmaceutical Chemistry from RGPV, Bhopal and PhD degree in Pharmaceutical Chemistry from Banasthali University, Rajasthan. Presently he is Professor and Head, Department of Pharmacy, Banasthali University, Rajasthan. He has published more than 100 research papers in International/National journals of repute. One of his most significant and recent publication is in *Nature-Scientific Reports (September 2015)*. He has obtained research projects worth Rs 150 Lacs from Indian Council of Medical Research, DST-CURIE, Centre of Excellence for Training and Research in Frontier Areas of Science and Technology (FAST). He has been bestowed with "Award for excellence in research" by European Institute of Scientific Research, Netherlands. More than ten research scholars have been awarded PhD degree under his direct supervision. He has delivered many key note Lectures in International/National Conferences. At present he is convener Indian Science Congress Association, Banasthali Chapter and also Life member of Indian Science Congress. He is member of Board of Studies, Faculty of Life Sciences and Academic Council of Banasthali University.

Contents

Preface .... (v)

Acknowledgement.. (vii)

List of Contributors .... (ix)

About the Editors .... (xi)

Chapter 1   Controlled Release and
Gastroretentive Drug Delivery Systems

Rajendra Awasthi, Vivek K. Pawar and Giriraj T. Kulkarni

1.1 Diffusion 2

    1.1.1 Fick's First Law of Diffusion..................... 2

    1.1.2 Fick's Second Law of Diffusion 3

1.2 Designing of Diffusion Controlled Matrix 3

    1.2.1 Classification of Diffusion Controlled
Drug Delivery Systems 6

    1.2.2 Reservoir Diffusion Systems 6

    1.2.3 Matrix Diffusion Systems 9

    1.2.4 Factors Affecting Drug Release
Rate from Monolithic Matrix Systems...... 10

1.3 Designing of Dissolution Controlled Matrix 11

1.4 Kinetic Modeling on Drug Release from
Diffusion and Dissolution Controlled Drug
Delivery Systems 13

    1.4.1 Zero Order Model 13

    1.4.2 First Order Model 14

    1.4.3 Higuchi Model 15

    1.4.4 Peppas' Model 16

    1.4.5 Krosmayer Peppas Model 16

    1.4.6 Hixson Crowell's Model............................ 17

    1.4.7 Selection of the Best Fit Model for
Release Data... 17

1.5 Design and Fabrication of Gastroretentive
     Dosage Forms 18
     1.5.1 Gastrointestinal Motility 19
     1.5.2 Factors Affecting Gastric Retention 20
     1.5.3 Formulation Approaches........................... 21
     1.5.4 High Density Systems............................... 21
     1.5.5 Swelling and Expandable Systems 21
     1.5.6 Mucoadhesive or Bioadhesive Systems.... 22
     1.5.7 Superporous Hydrogel based Systems...... 22
     1.5.8 Magnetic Systems 23
     1.5.9 Floating Drug Delivery Systems............... 24
            1.5.9. 1 Classification of Floating Drug
                       Delivery Systems...................... 24
            1.5.9.2 Effervescent Systems................. 24
            1.5.9.3 Non-Effervescent Systems 25
            1.5.9.4 Hydrodynamically Balanced
                       Systems..................................... 25
            1.5.9.5 Low-Density Systems................ 25
            1.5.9.6 Raft Forming Systems 25
     1.5.10 Advanced Technologies used to
             Develop Gastroretentive Systems 27
            1.5.10.1 Intragastric Floating
                        Gastrointestinal Drug
                        Delivery Systems...................... 27
            1.5.10.2 Inflatable Gastrointestinal
                        Drug Delivery Devices 28
            1.5.10.3 Intragastric Osmotically
                        Controlled Floating Drug
                        Delivery Devices 28
     1.5.11 Evaluation of Gastroretentive
             Drug Delivery Systems 30
            1.5.11.1 *In vitro* Evaluation.................... 31
            1.5.11.2 *In vivo* Evaluation.................... 32
     1.5.12 Future Recommendations 33
References.. 33

Chapter 2 Self-Emulsifying Drug Delivery Systems:
A Novel Drug Delivery Model

*Jaya Gopal Meher, M. Chaurasia, S. K. Paliwal and
Manish K. Chourasia*

2.1 Introduction.. 38

2.2 Excipients.. 41

    2.2.1 Oils.. 41

    2.2.2 Surfactants.. 42

    2.2.3 Co-solvents/Co-surfactants 45

    2.2.4 Pharmaceutical Additives 46

2.3 Formulation and Development 46

2.4 Factors Affecting Formulation and
Performance of SEDDS 53

    2.4.1 Excipients.. 53

    2.4.2 Physicochemical State of SEDDS and
Intended Dosage Form 55

2.5 Characterization 57

    2.5.1 Self-emulsification Efficiency 57

    2.5.2 Zeta Potential 57

    2.5.3 Size and Size Distribution................. 58

    2.5.4 Morphology.. 58

    2.5.5 Drug Content..................................... 59

    2.5.6 *In vitro* Drug Dissolution and
Ex Vivo Drug Permeation........................ 59

    2.5.7 *In vivo* Bio-Distribution 60

    2.5.8 Stability... 60

2.6 Fate of SEDDS *In vivo*.......................... 61

2.7 Safety and Toxicological Issues............ 63

2.8 Applications of SEDDS 64

2.9 Commercial SEDDS 69

2.10 Future Prospects and Challenges 70

References 73

Chapter 3   Colon Specific Drug Delivery Systems

Arvind Gulbake, Pramod Kumar, Prashant Khare and Nitin K. Jain

3.1   Introduction 78

3.2   Anatomy and Physiology of
       Gastro Intesitinal Tract 79

       3.2.1   The Stomach 79

       3.2.2   The Small Intestine 79

       3.2.3   The Large Intestine 80

3.3   Important Factors Considered for
       Colonic Drug Delivery 81

       3.3.1   Gastric Emptying 82

       3.3.2   Small Intestinal Transit 82

       3.3.3   Colonic Transit 82

       3.3.4   Gastrointestinal pH 83

       3.3.5   Colonic Microflora 83

       3.3.6   Disease state of Large Intestine 84

3.4   Drug Candidates for Colon Specific
       Drug Delivery 85

3.5   Formulation Approaches for Colon
       Specific Drug Delivery 85

       3.5.1   Timed Release/Delayed Release
               Dosage Forms 86

       3.5.2   Osmotic Controlled Drug Delivery 87

       3.5.3   pH Dependent Systems: Enteric Coating .. 89

               3.5.3.1 CODES^{TM} 92

       3.5.4   Prodrug Based Systems 93

       3.5.5   Pressure Based Drug Delivery Systems 94

       3.5.6   Microbial Triggered Approach 94

       3.5.7   Commensal Bacteria 95

       3.5.8   Hydrogel 96

       3.5.9   Redox-Sensitive Polymers 98

3.6   Colon Specific Polymeric Carrier Systems 98

       3.6.1   Biodegradable Polysaccharide Carriers 99

3.6.2 Microspheres based Systems 100

3.6.3 Nanoparticle based Systems.............. 101

3.6.4 Ligand Anchored Polymeric
Nanoparticles 102

3.7 Conslusion 103

References 104

Chapter 4   Targeting of Bioactives to Peyer's Patches

Piush Khare, Mohini Chaurasia, Prashant Khare,
S. K. Paliwal, Nitin K. Jain and Manish K. Chourasia

4.1 Introduction.. 108

4.1.1 Small Intestine 109

4.1.2 Peyer's Patches 110

4.1.3 M-Cells 112

4.2 Targeting of Therapeutics to Peyer's Patches...... 113

4.2.1 Uptake of Particles through
Peyer's Patch................................ 116

4.2.1.1 Size of the Micro/
Nanoparticles...................... 118

4.2.1.2 Species Difference and
Number of Peyer's Patches...... 119

4.2.1.3 Hydrophillic/Hydrophobic
Nature of the Microparticles.... 120

4.2.1.4 Type of Polymer...................... 120

4.2.1.5 Influence of Co-administered
Agents.................................. 120

4.2.1.6 Fluid Volume and Osmotic
Parameters 121

4.3 Role of Peyer's Patches in Design and
Development of Oral Vaccines.......................... 121

4.4 Targeting Strategies 124

4.4.1 Lectin Mediated Targeting.................... 124

4.4.2 Antibody Mediated Targeting................. 126

4.4.3 Other Targeting Ligands 126

4.5 Evaluation of the Uptake of Particles 127

    4.5.1 Microscopic Methods 128

    4.5.2 Electron Microscopy 128

    4.5.3 Fluorescent Activated Cell Sorter 129

    4.5.4 Radioactivity and Fluorometry 129

4.6 Models for Assessment of Uptake 129

4.7 Conclusion and Future Prospects 130

References 131

Chapter 5   Drug Delivery Systems based on Multiple Emulsions

Vinod K. Dhote, Kanika Dhote, Piush Khare and
Sharad P. Pandey

5.1 Introduction 137

    5.1.1 Multiple Emulsions 138

5.2 Formulation Considerations 139

    5.2.1 Pharmaceutical Oils 139

    5.2.2 Pharmaceutical Emulsifiers 140

    5.2.3 Surface Active Agents 140

    5.2.4 Preservatives 141

    5.2.5 Antioxidants and Humectants 141

5.3 Formulation of Multiple Emulsions 142

    5.3.1 Double Emulsification Technique (Two Step Technique) 143

    5.3.2 Phase Inversion Technique 144

    5.3.3 Membrane Emulsification Technique 145

5.4 Instability in Multiple Emulsions 145

5.5 Multiple Emulsion Stability Testing 148

5.6 Drug Release Mechanism from Multiple Emulsions (Vaziri and Warburton, 1994) 149

    5.6.1 Diffusion Mechanism 150

    5.6.2 Facilitated Diffusion (Carrier-Mediated Transport) 150

    5.6.3 Thinning of the Oil Membrane 150

    5.6.4 Photo-Osmotic Transport 150

5.6.5   Rupture of Oil Phase 150

5.6.6   Solubilization of Internal Phase in the
         Oil Membrane 150

5.6.7   Micellar Transport 150

5.7   Application of Multiple Emulsions..................... 151

References.. 154

Chapter 6   Site Specific Oral Drug Delivery Systems

Pankaj K. Singh and Priya Singh Kushwaha

6.1   Introduction.. 157

6.2   Designing of Oral Mucosal
       Drug Delivery System 160

6.3   Buccal Tablets.. 161

6.3.1   Mucoadhesion 162

6.3.1.1   The Electronic Theory 163

6.3.1.2   The Adsorption Theory 163

6.3.1.3   The Wetting Theory................ 163

6.3.1.4   The Diffusion Theory 163

6.3.1.5   The Fracture Theory 163

6.3.2   Basic Components of Mucoadhesive
         Buccal Tablets and Patches..................... 164

6.3.2.1   Drug Substance....................... 164

6.3.2.2   Mucoadhesive Polymers.......... 164

6.3.2.3   Permeation Enhancers 166

6.3.2.4   Backing Membrane................. 167

6.3.3   Advantages of Buccal Tablets and
         Buccal Patches 167

6.3.4   Formulation of Mucoadhesive
         Buccal Tablet 168

6.3.5   Evaluation of Buccal Tablets 169

6.3.5.1   Weight Variation 169

6.3.5.2   Thickness 170

6.3.5.3   Hardness 170

6.3.5.4   Friability 170

6.3.5.5   Drug Content 170

6.3.5.6   Stability Studies...................... 170

6.4   Buccal Patches 171

    6.4.1   Method of Preparation 171

        6.4.1.1   Solvent Casting...................... 171

        6.4.1.2   Direct Milling 171

    6.4.2   Evaluation of Buccal Patches.................. 172

        6.4.2.1   Surface pH 172

        6.4.2.2   Thickness.................................. 173

        6.4.2.3   Swelling Index...................... 173

        6.4.2.4   Common Parameters for Evaluation of Buccal Tablets and Buccal Patches 173

6.5   Osmotic Tablet.................................... 176

    6.5.1   Osmosis and its Principal...................... 176

    6.5.2   Historical Aspects of Osmotic Pumps..... 177

    6.5.3   Advantages of Osmotic Tablets 179

    6.5.4   Disadvantages 180

    6.5.5   Components of Osmotic Tablets............. 180

        6.5.5.1   Drug... 180

        6.5.5.2   Osmotic Agent....................... 180

        6.5.5.3   Semipermeable Membrane...... 181

        6.5.5.4   Plasticizers.............................. 182

        6.5.5.5   Hydrophilic and Hydrophobic Polymers 182

        6.5.5.6   Wicking Agents 183

        6.5.5.7   Flux Regulators...................... 183

    6.5.6   Classification of Osmotic Tablets........... 184

        6.5.6.1   Elementary Osmotic Pump...... 184

        6.5.6.2   Controlled Porosity Osmotic Pump 184

        6.5.6.3   Osmotic Bursting Osmotic Pump.. 185

6.5.6.4 Push Pull Osmotic Pump 185

6.5.6.5 Sandwich Osmotic Tablets 186

6.5.7 Marketed Osmotically Controlled Tablets 186

6.6 Pulsincap 187

6.6.1 Types of Pulsincaps 188

6.6.1.1 Osmosis Dependent Pulsincap... 189

6.6.1.2 Erodible or Rupturable Layer Dependent Pulsincap 189

6.6.1.3 Capsule Shell Dependent Pulsincap 190

6.6.1.4 pH Induced Pulsincap 190

6.6.1.5 Temperature Induced Pulsincap 190

6.6.1.6 Chemically Induced Pulsincap 190

6.6.1.7 Externally Induced Pulsincap .. 191

6.6.2 Evaluation of Pulsincap 191

6.6.2.1 Swelling Index 191

6.6.2.2 Lag Time and Drug Release 191

6.6.2.3 Water Uptake Study 191

6.6.2.4 Hardness 192

6.6.2.5 Thickness of Enteric Coated Layer 192

6.7 Lozenges 192

6.7.1 Classification of Lozenges 193

6.7.1.1 Medicated Lozenges 193

6.7.2 Commercially Available Lozenges 198

6.8 Medicated Chewing Gum 199

6.8.1 Advantages of MCG over Conventional Drug Delivery System 200

6.8.2 Disadvantages of MCG 200

6.8.3 Composition 201

6.8.4 Manufacturing and Evaluation................ 202

    6.8.4.1 Conventional/Traditional Method (Melting) 202

    6.8.4.2 Cooling, Grinding and Tableting Method 203

    6.8.4.3 Use of Directly Compressible Chewing Gum Excipients........ 204

6.8.5 Factors affecting Release of Active Ingredient 205

    6.8.5.1 Contact Time 205

    6.8.5.2 Physicochemical Properties of Active Ingredient................ 205

    6.8.5.3 Inter Individual Variability...... 206

    6.8.5.4 Composition of Gum Base 206

6.8.6 Evaluation of MCG................................ 206

    6.8.6.1 Uniformity of Mass (Weight Variation Test)........... 206

    6.8.6.2 Uniformity of Content 206

    6.8.6.3 *In-Vitro* Drug Release Study ... 207

6.8.7 Applications 208

6.8.8 Systemic Therapy.................................... 208

6.9 Egalet® Technology 209

6.9.1 Mechanism of Action.............................. 209

6.9.2 Manufacturing.. 210

    6.9.2.1 Egalet® Prolonged Release Tablets 212

    6.9.2.2 Egalet® Delayed Release 212

6.9.3 Factors Affecting Drug Release from Egalet® Tablets.................................. 213

    6.9.3.1 Erosion of Matrix.................... 213

    6.9.3.2 Agitation 214

    6.9.3.3 Surface Area of Tablet............. 214

    6.9.3.4 Immediate Release Layer (Lag Compartment) 214

6.10 Enterion Capsule Technology 215

    6.10.1 Discription of Technology 215

    6.10.2 Tracking the Enterion Capsule 217

    6.10.3 Application of the Technology 218

6.11 Hydrophilic Sandwich 218

References 219

Chapter 7   Coarse Dispersion

Sharad P. Pandey, Tripti Shukla, Vinod K. Dhote,
Kanika Dhote and Puneet Bhatnagar

7.1 Introduction 224

    7.1.1 Molecular Dispersion 224

    7.1.2 Colloidal Dispersion 225

    7.1.3 Coarse Dispersion 225

7.2 Fundamentals of Suspension System 227

    7.2.1 Advantages and Disadvantages of
        Suspension 227

    7.2.2 Properties of an Ideal Suspension 228

    7.2.3 Theoretical Consideration of Stable
        Formulation 228

    7.2.4 Particle Size and its Distribution 229

    7.2.5 Flocculated Suspensions 230

        7.2.5.1 Inter-Particle Collision 231

        7.2.5.2 Reduction of Electrical Charge .. 232

        7.2.5.3 Synthetic Bridging
               Flocculants 233

    7.2.6 Deflocculated Suspension 234

    7.2.7 Formulation of Stable Suspension 235

    7.2.8 Stability of a Suspension 238

        7.2.8.1 Chemical Stability 239

        7.2.8.2 Physical Stability 239

        7.2.8.3 Crystal Growth 239

7.2.9   Evaluation of Suspension 240

      7.2.9.1   Appearance 240

      7.2.9.2   Photomicroscopic Examination 240

      7.2.9.3   Organoleptic Properties (color, taste, odor) 240

      7.2.9.4   Sedimentation Rate, Volume, Resuspendability 241

      7.2.9.5   Viscosity 242

      7.2.9.6   pH Value 242

      7.2.9.7   Zeta Potential Measurement 242

      7.2.9.8   Freeze Thaw Cycling 243

      7.2.9.9   Drug Content Uniformity 244

      7.2.9.10   Dissolution Testing 244

7.3   Pharmaceutical Emulsions 245

      7.3.1   Advantages of Emulsions 246

      7.3.2   Theory of Emulsification 246

        7.3.2.1   Mono-Molecular Adsorption ... 247

        7.3.2.2   Multi-Molecular Adsorption 247

        7.3.2.3   Solid Particle Adsorption Theory 248

      7.3.3   Emulsion Type and Means of Detection ... 248

        7.3.3.1   Dilution Test 248

        7.3.3.2   Conductivity Test 249

        7.3.3.3   Dye-Solubility Test 249

        7.3.3.4   Fluorescence Test 250

        7.3.3.5 $CoCl_2$/Filter Paper Test 250

      7.3.4   Stability of Pharmaceutical Emulsions ... 250

        7.3.4.1   Chemical Instability 250

        7.3.4.2   Physical Instability 251

      7.3.5   Formulation of Emulsion 253

        7.3.5.1   Immiscible Phases 253

        7.3.5.2   Emulsifiers 253

7.3.5.3 Auxiliary Agents
(Emulsion Stabilizers) 255

7.3.5.4 Preservatives 256

7.3.5.5 Antioxidants 258

7.3.6 Method of Preparation of Emulsion 259

7.3.6.1 Dry Gum Method 259

7.3.6.2 Wet Gum Method 260

7.3.6.3 Bottle or Forbes Bottle
Method 260

7.3.7 Preparation of Emulsion at
Industrial Scale 260

7.3.7.1 Agitators/Mechanical Stirrers 261

7.3.7.2 Colloid Mill 261

7.3.7.3 Homogenizers 261

7.3.7.4 Ultrasonic Devices 262

7.3.8 Evaluation of Emulsions 262

7.3.8.1 Globule Size and its
Distribution 263

7.3.8.2 Electro-Kinetic Behavior 263

7.3.8.3 Drug Release Behavior 263

7.4 Sustained Release Suspensions 265

7.5 Conclusion 267

References 267

Chapter 8 Modified Release Drug Delivery Systems for Oral Route

Sharad P. Pandey, Vinod Dhote, Tripti Shukla and M. S. Sudheesh

8.1 Introduction 270

8.2 TIMERx Technology 274

8.2.1 Advantages of the System 276

8.2.2 Problems Associated with the
Formulation 277

8.2.3 Advancement 277

8.3 MASRx and COSRx: Modified Release Providing Systems 277

    8.3.1 MASRx Technology 278

    8.3.2 COSRx Technology 278

8.4 Smartrix® Technology 279

8.5 Geometrically Modified Core Containing Formulation: Procise Technology 281

    8.5.1 Advantages of Procise Technology 282

8.6 Ring Cap Technology 283

    8.6.1 Advantages 283

8.7 Pulsincap Technology 283

    8.7.1 Polymeric Hydrogel Capsule 284

    8.7.2 Gelatin Capsule having Impermeable Coating 285

    8.7.3 Hydrophilic Polymer Sandwiched in between the Layers of two Capsules 285

8.8 Spheroidal Oral Drug Absorption System 286

8.9 Egalet Technology 288

8.10 Conclusion 289

References 289

Chapter 9   Designing of Modulated Release Drug Delivery Systems by Pelletization Techniques

Vinod K. Dhote, Kanika Dhote, Sharad. P. Pandey, Tripti Shukla and Vandana Soni

9.1 Introduction 292

    9.1.1 History of Pelletization 293

    9.1.2 Advantages and Limitations 293

        9.1.2.1 Technological Advantages 293

        9.1.2.2 Therapeutic Advantages 294

        9.1.2.3 Limitations of Pelletization 294

    9.1.3 Rationale of using Pelletization 294

9.2 Pelletization Techniques 295

  9.2.1 Extrusion/Spheronization 296

    9.2.1.1 Advantages of Spheronization ... 297

    9.2.1.2 Dry Mixing 297

    9.2.1.3 Wet Massing 298

    9.2.1.4 Extrusion 298

  9.2.2 Roto Granulation 299

  9.2.3 Solution and Suspension Layering 299

  9.2.4 Dry Powder Layering 300

  9.2.5 Cryopelletization 300

  9.2.6 Spray Drying and Spray Congealing 301

  9.2.7 Freeze Pelletization 302

  9.2.8 Melt-Induced Agglomeration 302

  9.2.9 Melt Spheronization 302

  9.2.10 Fluid-Bed Granulation 302

  9.2.11 Bottom Spray Coating Process 303

  9.2.12 Tangential Spray Fluid Bed Granulation ... 304

  9.2.13 Suspension/Solution Layering Technique 304

  9.2.14 Innovative Technologies 305

    9.2.14.1 CPS™ Technology 305

    9.2.14.2 MicroPx™ Technology 306

    9.2.14.3 ProCell™ Technology 306

9.3 Factors Affecting Pelletization Process 307

  9.3.1 Moisture Content 307

  9.3.2 Rheological Characteristics 308

  9.3.3 Solubility of Excipients and Drug in Granulating Fluid 308

  9.3.4 Composition of Granulating Fluid 308

  9.3.5 Physical Properties of Starting Material 308

  9.3.6 Speed of the Spheronizer 308

  9.3.7 Drying Technique and Drying Temperature 309

  9.3.8 Extrusion Screen 309

9.4 Characterization of Pellets 309

   9.4.1 Particle Size Distribution 310

   9.4.2 Surface Area... 310

   9.4.3 Porosity 310

   9.4.4 Density 311

   9.4.5 Hardness and Friability 311

   9.4.6 Tensile Strength 311

   9.4.7 Disintegration Time 311

   9.4.8 *In vitro* Dissolution Studies..................... 311

9.5 Applications 312

   9.5.1 Taste Masking....................................... 312

   9.5.2 Immediate Release 312

   9.5.3 Sustained Release.................................. 313

   9.5.4 Chemically Incompatible Products 314

   9.5.5 Varying Dosage without Reformulation.... 314

9.6 Conclusion 314

References 315

Chapter 10 Colloidal Drug Delivery Systems

Vinod K. Dhote, Kanika Dhote, Tripti Shukla,
Sharad P. Pandey and Piush Khare

10.1 Colloidal Nanocarriers: General Considerations..... 318

   10.1.1 Colloidal Drug Delivery Systems 320

   10.1.2 Properties of an Ideal CDDS.................. 322

   10.1.3 Applications of CDDS 323

10.2 Colloidal Drug Carriers 324

   10.2.1 Liposomes.. 324

      10.2.1.1 Advantages of Liposomes 325

      10.2.1.2 Pharmaceutical Applications
            of Liposomes 326

   10.2.2 Polymer Micelles and Polymersomes..... 327

   10.2.3 Polymer Particles 328

   10.2.4 Solid Lipid Nanoparticles 328

   10.2.5 Microemulsion 329

10.3 *In-vivo* Fate of Colloidal Drug Carriers 330

10.4 Advantage and Successes 331

10.5 Conclusion 333

References 334

Chapter 11 *In-situ* Gel and Liquid Crystals as Potential Drug Delivery Systems

Ashish Parashar, Ankit Jain, Kamlendra Bhadoriya, Piush Khare and Punit Bhatnagar

11.1 Introduction.. 339

11.2 *In-Situ* Gelling System...................................... 340

   11.2.1 Physiological Stimuli Approach 341

      11.2.1.1 Temperature Induced............... 341

      11.2.1.2 pH Induced 342

   11.2.2 Physical Reaction Approach 342

   11.2.3 Chemical Changes in Biomaterial........... 343

      11.2.3.1 Ionic Crosslinking.................... 343

      11.2.3.2 Photo-Polymerization 343

      11.2.3.3 Enzymatic Cross Linking 343

11.3 Methods of Preparation of *In-Situ* Gel Systems... 344

   11.3.1 Solution Polymerization/Crosslinking 344

   11.3.2 Suspension Polymerization 344

   11.3.3 Polymerization by Irradiation 345

   11.3.4 Chemically Crosslinked Hydrogels 345

   11.3.5 Physically Crosslinked Hydrogels 345

11.4 In-Situ Gelling Polymers 345

   11.4.1 Pectin.. 346

   11.4.2 Gellan Gum.. 346

   11.4.3 Xyloglucan... 346

   11.4.4 Guar Gum.. 347

   11.4.5 Xanthum Gum....................................... 347

   11.4.6 Carbopol.. 347

   11.4.7 Synthetic Polymers 348

11.5 Evaluation and Characterizations of
In-Situ Gel System 348

    11.5.1 Clarity 348

    11.5.2 Texture Analysis 348

    11.5.3 pH of Gel... 348

    11.5.4 Sol-Gel Transition Temperature and
    Gelling Time 348

    11.5.5 Gel-Strength.. 349

    11.5.6 Viscosity and Rheology 349

    11.5.7 Fourier Transform Infrared
    Spectroscopy and Thermal Analysis....... 349

    11.5.8 *In-vitro* Drug Release Studies................. 349

11.6 Applications of *In-Situ* Polymeric
Drug Delivery System 350

    11.6.1 *In-Situ* Gel based Oral Drug Delivery..... 350

    11.6.2 Ocular Delivery.................................... 351

    11.6.3 Nasal Delivery 351

    11.6.4 Rectal and Vaginal Drug Delivery
    Systems 352

    11.6.5 Injectable Drug Delivery Systems 352

11.7 Liquid Crystals as Drug Delivery Systems.......... 353

    11.7.1 Classification of Liquid Crystals............. 355

        11.7.1.1 Lyotropic Liquid Crystals........ 355

        11.7.1.2 Thermotropic Liquid Crystals.... 356

    11.7.2 Characterization of Liquid Crystals 356

        11.7.2.1 Polarized Light Microscopy 357

        11.7.2.2 Transmission Electron
        Microscopy 357

        11.7.2.3 X-Ray Scattering Pattern......... 357

        11.7.2.4 Differential Scanning
        Calorimetry............................. 357

        11.7.2.5 Rheology................................ 357

        11.7.2.6 Determination of Vesicle Size.. 357

11.7.3 Applications of Liquid Crystals 358

11.7.3.1 Liquid Crystalline Drug Substances 358

11.7.3.2 Liquid Crystalline Formulations for Dermal Application 358

11.7.3.3 Liquid Crystalline Formulations for Sustained Drug Delivery 358

11.7.3.4 Liquid Crystals in Cosmetics... 358

11.8 Conclusion 359

References 359

Index 363

1 Controlled Release and Gastroretentive Drug Delivery Systems

Rajendra Awasthi[1], Vivek K. Pawar[2] and Giriraj T. Kulkarni[3]

[1]Department of Pharmaceutics, Laureate Institute of Pharmacy, Kathog, Kangra-177 101, India.

[2]Pharmaceutics Division, CSIR-Central Drug Research Institute, Lucknow-226 031, India.

[3]School of Pharmacy, ITM University, Gwalior-474 001, India.

Over the past decades we have witnessed the availability of wide range of controlled release dosage forms in the pharmaceutical market. There are several reasons for the attractiveness of these dosage forms, such as, reduced dosing frequency, patient compliance, improved dissolution profiles, and maintenance of the peak plasma concentration for prolonged time period. The performance of a controlled release delivery system depends on:

(a) Drug release from the dosage form (dissolution)

(b) Movement of the drug within the body

The dissolution process involves two steps, an initial detachment of drug molecule from the solid bulk surface to the adjacent liquid interface, followed by the diffusion of drug molecule from the solid-liquid interface into the bulk liquid medium. The dissolution of dosage form depends on the dosage form fabrication and physicochemical properties of the drug molecule. Movement of the drug within the body depends on pharmacokinetics of the drug.

Based on the formulation technologies, controlled release drug delivery systems can be classified as activation-modulated, diffusion controlled, dissolution controlled, feedback-regulated, site-targeted, or stimuli-sensitive delivery systems. Diffusion controlled or dissolution controlled systems are the most common controlled release systems. Diffusion controlled systems are either matrix type or reservoir type; whereas dissolution controlled systems are encapsulated systems, matrix systems or multi-layer matrix tablets. This chapter will consider the basic approaches used in the development and kinetic modeling of diffusion and dissolution controlled delivery systems. Further the chapter will give a laconic overview of various controlled release gastroretentive drug delivery systems.

1.1 Diffusion

Diffusion process is related to the intermixing of molecules as a result of random motion caused by molecular kinetic energy. Mixing of water soluble dye in a water filled beaker is the simplest example explaining the diffusion process. The dye molecules diffuse throughout the water beaker resulting in a uniform colour. At equilibrium, when a uniform colour exists throughout the water due to the equal distribution of dye molecules, no further net movement is observed (Fig. 1.1). The same case can be observed in the diffusion of drug molecule in our body. The process of transport of a drug through a polymer carrier can be well explained by Fick's laws of diffusion, which are derived by Adolf Fick in 1855. Fick's first and second law are applied to asses flux and drug concentration across the biological membrane.

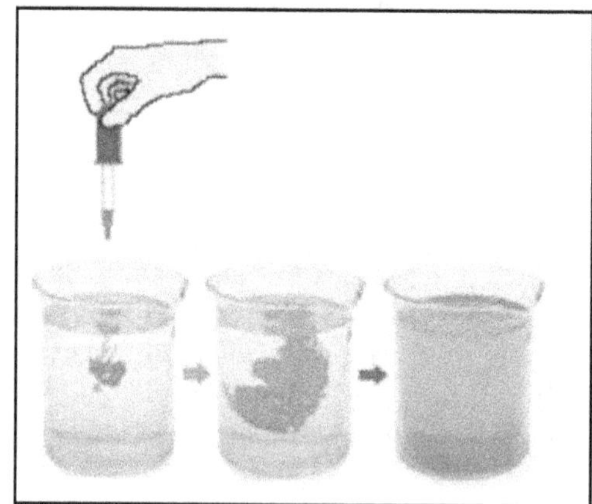

FIGURE 1.1 Process of colour diffusion in water system.

1.1.1 Fick's First Law of Diffusion

Fick's first law postulates that, under the assumption of steady state, the flux goes from a region of higher concentration to a region of lower concentration, with a magnitude that is proportional to the concentration gradient. This is a first order rate process as it depends on the concentration.

$$J = -D\frac{dc}{dx}$$

where, J is the amount of drug passing perpendicularly through a unit surface area per time, D is the diffusion coefficient, and dc/dx is the concentration gradient. The negative sign suggests that diffusion occurs in the direction opposite to the increasing concentration i.e., it is the opposite of the concentration gradient.

Diffusion coefficient is proportional to the squared velocity of the diffusing particles, which depends on the temperature and viscosity of the system, and the size of the drug particles according to the Stokes-Einstein relation.

1.1.2 Fick's Second Law of Diffusion

Fick's second law is used for unsteady state situations, i.e., when we wish to predict how drug concentration changes with time. This law is valid when the amount of initial drug per unit volume is smaller than the dimensional solubility of drug particle. It predicts the drug concentration change with time during the diffusion process. This law is based on the assumptions that the entire drug dissolves during diffusion process, but that does not apply in the real situations, there are always some drug particles left behind. It says that, the rate of change in drug concentration in a volume within the diffusional field is proportional to the rate of change in spatial concentration gradient at that point. The diffusion coefficient is represented as:

$$\frac{dc}{dt} = D\frac{d^2C}{dx^2}$$

Thus, it states that the change in concentration with time in a particular region is proportional to the change in concentration gradient at that point. The concentration gradient is greatest at the beginning, as the drug amount in the matrix is at maximum at the beginning and then decreases with the time as the drug diffuses from the system.

1.2   Designing of Diffusion Controlled Matrix

Diffusion controlled systems are characterized by diffusion rate dependent drug release through an inert insoluble polymeric barrier.

Examples of diffusion controlled solid dosage forms are single-unit tablets, mini-tablets in capsules and particulates systems like microspheres or beads. In general, the methods used for the tablet manufacture include dry granulation, wet granulation, direct compression, and thermoplastic pelletizing (e.g., high shear, melt-extrusion, spray-congealing). The processes for producing spherical particulate systems cover spray-granulation or spray-drying, spray-congealing, extrusion-spheronization, solvent evaporation and emulsification. The nature of coating substrate (e.g., size, tensile strength, etc.,) is an important factor which needs consideration while selecting coating technique such as pan coater or fluidized bed coater. Generally, use of conventional manufacturing processes and equipment is preferred. When a more complex process is required (e.g., multilayered tablets, compression coating, mixed beads, or minitablets), emphasis should be placed on increased process and product understanding throughout the development lifecycle to ensure successful development from lab scale to commercial scale. During the product development, an understanding of drug release mechanism and key properties of the rate controlling materials is important to assure batch-to-batch consistency. It is well known that, the polymers have inherently higher variability in physicochemical properties. Thus, it is important to understand the structural multifariousness and potential impact on product performance due to the polymers used. The same compendial grade of materials from different manufacturers/ source may influence the product performance due to the variation in its chemical properties. In general, it is usually recommended to select a synthetic or semi-synthetic polymer such as hydroxypropyl methylcellulose (HPMC) over a natural polymer (e.g., alginate) because the chemistry and properties of the natural polymers are often influenced by a number of factors (e.g., source, geographical area, etc.,) that are difficult to control.

The process of drug diffusion depends on the nature and type of the drug, polymer and dissolution medium used in the study. The drug dissolution from a spherical molecule can be explained using Stokes-Einstein equation ($D = kBT/6\pi a\eta$), where kB is the Boltzmann's constant, T is the absolute temperature in Kelvin, a is the molecule's radius, and η is the solvent viscosity.

This equation confirms that the large molecules diffuse more slowly than small ones and the diffusion process decreased with an increase in the viscosity of liquids. The factor kBT in Stokes-Einstein equation accounts for the Brownian motion of molecules caused by thermal agitation. In a polymeric system, the flow of polymer matrix is not like a liquid, and thus, the viscosity is not a correct parameter to predict diffusion of drug molecules.

The drug release from hydrophilic matrix after oral administration is based on diffusion of the drug through the hydrated polymer layer on the matrix surface (Paul & McSpadden, 1976). The molecules undergo collisions with each other, and results in thermal or Brownian motion. The theory of random walks shows that the average distance (root mean squared) that molecules travel by diffusion is proportional to the square root of time, i.e., average distance travelled $\sim \sqrt{Dt}$, where D is diffusion coefficient and t is time, a measure of the molecule's mobility in the medium.

The process of drug diffusion is a consequence of constant thermal movement of molecules, which results in a net transfer of drug molecules from a region of higher concentration to a region of lower concentration. The rate of diffusion from a matrix system is dependent on temperature, size, mass, and the viscosity of the microenvironment. Molecular movement of drug molecules increases with increase in temperature of the system leading to a higher average kinetic energy of the system (Lee, 1980).

$$\text{Kinetic energy (E)} = \frac{\text{Boltzmann's constant (k)} - \text{Temperature (T)}}{2}$$

$$= \frac{\text{Mass (m)} \times \text{Velocity (v)}}{2}$$

This equation shows that, an increase in temperature is exponentially correlated to velocity (v^2). Mass is also an important factor in the drug diffusion process. At a given temperature, mass of the molecule is inversely proportional to the velocity. The slower velocity of larger molecules is due to the more interaction of such molecules with the surrounding environment, which leads to slow particle diffusion. The environment viscosity also affects the diffusion process, since the rate of molecular movement is associated with the viscosity of the environment. In the case of a highly soluble drug, this may cause an initial burst release due to the presence of the drug on the matrix surface. Highly viscous gel layer thickness increases with time at the matrix surface due to the dissolution solvent permeation into the core of the matrix, which provides a diffusion barrier to drug release. The behaviour of such a gel layer is important in describing the release kinetics. After a certain time period this swelling of the polymer layer stops due to complete hydration of the matrix. At this stage, the polymer chains become completely relaxed and the gel layer cannot be maintained and leads to disentanglement and erosion of the matrix surface. At this stage a sharp change occurs in the rheological behaviour of the gel layer. This suggests that the polymer-polymer and polymer-solvent interactions are important in controlling the gel network and erosion.

1.2.1 Classification of Diffusion Controlled Drug Delivery Systems

The drug release from a porous polymeric controlled release system, following diffusional release, occurs primarily through the network of wet pores created by solid drug particles that are loaded in the polymer matrix. Based on the principle of drug diffusion, controlled release systems can be classified either as a reservoir system or as a matrix system. In case of nonporous systems, the drug release is controlled by the drug solubility in the polymer matrix and by the drug diffusivity through polymer matrix. Whereas, in case of porous matrix, drug solubility and polymer network tortuosity affect drug release. In addition, drug loading also influences the release profile, since high loading can complicate the release mechanism because of formation of more cavities due to the release of more drug at higher drug concentration. Thus, the formation of more porous matrix may lead to increased rates of drug release. In monolithic systems, the drug is dissolved or dispersed within a matrix system, depending on its solubility and the drug release kinetics depends on drug solubility. If the drug level in the polymer matrix is below its solubility limit, it can be dissolved in a polymer matrix, and if, it is present above its solubility limit, it is dispersed. For such systems, it is assumed that the dissolution rate of the drug is slower compared to the diffusion rate of the drug. The drug release from diffusion controlled reservoir/matrix systems requires various assumptions such as: the drug diffusion coefficient in a particular medium must be constant, there should be a pseudo-steady state during drug release from these systems, the dissolution of solid drug must occur prior to the drug release.

1.2.2 Reservoir Diffusion Systems

The basic application of these systems is to control the release of water-soluble drugs surrounded by an insoluble polymer membrane. Microencuplation of drug or other particles and press coating of tablets exemplifies reservoir type devices. A porous membrane is produced by adding soluble or leachable additive like water-soluble polymer, plasticizer etc., which resist drug diffusion at a predetermined rate upon contact with aqueous dissolution medium. The drug diffusion from reservoir device follows Fick's second law (unsteady-state conditions, concentration dependent flux). In case, the device contains dissolved drug, the process of drug release follows first order kinetics. It means, in such situation, the rate of release decreases exponentially with time as the concentration of the drug within the device decreases. In case, the device contains drug in the form of saturated suspension, the process of drug release follows zero order kinetics. Thus, the driving force for drug release is kept constant until the device is no longer saturated.

Drug release from the reservoir into external solution takes place in three steps:

(i)   dissolution of drug in polymer;

(ii)   diffusion of drug across the polymer membrane

(iii)   dissolution of the drug into external phase.

The drug release from these systems is based on various assumptions such as there is no bulk flow (no convection), no generation/consumption of drug, the drug is diluted within the material, and drug release is controlled by the thickness and composition of surrounding membrane. The drug release rate depends on drug solubility, film thickness, and pore characteristics. These systems are effective at achieving zero-order, or constant drug delivery. However, there is a risk of significant burst release due to the accidental dose dumping, which may occur if the controlling membrane ruptures. The burst release effect has been observed in membrane reservoir systems after storage for specified time duration. When placed in a release medium, the drug diffused to the surface of the membrane is released immediately, causing a burst effect. The amount of drug released with an initial burst, M_t, from these systems is estimated by:

$$M_t = \frac{Dc_0}{1}\left(1 + \frac{1^2}{6D}\right)$$

where D is the drug diffusion coefficient, C_0 is the drug concentration on the inside of the membrane, and 1 is the membrane thickness, with a given burst of $C_0 1/6$, but the release profile during burst stage $(t > 0)$ was not predictable. In order to maintain a constant release rate, the drug concentration difference must remain constant. This can be achieved by placing drug at the centre of the matrix.

The drug solubility in polymer and in dissolution media based on interfacial partitioning can be expressed using following equation:

Partition coefficient of the drug molecule from polymer to solution (K)

$$= \frac{\text{Solubility of drug insolution phase } (C_s)}{\text{Solubility of drug insolution phase } (C_p)}$$

With the above assumptions, the cumulative amount of drug released (Q) from a diffusion-controlled reservoir type drug delivery system with a unit surface area can be depicted as:

$$Q = \frac{C_p KD_d D_m}{KD_d h_m + D_m h_d} - \frac{D_d D_m}{KD_d h_m + D_m h_d} \int_0^t C_{b(t)} d_t$$

where D_m is diffusivity of the drug in a polymer membrane having thickness h_m, D_d is diffusivity of hydrodynamic diffusion layer with thickness h_d, C_b is concentration of drug in reservoir, and t is time.

Under a perfect sink condition, $C_{b(t)} \cong 0$ or $C_s \gg C_{b(t)}$, above equation reduced to

$$Q = \frac{C_p KD_d D_m}{KD_d h_m + D_m h_d} t$$

This shows that drug release can be a constant, with the rate of drug release being

$$\frac{Q}{t} = \frac{C_p KD_d D_m}{KD_d h_m + D_m h_d}$$

The rate of drug release depends on the polymer membrane layer or hydrodynamic diffusion layer. If, the release of drug is dependent on polymer membrane layer, in such case, $KD_d h_m \gg D_m h_d$, and above equation becomes:

$$\frac{Q}{t} = \frac{C_p D_m}{h_m}$$

This shows that the rate of drug release is directly proportional to its solubility and inversely proportional to the polymer membrane thickness.

Transdermal delivery system is a typical example of the reservoir system. It consists of a backing layer, a rate-limiting membrane, a protective liner, and a drug reservoir compartment. The drug release from reservoir compartment is controlled through a rate-controlling polymer membrane. The drug release from such systems can be varied by selecting a proper polymer at different concentrations. The first transdermal system for systemic delivery, a three-day patch that delivers scopolamine to treat motion sickness, was approved in the United States in 1979.

Ocusert® is a commercially available reservoir system which delivers Pilocarpine to treat glaucoma. It is placed in the lower eye lid to administer drug for one week duration. This product was not successful due to patient compliance, as patients felt more comfortable using the regular drops compared to placing a foreign object in the eye. These devices are five times more expensive than regular drops (Malcolm *et al.*, 2012).

Norplant® is another commercially available reservoir system consisting of 6 silicone rods containing 36 mg of levonorgestrel dissolved in the polymeric matrix. Norplant® is implanted under the upper arm skin. These systems are able to delivers hormone for up to five years (Malcolm *et al.*, 2012). Currently this has been discontinued from the market due to multiple lawsuits in the USA.

1.2.3 Matrix Diffusion Systems

A matrix system, described as monolithic device, is designed by homogenous dispersion or dissolution of solid drug in an inert polymeric mix. These systems are favoured over other systems for their simplicity, low manufacturing costs, and lack of accidental dose dumping. These systems are easier to produce than the reservoir systems and can deliver high molecular weight drugs. The release property of the device depends upon the porous or nonporous nature of the matrix. Diffusional release of the drug is normally governed by Fick's first and second laws.

Mathematically, the rate of drug release in diffusion-controlled matrix systems can be described by Fick's first law of diffusion, which is expressed as:

$$J = -D\frac{dC}{dX}$$

where J is diffusion flux, D is the diffusivity of drug molecule, and dC/dX is concentration gradient of the drug molecule across diffusional barrier with thickness dX.

The drug release from a monolithic porous system is Fickian diffusion based on Fick's second law. Fick's second law describes how the concentration (c) within the diffusion volume changes with respect to time.

$$\frac{dC}{dX} = D.\Delta C$$

In such systems, the release rate is proportional to the square root of time and the release rate is dependent on the diffusion length. For the first 60% of released drug, the release corresponds to the early time approximation of Fick's second law, which is expressed as:

$$\frac{dM_t}{dt} = \sqrt{2M_0 \frac{D}{\pi l^2 t}}$$

where l is the thickness of a slab, M_o is the amount of drug dissolved, and M_t is the amount released at time t.

The release kinetics of diffusion controlled systems follows first order kinetics according to the following equation:

$$\frac{dM_t}{dt} = \sqrt{\frac{8DM_0}{1^2} \exp \frac{\pi^2 Dt}{1^2}}$$

Thus, a first order linear release profile is obtained for a drug releasing from a porous polymeric matrix. A simple mathematical model (Higuchi's model) is applied for the examination of drug release from a spherical system or a planar surface following diffusional release mechanism. For matrix systems, because of the changing thickness of the depletion zone, release kinetics is a function of the square root of time. Higuchi described the drug release from an insoluble homogeneous planar matrix system as a square root of time dependent process based on Fickian diffusion:

$$Q = \sqrt{(2C - C_s) DtC_s}$$

where Q is the amount of drug released at time t, D is the diffusitivity of the drug, C is the drug initial drug concentration, and C_s is the solubility of the drug in the matrix.

1.2.4 Factors Affecting Drug Release Rate from Monolithic Matrix Systems

1. Initial drug loading, solubility and dissolution rate
2. Boundary conditions

    (i)   The sink condition

    (ii) Stagnant layers and external mass-transfer resistances

    (iii) Dissolution media of finite volume

3. Drug and matrix diffusion coefficients
4. Drug molecular weight and size
5. Matrix pore size
6. Tortuosity of interconnecting channels within matrix
7. Matrix swelling
8. Osmotic pressure gradients
9. Ionic exchanges
10. Local electromagnetic force fields
11. Matrix erosion and drug solubility.

1.3   Designing of Dissolution Controlled Matrix

The dissolution process involves two basic steps, containing, and initial separation of drug molecules from the solid surface to the adjacent interface of the dissolution medium followed by their diffusion from the interface into the bulk dissolution medium. It is possible to develop a controlled release system of highly water soluble drug by decreasing the drug dissolution rate by coating the drug with slowly dissolving materials, or by incorporating it into tablet with a slowly dissolving carrier. Encapsulated dissolution systems can be prepared either by coating particles or granules of drug with varying thickness of slowly soluble polymers, or by micro-encapsulation. These coated particles can be compressed into tablets called as SPACETABS or placed in capsules as in SPANSULES. After the dissolution or erosion of the coating, drug molecules become available for absorption. Release of the drug at a predetermined time is accomplished by controlling the thickness of coating. In Spansule®, drug molecules are enclosed in beads of varying thickness to control the time and amount of drug release (Shen *et al.*, 2003). The encapsulated particles with thin coatings will dissolve and release the drug first, while a thicker coating will take longer to dissolve and will release the drug at a later time. Coating-controlled delivery systems can also be designed to prevent the degradation of the drug in the acidic environment of the stomach. Such systems are generally referred as enteric-coated systems. Most of the formulations relying on dissolution to release the drug fall into three categories:

1. Encapsulated dissolution systems
2. Matrix dissolution systems
3. Multi-layer matrix tablet

Dissolution of drug from dosage form occurs till the surrounding dissolution medium is not saturated. The process of drug dissolution involves two steps. In the first, solid dissociate from the matrix surface and surround itself with dissolution medium. In second step, the solvated drug diffuses away from the matrix surface. The first step is more rapid than the second step, unless the drug is highly insoluble.

The fundamental principle for surface action phenomenon of drug dissolution in a liquid media was proposed by Noyes-Whitney in 1897. According to the Noyes–Whitney equation, the amount dissolved per unit area per unit time i.e., rate of drug dissolution (dC/dt) can be expressed as:

$$\frac{dC}{dt} = \frac{DA}{h\,(C_0 - C_t)}$$

where D is the diffusion coefficient of drug in diffusion layer, h is thickness of diffusion layer, A is surface area of drug particles, C_0 is saturation concentration of the drug in diffusion layer, C_t is the concentration of drug in bulk fluid at time t.

The rate of drug dissolution is directly proportional to the surface area of the drug particle. When C_t is less than 15% of the saturated solubility, C_t has a negligible influence on the dissolution rate of the solid. Under such conditions, the dissolution of the solid is said to be occurring under sink conditions. In general, the surface area (A) and thickness (h) of hydrodynamic diffusion layer are not constant except when the quantity of material present exceeds the saturation solubility, or initially, when only small quantities of drugs have dissolved. Factors affecting dissolution kinetics include particle size, solubility of polymers, viscosity of the hydrated polymer, diffusion coefficient (diffusivity), hydrodynamics of the stirring solvent, and diffusion of dissolved drug molecules through the hydrated polymer layer, and pH of the dissolution medium for enteric-coated controlled release systems.

In case of dissolution of powdered drug, a cube-root relationship is observed between the amount of remaining solid mass and time. This relationship is known as Hixson-Crowell cube-root law and represented by the equation:

$$W_0^{1/3} - W_t^{1/3} = \kappa t$$

where W_0 is the initial amount of drug in the pharmaceutical dosage form, Wt is the remaining amount of drug in the pharmaceutical dosage form at time t and κ (kappa); a constant incorporating the surface-volume relation. For dissolution of solid particles, this law assumes that the thickness of the diffusion layer is constant during the dissolution process; however this is not necessarily true.

In case of system coated with water soluble polymers, the first step of dissolution is hydration of polymer layer followed by dissolution (disentanglement) of the hydrated polymer. Esters of phthalic acid (weak acids containing carboxyl groups) are commonly used as enteric coating polymer. These polymers contain carboxylic acid groups which are un-ionized at gastric pH (pH 1.2 to 4.8) but become ionizedat intestinal pH (pH 6-7.5). The dissolution of enteric coating in alkaline pH is depended upon the ionization of polymers utilized. Enteric coating disrupt at higher pH due to the repelling effect of ionized polymers. Rapid dissolution of enteric coated systems requires higher pKa values of polymers compared to pH values of the dissolution media.

1.4   Kinetic Modeling on Drug Release from Diffusion and Dissolution Controlled Drug Delivery Systems

Kinetic modeling of drug release from diffusion and dissolution controlled drug delivery systems is helpful to speed up the process of product development and to better understand the mechanisms that are governing drug release from the developed delivery systems.

1.4.1 Zero Order Model

The process that takes place at a constant rate, independent of drug concentration is called as zero order kinetics. It means that, the rate of process cannot be increased with an increase in drug concentration. This ideal delivery is particularly important in certain classes of drugs, such as, antibiotic, ant-diabetic, anti-hypertensive, antidepressants etc.

Mathematically, the process of drug dissolution from dosage forms that do not disaggregate and allow a slow drug release (assuming that the area does not change and no equilibrium conditions are obtained) can be represented by the equation:

$$Q_t = Q_0 - K_0 t$$

where, Q_t is the amount of drug dissolved in time t, Q_0 is the initial amount of drug in the solution (most times, $Q_0 = 0$) and K_0 is the zero order release rate constant. The rate constant for zero order process is expressed in terms of mg/min.

To study the release kinetics, data obtained from *in vitro* drug release studies are plotted as the cumulative amount of drug released against time. This plot yields a straight line whose slope is $- K_0$. The half life of the drug following zero order kinetics can be calculated as 0.5 Q_0/K_0. This indicates that, the half life of drug depends on initial drug concentration. This model can be applied for the determination of drug release kinetics from transdermal systems, IV infusion and matrix tablets containing low soluble drugs (Varelas *et al.*, 1995).

1.4.2 First Order Model

This model was first proposed by Gibaldi and Feldman in 1967 to describe the process of absorption and elimination of drugs (Gibaldi & Feldman 1967). However, theoretical conceptualization of this model is a difficult task. The release of the drug which followed first order kinetics can be expressed by the equation:

$$\frac{dC}{dt} = -Kc$$

where K is the first order rate constant expressed in units of time^{-1}.

Above equation can be expressed as:

$$\log C = \log C_0 - \frac{K_t}{2.303}$$

where C_0 is the initial concentration of drug, k is the first order rate constant, and t is the time. The above equation shows that, the first order processes are directly proportional to the drug concentration, it means, the rate of process increases linearly with an increase in drug concentration. The data obtained from the *in vitro* release study of a porous matrix system containing water soluble drug are plotted as log cumulative percentage of drug remaining against time which yield a straight line with a slope of $- K/2.303$. The rate constant for first order kinetics is expressed as min^{-1} or hour^{-1}. The half life of the drug following first order kinetics can be calculated as 0.693/K. This indicates that, the half life is concentration independent and it is constant. This model is mainly applicable to determine the release kinetics of dosage form those containing water soluble drugs in a porous matrix (Mulye & Turco, 1995).

1.4.3 Higuchi Model

A square root time dependent diffusion controlled drug release process of water soluble drugs from a hydrophilic matrix or suspensions based on Fick's first law was described by Takeru Higuchi in 1961 (Higuchi, 1961). He divided the matrix into two regions. In one region (depletion zone) all drugs are dissolved and a concentration gradient exists, and in the other region solid and dissolved drug coexist, making the dissolved drug concentration constant. This model is based on various hypotheses, such as, the drug is equally spread in the matrix, diffusion is unidirectional due to the negligible edge effect; the drug concentration in the matrix is initially much higher than the solubility of the drug; the thickness of the dosage form is much larger than the size of the drug molecules; the swelling and dissolution of the matrix is negligible; the diffusivity of the drug is constant; and perfect sink conditions are attained (Higuchi, 1963).

Initially, this equation was valid only for planar matrix systems, and later it was modified to consider different geometrical shapes and matrix characteristics including porous structures. Following equation was obtained to study the dissolution from a planar system having a homogeneous matrix:

$$Q = \sqrt{(2C - C_s)DtC_s}$$

where Q is the amount of drug released at time t, C is the drug initial drug concentration, C_s is the drug solubility in the matrix media and D is the diffusivity of the drug molecules in the matrix.

Assuming that diffusion coefficient and other parameters remain constant during the release, the above equation reduces to:

$$Q = \sqrt{Kt}$$

Thus, for diffusion controlled release mechanism, a plot of cumulative percentage of drug released against the square root of time will result in a straight line. The linearity of the plots is confirmed by the calculation of correlation coefficient. The equation was derived under pseudo-steady state assumptions and cannot be applied to real controlled release systems. According to the Higuchi's model, the data obtained from *in vitro* dissolution study are plotted as a cumulative percentage drug release against the square root of time (Awasthi & Kulkarni, 2014a). This relationship can be applied to depict the drug dissolution from several modified release pharmaceutical dosage forms, such as transdermal systems and matrix tablets containing water soluble drugs.

1.4.4 Peppas' Model

According to logarithmic form of Peppas' equation, the rate of drug release can be expressed as:

$$Q = Kt^n$$

the logarithmic form of the above equation is

$$\log Q = \log K + n \log t$$

where Q is the amount of drug released, 't' is the time and 'n' is the slope of the linear plot. If the value of n is less than or equal to 0.5, the mechanism of drug release is diffusion without swelling. If the value is greater than 0.5 and less than 1, the release through diffusion with swelling and if it is above 1, the release mechanism is anomalous diffusion, not confirming to any Fick's laws (non-Fickian)(Awasthi & Kulkarni, 2014a; Peppas, 1985; Ritger & Peppas, 1987a,b).

1.4.5 Krosmayer Peppas Model

(Korsmeyer et al. 1983) derived a semi-empirical model, which described the drug release from a polymeric system. According to the Korsmeyer-Peppas model, first 60% drug release data are fitted to find out the mechanism of drug release. This model is generally applied to analyze the drug release from a polymeric dosage form, where the release mechanism is not well recognized or when more than one type of release process could be involved (Peppas & Korsmeyer, 1986). To study the release kinetics, data obtained from *in vitro* drug release studies were plotted as log cumulative percentage drug release versus log time.

$$\frac{M_t}{M_\infty} = Kt^n$$

Where M_t/M_∞ is a fraction of drug released at time t, K is the release rate constant and n is the release exponent. The n value is used to characterize different release for cylindrical shaped matrices.

In case of cylindrical tablets, $0.45 \leq n$ corresponds to a Fickian diffusion mechanism, $0.45 < n < 0.89$ to non-Fickian transport, $n = 0.89$ to Case II (relaxational) transport, and $n > 0.89$ to super case II transport.

This model is based on following assumptions:

1. Drug release occurs in an one dimensional way.
2. The length to thickness ratio of system should not be less than 10.
3. The equation is applicable for small values of time (t) and the portion of release curve where $M_t/M_\infty < 0.6$ should only be used to determine the exponent n.

1.4.6 Hixson Crowell's Model

(Hixson and Crowell 1931) reported that the particles' regular area is proportional to the cube root of its volume. This model describes the drug release from systems where there is a change in surface area and diameter of delivery system, such as, particles or tablets. They derived the equation:

$$W_0^{1/3} - W_t^{1/3} = \kappa t$$

where W_0 is the initial amount of drug in the pharmaceutical dosage form, W_t is the remaining amount of drug in the pharmaceutical dosage form at time t and κ (kappa) is a constant incorporating the surface-volume relation.

The equation describes the release from systems where there is a change in surface area and diameter of particles or tablets. To study the release kinetics, data obtained from *in vitro* drug release studies were plotted as the cube root of drug percentage remaining in the matrix versus time. This expression applies to pharmaceutical dosage forms where the dissolution occurs in planes that are parallel to the drug surface. In case, if the tablet dimensions diminish proportionally, in such a manner that the initial geometrical form keeps constant all the time (Niebergall *et al.*, 1963).

1.4.7 Selection of the Best Fit Model for Release Data

Based on the statistical treatments, determination of correlation coefficient 'r^2' is the most widely used method to assess the fit of the model equation. The model having r^2 values less than 1 but, closest to 1 is considered as best fit model. However, this approach can be applied only when the parameters of the model equations are similar. But when the parameters of the comparing equations increased; an adjusted coefficient (r^2 adjusted) is used for selecting best fit model using following equation:

$$r^2_{adjusted} = 1 - \frac{n-1}{n-p}(1-r^2)$$

where, n is the number of dissolution data points and p is the number of parameters in the model. Hence, the best model is the one with the highest adjusted coefficient of determination. Similarly, other statistical tools like Analysis of Variance (ANOVA) and Multivariate analysis of variance (MANOVA) are used for the selection of best fit models (Costa & Lobo, 2001).

1.5   Design and Fabrication of Gastroretentive Dosage Forms

The goal in designing controlled release drug delivery system is to control the drug concentration in target tissue, reducing the number of administrations and to improve the efficacy of drugs. However, a controlled release dosage form offers limited advantages for drugs that have an absorption window in the stomach or solubility dependent absorption. In order to increase the bioavailability of this type of drug, the residence time of the controlled-release dosage form in the stomach needs to be prolonged (Streubel, 2006). Gastroretentive controlled drug delivery systems have found to produce more significant improvement in pharmacotherapy of drugs having narrow absorption window in the gastrointestinal tract. Several attempts have been made to improve the bioavailability of drugs by increasing the residence time of dosage form in the gastric region. Over the last two decades, numerous gastroretentive systems such as high density, floating, expandable, mucoadhesive or bioadhesive, magnetic, dual working systems and superporous systems have been designed to prolong the gastric retention time (Pawar *et al.*, 2011). Fig. 1.2 describes localization mechanisms of the different gastroretentive dosage forms and Table. 1.1 presents list of marketed formulations based on gastric retention technology.

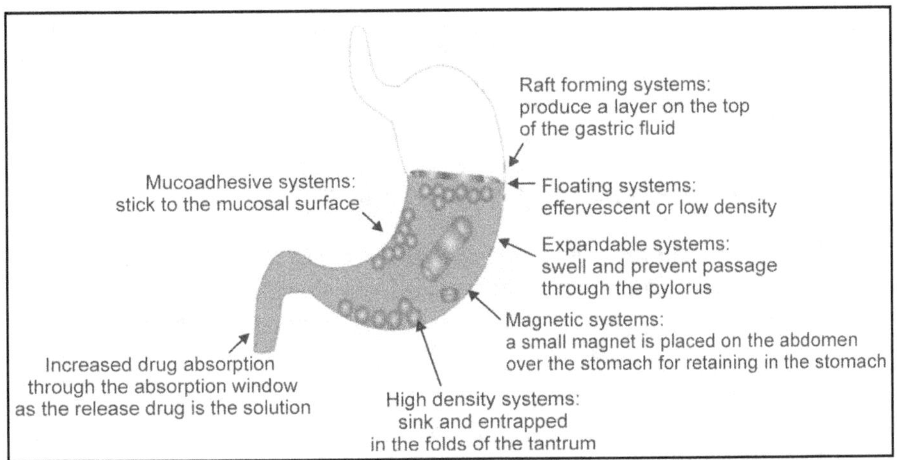

FIGURE 1.2   Localization mechanisms of the different gastroretentive dosage forms.

After administration, these systems remain in the stomach for a determined time period and can maintain the drug concentration at the target site. Gastric floating drug delivery system is particularly useful for drugs that are primarily absorbed in the duodenum and upper jejunum segments. The major advantage of these systems is that the released drug will have whole surface area of stomach and small intestine for absorption. These systems are not suitable for those drugs which cause gastric lesions, such as non steroidal anti-inflammatory agents.

1.5.1 Gastrointestinal Motility

Two distinct patterns of gastrointestinal motility and secretion exist corresponding to the fasted and fed states. The fasted state is associated with various cyclic events which is called the interdigestive myoelectric cycle or migrating myoelectric complex (MMC). MMC is divided into four consecutive phases: phase I (basal phase) occurs for 40 to 60 min with rare contractions, phase II (preburst phase) lasts for 40 to 60 min with intermittent action potential and contractions, phase III (burst phase) occurs for 4 to 6 min with intense and regular contractions for short period, and phase IV lasts for 5 min; a transitional phase that occurs between phases III and I of two consecutive cycles. Due to intense waves of phase III, all the material is swept out of the stomach to the small intestine. Phase III waves are also known as the 'housekeeper' waves. In the fed state, the gastric emptying rate is slowed since the onset of MMC is delayed. The motor activity after meal ingestion is induced after 5-10 min and it persists as long as food remains in the stomach. The large amount of food ingested is corresponds to the longer period of fed activity (2-6 h) with phasic contractions similar to Phase II of MMC (Takahashi, 2012).

1.5.2 Factors Affecting Gastric Retention

1. ***Density of the drug delivery system:*** Gastric retention time (GRT) is a function of buoyancy of dosage form which is dependent on the density of the system. Density of dosage form should be less than the gastric contents (Awasthi *et al.*, 2010).

2. ***Size and shape of dosage form:*** Dosage form units with a diameter greater than 7.5 mm are reported to have an increased GRT. Tetrahedron and ring shaped devices with a flexural modulus of 48 and 22.5 kilo pounds per square inch are reported to have better retention at 24 h compared with other shapes (Timmermans & Moes, 1994).

3. ***Single or multiple unit dosage forms:*** Multiple unit formulations show more predictable release profile and insignificant impairing of formulation performance due to the failure of units. They allow co-administration of units with different release profiles and permit larger margin of safety against dosage form failure compared to single unit dosage forms (Newton, 2010).

4. ***Fed or unfed state of the stomach:*** Under fasting conditions, the gastric motility is characterized by periods of strong motor activity or MMC that occurs every 1.5 to 2 h. The MMC sweeps undigested material from the stomach. The GRT of the unit can be expected to very short when timing of formulation administration coincides with MMC (Mazer *et al.*, 1988).

5. ***Nature of meal:*** Feeding of indigestible polymers or fatty acid salts can change the motility pattern of the stomach to a fed state, thus decreasing the gastric emptying rate.

6. ***Caloric content:*** GRT can be increased by 4 to 10 h with a meal having high proteins and fats content.

7. ***Frequency of feed:*** The GRT can increase by over 400 minutes when successive meals are given compared with a single meal leading to low frequency of MMC.

8. ***Age:*** Elderly people, especially those over 70, have a significantly longer GRT (Mojaverian *et al.*, 1988).

9. ***Posture:*** GRT can vary between supine and upright ambulatory states of the patient (Mojaverian *et al.*, 1988).

10. ***Gender:*** Mean ambulatory GRT in males (3.4 ± 0.6 h) is less compared with their age and race matched female counterparts (4.6 ± 1.2 h), regardless of the weight, height and body surface (Mojaverian *et al.*, 1988).

1.5.3 Formulation Approaches

Formulation approaches used for the development of gastroretentive systems are classified into the six categories based on formulation variables and mechanism of gastric retention. These systems have different principles of working and have their own merits and demerits.

1. High density systems
2. Swelling and expandable systems
3. Mucoadhesive or bioadhesive systems
4. Superporus hydrogel based systems
5. Magnetic systems
6. Floating systems

1.5.4 High Density Systems

The density of gastric content is close to the density of water (~1.004 g/cm^3), whereas the density of these systems, is about 3 g/cm^3. These systems are retained in the stomach due to high density, and are capable of withstanding its peristaltic movements. This phenomenon is confirmed by various clinical studies (Hejazi & Amiji, 2002; Timmermans & Moes, 1994). The manufacturing of high density systems is technically difficult with a large amount of drug, because weight of the matrix decreases progressively as the drug gets released. Thus, the duration of gastric retention also reduce. High density systems have not been significantly able to extend the gastric residence time (Rouge *et al.*, 1998).

1.5.5 Swelling and Expandable Systems

The initial size of an ideal expandable system should be minimum possible to facilitate easy swallowing. Once the dosage form reaches stomach, the size of the dosage form should significantly increase rapidly and thus prevent premature passage through the pyloric sphincter. For these systems, some amount of gastric fluid in the stomach is must as the swelling takes place due to the fluid absorption by the system. Superporous hydrogels can reduce this problem to a certain limit as they have high swelling capacity. The desired expansion can be achieved by swelling due to the osmosis or unfolding of polymeric chains. An expandable system based on unfolding mechanism has been reported for veterinary applications. The size of the expandable system needs to decrease after the complete drug release for easy evacuation from the stomach. The system should be designed in such a way that it gets eliminated from the body after completion of drug release. In terms of safety, these systems should not interfere with gastric motility, must be biodegradable, and must not cause any local damage to the gastric mucosa (Hou *et al.*, 2003).

1.5.6 Mucoadhesive or Bioadhesive Systems

Adhesion of the delivery system to the stomach mucosal membrane is an attractive approach to prolong the gastric retention time of dosage form in the stomach. The gastric mucoadhesion of the dosage form may follow any of the mechanisms reported for mucoadhesion, such as absorption, diffusion, electron transfer, orwetting. The bioadhesion of polymers to the mucus membrane is achieved by the formation of electrostatic and hydrogen bonding at the mucus-polymer boundary. These formulations utilize materials such as, polyacrylic acids (Carbopol), chitosan, cholestyramine, dextrin, gliadin, HPMC, polyethylene glycol, sodium alginate, sucralfate, tragacanth, etc., which enables the device to adhere to the gastric mucosal wall. It has been established that the anionic polymers have better mucoadhesion property than neutral or cationic polymers (Huang *et al.*, 2000). It seems that the mucoadhesive polymers are unable to effectively control gastrointestinal transit of the dosage form. It is very difficult to maintain effective mucoadhesion, due to continuous renewal of gastric mucosa, resulting in unpredictable adherence of delivery system to the gastric mucosa. These systems can cause local side-effects, such as gastric irritation, due to the prolonged contact of system with gastric mucosa (Chun *et al.*, 2005).

1.5.7 Superporous Hydrogel based Systems

Hydrogels have been used in pharmaceutical products due to their biodegradable and biocompatible property. These are cross linked network of hydrophilic polymers that are insoluble in water. Hydrogels have the ability to swell by absorbing water or gastric fluid (Fig. 1.3). The rate of swelling of conventionally available hydrogels is very slow, and hence, there are chances of premature evacuation of the delivery system through the pyloric sphincter. Therefore, such conventional hydrogels are commonly not preferred in the development of gastroretentive drug delivery systems. Superporous hydrogels had pore size >100 μm and swell very fast due to rapid water uptake, hence, superporous hydrogels are important in the development of gastroretentive drug delivery systems. Superporous hydrogels are water insoluble, thus, can retain their mechanical strength. Examples of commonly used materials for forming superporous hydrogels are poly (acrylamide-co-acrylic acid)/ polyethyleneimine polymer networks, polymerized vinyl monomers, or acrylate derivatives, sucrose and croscarmellose sodium (Qiu & Park, 2003).

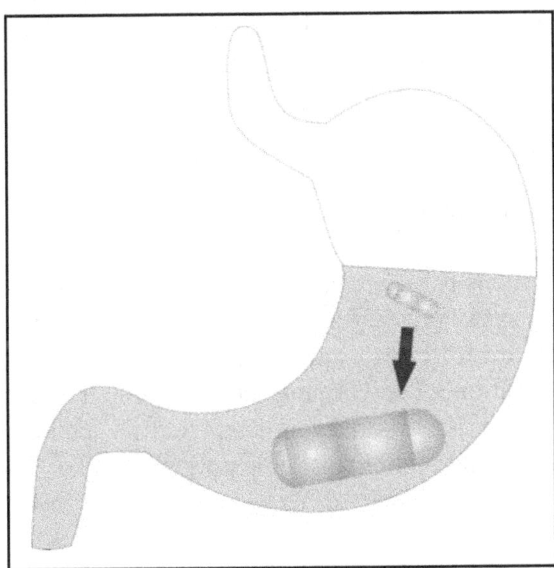

FIGURE 1.3 Expansion of a superporous hydrogels based gastroretentive system upon contact with gastric fluid.

1.5.8 Magnetic Systems

Magnetic systems contain a small internal magnet (iron powder) and an extracorporal magnet placed on the abdomen over the position of the stomach, which control the gastrointestinal transit of the dosage form. A number of human studies on gastroretention properties have been reported by many researchers based on magnetic systems. The images are taken by very sensitive bio-magnetic measurement equipments. The major drawback of these systems is that the effectiveness of the therapy depends on the position of the external magnet, which might compromise patient compliance. The prolonged retention of these systems in human stomach has been proved by magnetic resonance imaging of the dosage forms (Groning *et al.*, 1998).

1.5.9 Floating Drug Delivery Systems

These are low-density systems which float over the gastric fluids and thus increase the retention time at the site of drug absorption, particularly in the stomach. These delivery systems are formulated by the incorporation of carbonate or bicarbonate salts in the swellable polymer matrix. Here, the density of dosage form decrease due to the entrapment of carbon dioxide gas within the polymer matrix, which is responsible for buoyancy (Mouzam *et al.*, 2011). These systems release the medicament in a controlled manner while the system floats over the gastric fluid, which results in increased bioavailability of the drug with reduced fluctuation in plasma concentration.

1.5.9.1 Classification of Floating Drug Delivery Systems

Floating systems can be classified based on the mechanism of buoyancy. Major classes of floating drug delivery systems are effervescent systems, noneffervescent systems, low density systems, and raft forming systems. The first category of floating systems is effervescent systems which are obtained by the incorporation of bicarbonate salt which is responsible for gas generation or by volatilization of an organic solvent which make hollow cavity. The other category is non-effervescent systems which are formulated by using gel-forming and highly swellable polymers.

1.5.9.2 Effervescent Systems

These systems are prepared by using swellable polymers such as methylcellulose and a gas forming agent like carbonate or bicarbonate salt with or without tartaric acid/citric acid. The coated resin beads containing bicarbonate are the most common systems prepared by this approach. In this system, the insoluble but permeable coating allows water to permeate through it, releasing carbon dioxide gas, causing the system to float when comes in contact with gastric environment. Other materials and approaches used are light mineral oils, mixture of cellulose derivatives and Carbopol along with $NaHCO_3$, polypropylene foam powder, mixture of alginate and bicarbonate salt, and systems based on ion exchange resin technology (Rubinstein & Friend, 1994).

1.5.9.3 Non-Effervescent Systems

These delivery systems are developed by using a high level of gel-forming, highly swellable polymers. HPMC is most commonly used for the preparation of non-effervescent floating systems, although agar, carrageenans, hydroxyethylcellulose (HEC), hydroxypropylcelulose (HPC), and sodium carboxymethycellulose (NaCMC) are also used. The penetration of fluid inside the device and consequent drug release is controlled due to the hydration of gel forming polymers and formation of gel barrier when comes in contact with the gastric fluid. The buoyancy of the dosage form depends on the density of swollen polymeric matrix, which can be reduced due to the entrapped air within the matrix (Nakamichi *et al.*, 2001).

1.5.9.4 Hydrodynamically Balanced Systems

Hydrodynamically Balanced Systems (HBS) are able to prolong the retention time for a long period by maintaining their low apparent density due to the hydration of polymer and formation of gel barrier (Erni & Held 1987).

1.5.9.5 Low-Density Systems

The major drawback of floating systems based on the mechanism of gas generation is that they have a floating lag time. Due to this, the system may undergo premature evacuation. The system having density lower than the gastric fluid does not have this kind of problem. Floatation can also achieve by the volatilization of an organic solvent (e.g., dichloro-methane). These are particulate systems such as microspheres or microballoons. They are characteristically free flowing powders with a size less than 200 µm. In these systems, low density materials are used as drug carrier. A buoyant system can also be developed by using a fluid-filled globular shell that floats in the stomach. A drug-polymer solution is used for further coating of these systems. Finally, the product remains buoyant for a prolonged time period over the gastric content with a constant and controlled drug release (Sharma & Pawar, 2006). For easy administration and accurate dose, these systems can be compressed into fast disintegrating tablets.

1.5.9.6 Raft Forming Systems

These are boat like systems, which float over the gastric fluid in the form of a continuous layer which is known as raft. The raft forming systems involve the formulation of effervescent floating liquid with *in situ* gelling properties, which has been assessed for sustaining drug delivery and targeting. The raft floats on the gastric fluid because it has bulk density less than the gastric fluid created by the liberation of carbon dioxide gas and act as a barrier to prevent the gastric reflux. When the system floats on the gastric fluid, the drug is released slowly in a controlled manner. After complete release of the drug, the residual system is emptied from the stomach. Raft forming systems have received much attention for the delivery of antacids and drug delivery for the treatment of gastrointestinal infections and disorders. These systems are designed by using a polymer having gel forming property. Carbonate or bicarbonate salts are also used as co-excipients in the formulation of these systems. When the system comes in contact with the gastric content, it forms a viscous gel. The presence of bicarbonate salts is responsible for gas generation. The system floats due to the entrapment of carbon dioxide gas within the viscous gel. Antacids such as aluminium hydroxide and antibiotics such as amoxicillin can be good candidates for incorporation in these systems (Rajinikanth & Mishra, 2008).

The conceptualization of the raft forming systems depends on the physicochemical properties of the drug molecule and the diseased condition for which treatment is required. Physicochemical and pharmaceutical factors include molecular weight, lipophilicity, molecular charge, pH, gelation temperature, viscosity, osmolarity, and spreadability whereas physiological factors include membrane transport and pH of tissue fluid. To achieve desired gastric retention of the system, the dosage form must be able to satisfy the following criteria:

1. The drug should be released in a controlled manner from the system while maintaining buoyancy for a prolonged period of time.

2. The dosage form must be able to withstand the force exerted by peristaltic waves, constant contractions, grinding and churning moments in the stomach.

3. Dosage form should maintain specific gravity lower than gastric fluid (1.004–1.01 g/cm^3).

4. Easy to administer.

5. After complete release of drug, the device should be easily evacuated from the stomach.

Various mechanisms for raft formation which have been reported are summarized below (Hampson *et al.*, 2005):

1.5.9.6.1   Raft Formation based on Chemical Mechanism

Here, ion sensitive polysaccharides such as carrageenan, gellan gum, pectin, and sodium alginate undergo phase transition in the presence of various ions such as K^+, Ca^+, Mg^+, and Na^+.

1.5.9.6.2   Raft Formation based on pH Dependent Gelling

In the development of such systems, various pH dependent polymers such as Carbopolor its derivatives, polyvinylacetal diethylaminoacetate, mixtures of poly (methacrylic acid) and poly(ethylene glycol) are used which organise into a *in situ* gel system (sol to gel) with respect to change in pH.

1.5.9.6.3   Raft Formation based on Temperature Dependent Gelling

This approach is based on the use of polymers which undergo temperature induced phase transition. Hydrogels such as pluronics [(poly(ethylene oxide)-poly(propylene oxide)-poly(ethylene oxide)] (PEO–PPOPEO Triblock), polymer networks of poly(acrylic acid) and polyacrylamide (PAAm) or poly(acrylamide-co-butyl methacrylate) are commonly used for the development of such systems. These hydrogels are liquid at room temperature (~25°C) and undergo gelation upon contact with body fluids (37 ± 2°C).

1.5.10   Advanced Technologies used to Develop Gastroretentive Systems

Various advanced approaches have been reported to increase the gastrointestinal transit time of the drug delivery systems in the stomach.

1.5.10.1   Intragastric Floating Gastrointestinal Drug Delivery Systems

These systems are composed of a drug reservoir encapsulated in a microporous compartment with apertures along its top and bottom surfaces. The walls of the drug reservoir compartment are properly sealed to avoid any direct contact of the undissolved drug with the mucosal surface. The intragastric floating can be achieved using low-density materials (e.g., fatty acids) and gas-forming agent. These systems can be prepared by simple ionotropic gelation method (Harrigan, 1977).

1.5.10.2 Inflatable Gastrointestinal Drug Delivery Devices

These devices are composed of an inflatable chamber containing a volatile liquid such as dichloromethane which gasified at 37°C to cause the chamber to inflate in the stomach. The inflatable chamber also contains a biodegradable polymer filament. These systems contain a copolymer of polyvinyl alcohol and polyethylene that gradually dissolves in the gastric fluid. Dissolution of this copolymer is responsible for the release of gas from the system after an extended period of time to permit the spontaneous ejection of the system from the stomach (Michaels, 1974).

1.5.10.3 Intragastric Osmotically Controlled Floating Drug Delivery Devices

These are hollow deformable polymeric capsule shells. The capsule is divided into two compartments separated by using a membrane that allows selective transport across it. The drug is enclosed in the inner reservoir, which is covered by an outer osmotically active compartment. The osmoticlally active compartment generally contains a volatile liquid such as dichloromethane that vaporizes at the body temperature. Vaporization of liquid increases the size of unit to inflate. The device contains a bioerodible plug that allows the vapours to escape from the device and bring it back to the original position after a prolonged period of time for easy removal from the body (Michaels *et al.*, 1975). This device consists of two basic compartments:

1. ***Drug reservoir compartment:*** This compartment is enclosed by a pressure responsive collapsible bag, which is impermeable to vapour and liquid and has a drug delivery orifice.

2. ***Osmotically active compartment:*** This compartment contains an osmotically active salt and is enclosed within a semipermeable housing. In the stomach, gastric fluid is continuously absorbed through the semipermeable membrane into the osmotically active compartment to dissolve the osmotically active salt. An osmotic pressure is created, which acts on the collapsible bag and, in turn, forces the drug reservoir compartment to reduce its volume and activate the release of a drug through the delivery orifice.

TABLE 1.1

List of marketed formulations based on gastric retention technology

Manufacturer	Dosage form	Brand Name	Active Drug	Technology
Hoffmann-LaRoche, USA	Capsule	Valrelease®	Diazepam	Floating capsule
Roche Products, USA	Capsule	Madopar®	Benserazide, Levodopa	HBS
Glaxosmithkline, India	Liquid	Liquid Gaviscon	Aluminium hydroxide, Magnesium carbonate	Effervescent floating preparation
Pierre Faber Drug, France	Liquid	Topalkan	Aluminium-magnesium antacid	Floating liquid alginate preparation
Ranbaxy, India	Colloidal gel	Conviron	Ferrous sulphate	Colloidal gel forming floating drug delivery system
Pharmacia, USA	Capsule	Cytotech	Misoprostol	Bilayer floating capsule
Ranbaxy, India	Tablet	Cifran OD	Ciprofloxacin	Gas-generating floating form
Pierre Fabre Drug, France	Liquid	Almagate float coat	Aluminium-magnesium antacid	Floating liquid formulation
Glaxosmithkline, Philadelphia	Effervescent floating form	Coreg CR	Carvedilol	Osmotic system
Bayer, USA	Tablet	Cipro XR	Ciprofloxacin hydrochloride and betaine	Erodible matrix based system
Sun Pharma, India	Tablet	Baclofen GRS	Baclofen	Coated multi-layer floating & swelling system
Sun Pharma, India	Tablet	Prazopress XL	Prazosin HCl	Effervescent and swelling-based floating system
Ranbaxy, India	Tablet	Zanocin OD	Ofloxacin	Effervescent floating system
Ranbaxy, India	Tablet	Riomet OD	Metformine HCl	Effervescent floating system
Depomed, USA	AcuForm	ProQuin XR	Ciprofloxacin	Polymer-based swelling technology.
Depomed, USA	AcuForm	Glumetza	Metformin HCl	Polymer-based swelling technology
Depomed, USA	AcuForm	Metformin GR	Metformin HCl	Polymer-based swelling technology

TABLE 1.1 Contd...

Manufacturer	Dosage form	Brand Name	Active Drug	Technology
Galenix, France	Tablet	Metformin HCl LP	Metformin HCl	Minextab Floating
Galenix, France	Tablet	Cafeclor LP	Cefaclor	Minextab Floating
Galenix, France	Tablet	Tramadol LP	Tramadol	Minextab Floating
Sato Pharma, Japan	Tablet	Inon Ace Tablets	Siméthicone	Foam based floating system
Depomed, USA	AcuForm	Gabapentin GR	Gabapentin	Polymer-based swelling technology

1.5.11 Evaluation of Gastroretentive Drug Delivery Systems

In today's world, the quality product is a key strategic factor to meet the global regularity requirements for better realization of organizational goals such as better customer care and increased profitability. In recent years, the quality control measurements have received much attention of researchers from the academia and industries. The quality product can be obtained by a critical product evaluation process. In this respect, the evaluation should start during the preformulation stage and continued till the finished product is delivered. The preformulation studies focus on those physiochemical properties of the formulation ingredients that affect the drug performance and development of an efficacious dosage form. A thorough understanding of these properties, ultimately provide a rationale for formulation design. Drug identification test and drug-exicipients compatibility studies are done in this phase to provide a useful support in the development of dosage forms. The preformulation studies includes following tests:

1. Drug identification tests such as solubility, melting point, physical appearance etc.

2. Fourier transform infrared spectroscopy for drug identification and to investigate the possible interaction between drug and excipients.

3. Differential scanning calorimetry to examine the thermal behavior of drug alone or in combination with excipients.

4. X-ray diffraction studies to examine the physical state (amorphous or crystalline) of drug alone or in combination with excipients.

1.5.11.1 *In vitro* Evaluation

The density of dosage form is a major factor affecting the performance of such delivery systems, thus it is an important parameter to be evaluated during product development. To float on the gastric fluid, a system should have a density lower than the gastric fluid ($\sim$1.004 g/cm^3). True density can be determined using liquid displacement or photographic counting method. The percentage buoyancy (buoyancy lag time and buoyancy duration) can be determined by taking a predetermined amount of dosage form in 100 ml of suitable medium such as 0.1 N hydrochloric acid (pH 1.2). In case of multiparticulate systems, floated and settled particles are collected separately after predetermined time intervals. The fractions (floating and settled) are weighed and the buoyancy can be determined using following formula:

$$\text{Buoyancy (\%)} = \frac{\text{Weight of floating units}}{\text{Weight of floating units} + \text{Weight of settled units}} \times 100$$

As the morphology of the system has an influence on the drug encapsulation and drug release behaviour, the detailed observations of surface and cross-sectional characters of the micro-particles could be estimated by scanning electron microscope.

The percentage encapsulation (in the case of multiparticulate systems) is determined by suspending the powered microparticles in a suitable medium. After suitable time period, filtrate is analyzed for drug content using an analytical technique after suitable dilution. The percentage drug encapsulation can be determined by dividing the actual amount of drug present in the microparticles to theoretical amount of drug added to the formulation.

In vitro drug release from gastroretentive systems is generally performed in simulated gastric fluid at 37°C. Determination of drug release from the system at slightly higher pH, such as phosphate buffer pH 6.8, is also recommended due to the variation in gastric pH based on fasting or fed conditions. Dissolution tests generally are performed using USP II dissolution apparatus. USP 28 states ''the dosage unit is allowed to sink to the bottom of the vessel before rotation of the blade is started''. A small, loose piece of non-reactive material with not more than a few turns of a wire helix may be attached to the dosage units that would otherwise float. It is described that the drug release rate is reduced when helical wire is used. This limitation can be overcome by the method reported by (Soppimath et al., 2001). Briefly, the floating drug delivery system is fully submerged under a ring or mesh assembly. Recently, a custom-built stomach model has been reported for simultaneous depiction of buoyancy and drug release profiles (Eberle *et al.*, 2014).

1.5.11.2 *In vivo* Evaluation

1.5.11.2.1 γ-Scintigraphy

In vivo buoyancy behaviour of gastroretentive systems can be examined using γ-scintigraphic technique. This technique is based on the incorporation of a radioisotope (such as 99 mTc-DTPA) within the dosage form. The radioisotope labelled formulation is administered to the suitable animals or human volunteers. Major draw-backs of this technique are ionization radiations, limited topographic information, low resolution, and high cost (Goole *et al.*, 2008; Wilding *et al.*, 2001).

1.5.11.2.2 Radiology

Radiology is a simplest technique used for estimation of *in vivo* gastroretention. However, this technique has not gained popularity due to exposure to X-rays. Radiographs are taken at various periodic time intervals after administration of the dosage form (Baumgartner *et al.*, 2000).

1.5.11.2.3 Gastroscopy

Optic-fibers and a video camera are used for visual observation of dosage form in the stomach. Poor results may be obtained due to the presence of food in the stomach.

1.5.11.2.4 Ultrasonography

Ultrasonic waves are used to produce images of body structures. The waves travel through tissues and are reflected back where density differs. The reflected echoes are received by an electronic apparatus that measures their intensity level and the position of the tissue reflecting them. The results can be displayed as images or as a moving picture (Hendee, 1994).

1.5.11.2.5 Magnetic Resonance Imaging

Magnetic Resonance Imaging (MRI) is a non-invasive technology uses magnetic field, radio frequency pulses, and a computer to produce a detailed image of the buoyant formulation during *in vivo* conditions. This technique does not use ionization radiation as is observed with γ-scintigraphy. Harmless paramagnetic and supra-magnetic imaging contrast agents are applied to obtain better results (Dorozynski *et al.*, 2007).

1.5.11.2.6 Pharmacokinetics

These investigations involve analysis of blood samples at specified time intervals after dose administration. Pharmacokinetic parameters including maximum plasma concentration (C_{max}), time to reach maximum plasma concentration (T_{max}) and area under the curve (AUC) are investigated to assess the *in vivo* performance of these drug delivery systems.

1.5.12 Future Recommendations

The expected gastric retention, especially with low calories or fasted conditions is compromised. To provide evidence that a gastroretentive technology actually works, development and *in vivo* testing of the system should be carried out by considering following parameters (Awasthi and Kulkarni, 2014b):

1. The size, shape and surface morphology of dosage form should be monitored. The delivery system should not break into parts during the testing and should release the drug at a constant rate for prolonged period of time.
2. The buoyancy can be controlled either by controlling water penetration inside the delivery system or by modifying the swelling property of the system.
3. The analysis of the position of dosage form, to determine the buoyancy behaviour, should be done using an imaging technique.
4. The effect of caloric content of the meal should be carefully monitored during the product development. At least 6 h break should be given between two successive meals.

References

Awasthi R, and Kulkarni G.T (2014a). Development of novel gastroretentive drug delivery system of gliclazide: hollow beads. *Drug Dev Ind Pharm* **40:** 398-408.

Awasthi R, and Kulkarni G.T (2014b). Decades of research in drug targeting to the upper gastrointestinal tract using gastroretention technology: Where do we stand? *Drug Delivery* Early Online: 1-17. DOI:10.3109/10717544. 2014.936535.

Awasthi R, Pawar V. K, and Kulkarni G.T (2010). Floating microparticulate systems: an approach to increase gastric retention. *Indian Journal of Pharmaceutics* **1:** 17-26.

Baumgartner S, Krist J, Vreer F, Vodopivecb P, and Zorko B (2000). Optimisation of floating matrix tablets and evaluation of their gastric residence time. *Int J Pharm* **195:** 125-135.

Chun M.K, Sah H. and Choi H.K (2005). Preparation of mucoadhesive microspheres containing antimicrobial agents for eradication of *H. pylori*. *Int J Pharm* **297:** 172-179.

Costa P, and Lobo J.M.S (2001). Modeling and comparison of dissolution profiles. *Eur J Pharm Sci* **13:** 123-133.

Dorozynski P, Kulinowski P, Jachowicz R, and Jasinski A. (2007). Development of a system for simultaneous dissolution studies and magnetic resonance imaging of water transport in hydrodynamically balanced systems: a technical note. *AAPS Pharm Sci Tech* **8:** E1-4.

Eberle V.A, Schoelkopf J, Gane P.A.C, Alles R, Huwyler J, and Puchkov M (2014). Floating gastroretentive drug delivery systems: comparison of experimental and simulated dissolution profiles and floatation behavior. *Eur J Pharm Sci* **58:** 34-43.

Erni W, and Held K. (1987). The hydrodynamically balanced system: a novel principle of controlled drug release. *Eur Neurol* **27:** 21-27.

Gibaldi M, and Feldman S (1967). Establishment of sink conditions in dissolution rate determinations - theoretical considerations and application to nondisintegrating dosage forms. *J Pharm Sci* **56:** 1238-1242.

Goole J, Gansbeke B.V, Pilcer G, Deleuze Ph, Blocklet D, Goldman S, Pandolfo M, Vanderbist F, and Amighi K (2008). Pharmacoscintigraphic and pharmacokinetic evaluation on healthy human volunteers of sustained-release floating minitablets containing levodopa and carbidopa. *Int J Pharm* **364:** 54-63.

Groning R, Berntgen M, and Georgarakis M (1998). Acyclovir serum concentrations following peroral administration of magnetic depot tablets and the influence of extracorporal magnets to control gastrointestinal transit. *Eur J Pharm Biopharm* **46:** 285-291.

Hampson F.C, Farndale A, Strugala V, Sykes J, Jolliffe I.G, and Dettmar P.W (2005). Alginate rafts and their characterization. *Int J Pharm* **294:** 137-147.

Harrigan R.M (1977). Drug delivery device for preventing contact of undissolved drug with the stomach lining. United States patent US 4, 055, 178. October 25.

Hejazi R, and Amiji M (2002). Stomach-specific anti *H. pylori* therapy I: Preparation and characterization of tetracycline of a floationg multiple-unit, capsule, a high-density loaded chitosan microcapsules. *Int J Pharm* **235:** 87-94.

Hendee WR. (1994). Fundamentals of diagnostic imaging: characteristics of the radio-graphic image. In: Putman CE, Ravin CE, eds. Textbook of diagnostic imaging, Vol. 1. Philadelphia: WB Saunders Co., 9-10.

Higuchi T (1961). Rate of release of medicaments from ointment bases containing drugs in suspensions. *J Pharm Sci* **50**: 874-875.

Higuchi T (1963). Mechanisms of sustained action mediation. Theoretical analysis of rate of release of solid drugs dispersed in solid matrices. *J Pharm Sci* **52**: 1145-1149.

Hixson A.W, and Crowell J.H (1931). Dependence of reaction velocity upon surface and agitation. *Ind Eng Chem* **23**: 923-931.

Hou S.Y, Cowles V.E, and Berner B (2003). Gastric retentive dosage forms: a review. *Crit Rev Ther Drug Carrier Syst* **20**: 459-497.

Huang Y, Leobandung W, Foss A, and Peppas N.A (2000). Molecular aspects of muco- and bioadhesion: tethered structures and site-specific surfaces. *J Control Release* **65**: 63-71.

Lee P, (1980). Diffusional release of a solute from a polymeric matrix: Approximate analytical solutions. *J Membrane Sci* **7**: 255-275.

Malcolm R.K, Fetherston S.M, McCoy C.F, Boyd P, and Major I (2012). Vaginal rings for delivery of HIV microbicides. *Int J Womens Health* **4**: 595-605.

Mazer N, Abisch E, Gfeller J.C, Laplanche R, Bauerfeind P, Cucala M, Lukachich M, and Blum A (1988). Intragastric behavior and absorption kinetics of a normal and "floating" modified-release capsule of isradipine under fasted and fed conditions. *J Pharm Sci* **77**: 647-657.

Michaels A.S (1974). Drug delivery device with self-actuated mechanism for retaining device in selected area, United States patent US 3, 786, 813. January 22.

Michaels A.S, Bashwa J.D, and Zaffaroni A (1975). Integrated device for administering beneficial drug at programmed rate. United States patent US 3, 901, 232. August 26.

Mojaverian P, Vlasses P.H, Kellner P.E, and Rocci M.L (1988). Effects of gender, posture, and age on gastric residence time of an indigestible solid: pharmaceutical considerations. *Pharm Res* **10**: 639-644.

Mouzam M.I, Dehghan M.H.G, Asif S, Sahuji T, and Chudiwal P (2011). Preparation of a novel floating ring capsule-type dosage form for stomach specific delivery. *Saudi Pharmaceutical Journal* **19**: 85-93.

Mulye N.V, and Turco S.J (1995). A simple model based on first order kinetics to explain release of highly water soluble drugs from porous dicalcium phosphate dihydrate matrices. *Drug Dev Ind Pharm* **21**: 943-953.

Nakamichi K, Yasuura H, Fukui H, Oka M, and Izumi S (2001). Evaluation of a floating dosage form of nicardipine hydrochloride and hydroxypropylmethylcellulose acetate succinate prepared using a twin-screw extruder. *Int J Pharm* **218:** 103-112.

Newton M.J (2010). Gastric emptying of multi-particulate dosage forms. *Int J Pharm* **395:** 2-8.

Niebergall P.J, Milosovich G, and Goyan, J.E (1963). Dissolution rate studies. II. Dissolution of particles under conditions of rapid agitation. *J Pharm Sci* **52:** 236-241.

Paul D, and McSpadden S (1976). Diffusional release of a solute from a polymer matrix. *J Membrane Sci* **1:** 33-48.

Pawar V.K, Kansal S, Garg G, Awasthi R, Singodia D, and Kulkarni G.T (2011). Gastroretentive dosage forms: A review with special emphasis on floating drug delivery systems. *Drug Deliv* **18:** 97-110.

Peppas N.A (1985). Analysis of Fickian and non-Fickian drug release from polymers. *Pharm Acta Helv* **60:** 110-111.

Peppas N.A, and Korsmeyer R.W (1986). Dynamically swelling hydrogels in controlled release applications. In: Peppas N.A (Ed.), Hydrogels in Medicine and Pharmacy, Vol. 3, Boca Raton: CRC Press. pp. 109-136.

Qiu Y, and Park K (2003). Superporous IPN Hydrogels Having Enhanced Mechanical Properties. *AAPS Pharm Sci Tech* **4** (4) Article 51. Available from http://www.pharmscitech.org.Accessed on 04 June 2010.

Rajinikanth P.S, and Mishra B (2008). Floating *in situ* gelling system for stomach site-specific delivery of clarithromycin to eradicate *H. pylori. J Control Release***125:** 33-41.

Ritger P.L, and Peppas N.A (1987a). A simple equation for description of solute release. I. Fickian and non-Fickian release from non-swellable devices in the form of slabs, spheres, cylinders or discs, *J Controll Release* **5:** 23-36.

Ritger P.L, and Peppas N.A (1987b). A simple equation for description of solute release II. Fickian and anomalous release from swellable devices. *J Control Release* **5:** 37-42.

Rouge N, Allemann E, Gex-Fabry M, Balant L, Cole E.T, Buri P, and Doelker E (1998). Comparative pharmacokinetic study of a floating multiple-unit capsule, a high density multiple-unit capsule and an immediate-release tablet containing 25 mg atenolol. *Pharm Acta Helbetiae* **73:** 81-87.

Rubinstein A, and Friend D.R (1994). Specific delivery to the gastrointestinal tract In: Domb AJ, ed. Polymeric site-specific pharmacotherapy. Chichester: Wiley. p. 282-283.

Shen S.I, Jasti B.R, and Li X (2003). Design of controlled-release drug delivery systems. In: Kutz M (Ed.), Biomedical engineering and design Handbook, Vol 2, Chapter 22, New York: McGraw-Hill Professional.

Sharma S, and Pawar A (2006). Low density multiparticulate system for pulsatile release of meloxicam. *Int J Pharm* **313:** 150-158.

Soppimath K.S, Kulkarni A.R, and Aminabhavi T.M (2001). Development of hollow microspheres as floating controlled-release system for cardio-vascular drugs: preparation and release characteristics. *Drug Dev Ind Pharm* **27:** 507-515.

Streubel A, Siepmann J, and Bodmeier R (2006). Drug delivery to the upper small intestine window using gastroretentive technologies. *Curr Opin Pharmacol* **6:** 501-508.

Takahashi T (2012). Mechanism of interdigestive migrating motor complex. *J Neurogastroenterol Motil* **18:** 246-257.

Timmermans J, and Moes A.J (1994). Factors controlling the buoyancy and gastric retention capabilities of floating matrix capsules: new data for reconsidering the controversy. *J Pharm Sci* **83:** 18-24.

Varelas C.G, Dixon D.G, and Steiner C (1995). Zero-order release from biphasic polymer hydrogels. *J Controll Release* **34:** 185-192.

Wilding I.R, Coupe A.J, and Davis S.S (2001). The role of gamma-scintigraphy in oral drug delivery. *Adv Drug Deliv Rev* **46:** 103-124.

2   Self-Emulsifying Drug Delivery Systems: A Novel Drug Delivery Model

Jaya Gopal Meher[1], M. Chaurasia[2], S. K. Paliwal[3] and Manish K. Chourasia[1]

[1]Pharmaceutics Division, CSIR-Central Drug Research Institute, Lucknow-226 031, India.

[2]Amity Institute of Pharmacy, Amity University, Lucknow-226 028, India.

[3]Department of Pharmaceutical Sciences, Banasthali University, Banasthali-304 022, India.

2.1   Introduction

Drug delivery sciences face some basic questions in the formulation development process and the most important among them are

(i) How the therapeutic efficacy of the drug molecules can be augmented?

(ii) How the toxic/adverse effect of drug molecules can be minimized maintaining the desired therapeutic response?

These questions are relevant to both the existing drug molecules as well as the new chemical entities. When the first question is being concerned, bioavailability comes to the picture which is dependent on both solubility and permeability of the drug molecules. Majority (approximately 40%) of the new chemical entities discovered in last few decades exhibit poor solubility leading to high intra-/inter-subject variability, and inadequate dose proportionality (Lukyanov and Torchilin, 2004). Hence, improvement of solubility and bioavailability of these drug molecules remain the prime objective of formulation scientists. Several strategies *viz.* particle size reduction, salt formation, complexation with carrier molecules, pro-drug development etc., are adopted to enhance solubility as well as bioavailability. Self-emulsifying drug delivery system (SEDDS) is one of the prominent alternatives which has gained industrial viability (Singh et al., 2011).

SEDDS are isotropic mixtures of drug molecules (lipophilic), oils (lipids), surfactants, and co-solvents/-emulsifiers. SEDDS may be in solid, liquid or semi-solid form and when come in contact with aqueous media (gastric fluid) with mild agitation (gastric motility), form a fine emulsion. The formation of emulsion may be either micro-/nano-emulsion based on the preparation procedure as well as excipients used. The solid-SEDDS have added advantages of comparatively better stability, ease of handling, packaging, transporting, storage and manufacturing. Based on the size of the oil droplets formed, these SEDDS may be self-micro-emulsifying drug delivery system (SMEDDS; size: 100-300 nm) or self-nano-emulsifying drug delivery system (SNEDDS; size: < 50 nm). Formation of emulsion increases the exposed surface area and facilitates the absorption and bioavailability of the lipophilic drug molecules from the gastro intestinal tract. The SEDDS can be delivered as a capsule (soft/hard gelatin) or even as a drinking emulsion for oral drug delivery (Kohli et al., 2010). SEDDS can be classified in different categories and a systematic classification has been depicted in Table 2.1.

TABLE 2.1

A systematic approach of classification of SEDDS

Types	Description
	Based on size of the emulsified droplets size
SEDDS	The emulsified droplets are not defined but vary usually in the range of 1-5 µm.
SMEDDS	The emulsified droplets are in the size of 100-300 nm.
SNEDDS	The emulsified droplets are in the size < 50 nm.
	Based on the physical state of SEDDS
Solid SEDDS	These are in the tablet, pallets, granule or lyophilized powder form. From the stability point of view solid SEDDS are better than other two form of SEDDS.
Semi-solid SEDDS	These are in semi-solid paste/admixture form depending on the type of excipients used. Usually these are delivered as a soft/hard gelatin capsule.
Liquid SEDDS	These are the conventionally manufactured SEDDS which are simple (isotropic) admixture of oils, surfactants and co-surfactants.
	Based on excipients and functional features
Type 1 SEDDS	Oil: 40-80%, surfactants: 20-40% (HLB < 12), co-solvent - 0, droplet size: 100-250 nm, emulsification capacity - low, solvent capacity - low, loss of solvent capacity on dilution - none to slight.

TABLE 2.1 *Contd...*

Types	Description
	Based on excipients and functional features
Type 2 SEDDS	Oil: 40-80%, surfactants: 20-40% (HLB > 12), co-solvent: 0-40%, droplet size: 100-250 nm, emulsification capacity - medium, solvent capacity -medium, loss of solvent capacity on dilution - moderate.
Type 3 SEDDS	Oil: < 20%, surfactants: 20-50% (HLB > 11), co-solvent: 50-100%, droplet size: ~100 nm, emulsification capacity - high, solvent capacity -high, loss of solvent capacity on dilution - none to slight.
Type 4 SEDDS	Oil: < 20%, surfactants: 20-60% (HLB ~10), co-solvent: 60-100%, droplet size: < 50 nm, emulsification capacity - high, solvent capacity - high, loss of solvent capacity on dilution - none to slight.

The prerequisite for a drug molecule to be delivered as SEDDS is low water solubility and high lipid solubility. Usually the BCS class II and IV drugs are suitable to be formulated as SEDDS. Majority of the chemotherapeutic agents are thus the eligible candidates for SEDDS. Precipitation of drug is very often seen upon dilution with water and must be taken seriously in the formulation development program. After being emulsified the drug must not be partitioned more into the aqueous phase, which may lead to precipitation and finally poor bioavailability (Tang et al., 2008). There are many proposed theories for the improved bio-availability of the SEDDS and more than one among them are predicted to be involved in this process. These theories include

(i) lymphatic uptake of the emulsified droplets containing drug molecules,

(ii) formation of bile salt micelles,

(iii) down regulation of the p-glycoprotein induced efflux of drug molecules and

(iv) reduction of the gastrointestinal metabolism of the drug molecule (Faisal et al., 2013; Yan et al., 2012).

Before proceeding for formulation and development some issues such as choice of excipients, physicochemical properties of drug molecule, solubility of drug in excipient, optimization of formulation, scale up, and production of the drug product must be discussed and properly planned. Scale up is a chief issue of concern for any novel drug delivery system.

Many of these delivery systems get confined only to laboratory scale and unless being scaled up to the industrial measure any drug delivery system cannot be considered as a successful model. SEDDS could be scaled up to the industrial scale and many products are commercially available for therapeutic use which is discussed in section 9. Such success advocates the feasibility of SEDDS and puts an end to all postulations regarding its failure as an effective drug delivery tool.

2.2   Excipients

Excipients have very crucial role to play in SEDDS. The selection and utilization of suitable excipients at appropriate concentration determine the development of a suitable product. Excipients must be able to develop a fine emulsion (micro-/nano-emulsion) upon contact with water (aqueous medium) and at the same time it must not also exhibit any undesirable side effect or toxic effect. The drug-excipient compatibility must be ensured before proceeding for product development. Many sophisticated analytical tools may be employed for this purpose and now-a-days many excipient manufacturing companies provide detailed information (material safety data sheet, excipient information etc.) which can be used. Many regulatory authorities publish list of recommended excipients which are also called as generally recognized as safe (GRAS) excipients can be used at their allowable concentration. SEDDS has 3 major components viz. oil (lipid), surfactant and co-solvent. Apart from these, there may be some additives such as antioxidant, chelating agent, stabilizer and preservatives etc. As a rule the number and quantity of excipients should be minimum as possible. Some excipients play role in the formation of emulsion and other show major role in the absorption of drug to the biological system.

2.2.1 Oils

For any emulsion formulation, oil is the integral component which gets emulsified with the surfactant and water forming an emulsion. For SEDDS also oils are very much essential and must be chosen with proper rationale. Edible oils are preferred for SEDDS formulations and are also suitable for various routes of administration such as oral, topical or parenteral routes. However, oils causing irritation should not be employed for oral formulations. Usually SEDDS forms an oil in water emulsion upon dilution and the oil is intended to carry the water insoluble drug(s). As it behaves like the carrier of the drug, it must have good solubilizing capacity for the drug. These oils or lipids may be either long chain or medium chain fatty acid esters (triglycerides). Functionalized triglycerides are preferred these days for their ability to accommodate high quantity of drug and to provide comparatively better stability than non-functionalized triglycerides. The spectrum of oils/lipids used in SEDDS is wide which includes phospholipids (phosphatidyl choline, phosphatidyl inositol, phosphatidyl ethanolamine, phosphatidic acid etc.), fatty alcohols (cetyl alcohol, stearyl alcohol, cetostearyl alcohol, lanolin alcohols, oleyl alcohol etc.), oils (cod liver oil, corn oil, cottonseed oil, safflower oil, sesame oil, soybean oil, olive oil, peanut oil etc.). Presently many functionalized oils are available which are either esterified/co-processed/combined with other ingredients and increase the solvent capacity as well as surfactant properties. Examples of such ingredients include Labrafil® (apricot kernel oil and PEG 300), Gelucire® (corn oil and PEG 300), Capmul® (glycerylmonocaprylocaprate), Maisine™ (glycerylmonolinoleate) etc. (Gursoy et al., 2003; Kohli et al., 2010; Prasad et al., 2013).

It is already known that edible oils are taken up by the lymphatic system of GIT up to a considerable extent. So it is possible that digestible oils carrying drug molecules may be taken up by the lymphatic system and directly influence bioavailability. Further it depends on the emulsification efficiency, digestibility, stability and solubilizing ability of oils on the amount of drugs to be transported by lymphatic system. It is evident that medium chain fatty acid esters containing drug gets rapidly absorbed from intestine and reach liver by hepatic portal system. By this way also the poorly soluble drugs get absorbed from the GIT and get distributed to the target site. The fatty acid esters are digested in the hepatocytes' mitochondria releasing carbon dioxide, water and energy (Gao et al., 2009; Lukyanov and Torchilin, 2004).

2.2.2 Surfactants

One of the general fact in drug delivery is that surfactants manage conflicts between the two immiscible phases viz. aqueous and oil phase. As in case of conventional emulsion a perfect combination of surfactant is responsible for the long term stability and efficacy of the SEDDS. The use of combination of surfactants is common and it is well known that the combination of surfactants could provide a rigid layer surrounding the oil globule helping to keep away other oil globules in the emulsion whereas a single surfactant may not be able to perform the same leading to degradation of emulsion (Rosen and Kunjappu, 2012). Combination of surfactants with considerable difference in HLB values is preferable as it could develop an appropriate packing arrangement around the emulsified oil globules. Fig. 2.1 gives a diagrammatic representation of the above discussed matter. Non-ionic surfactants self-assemble forming micelles, in to lamellar, hexagonal and sponge like bi-continuous morphologies (Lachman L. et al., 1990). In the micro-/ nano-emulsions the rigid layer of surfactant form an extended interface between oil-water and its local curvature determines the structure of emulsion. Exhaustive chemistry involved in this process is beyond the scope of this book, and readers are encouraged to go through related literature. The concept of using combination of surfactants is also applicable to SEDDS.

In case of liquid/semi solid SEDDS, the isotropic mixture of oils, surfactants and co-solvents remains in the liquid state and possibility of destabilization is more. At the same time solid SEDDS is considered to be comparatively stable. This phenomenon may be assumed due to the increased/facilitated rate of reaction of excipients and drug in the liquid/semisolid state, which might be less or even absent in solid SEDDS. Surfactants may influence the biological membranes and thus alter drug absorption. The quality and quantity of surfactants collectively decide the availability of the drug in the emulsified state, or else precipitation of drug in aqueous environment may occur leading to poor bioavailability (Rowe et al., 2009). However, mere theoretical assumptions may be not enough and practical experience in this regard is useful in selecting suitable surfactant combination for the development of SEDDS.

The usual concentration of surfactant in the SEDDS is 30-60%. It is noteworthy that the concentration of surfactant is high in this case in comparison to the conventional/novel emulsions. In regular emulsion an additional mechanical/temperature is applied to achieve emulsification, whereas SEDDS are intended to be emulsified *in situ* and no such additional forces are applied. This is the primary reason for high concentration of surfactant in SEDDS. Sometimes, high concentration of surfactants may cause gastric irritation and their safety must be assured earlier. Literature reveals that non-ionic surfactants with HLB 12-15 is most suitable in formulation of SEDDS (Tang et al., 2008). This may be attributed to the fact that most SEDDS are oil in water type emulsions, necessitating higher ranges of HLB. There is a vast number of surfactants available including non-ionic surfactants viz. cetomacrogol (polyoxyethylated glycol monoethers), Spans (sorbitan esters) and Tweens (polysorbates), anionic surfactants (potassium laurate, sodium lauryl sulphate), cationic and amphoteric surfactants. Other examples include oleic acid, lauric acid, capric acid, heptanoic acid, stearic acid, sodium cholate, and glycocholate. The growing demand of surfactant for various purposes has led to the development of functionalized polymers such as Labrafil 1944 Cs, Lauroglycol 90, Peceol, Plurololeique CC497,

Labrafil M 2125 Cs, Labrasol, and Capryol 90 (Holmberg et al., 2003; Rowe et al., 2009). Utilization of HLB theory in the formulation of SEDDS has been discussed in many scientific research papers, but a systematic approach in this regard is yet to be established.

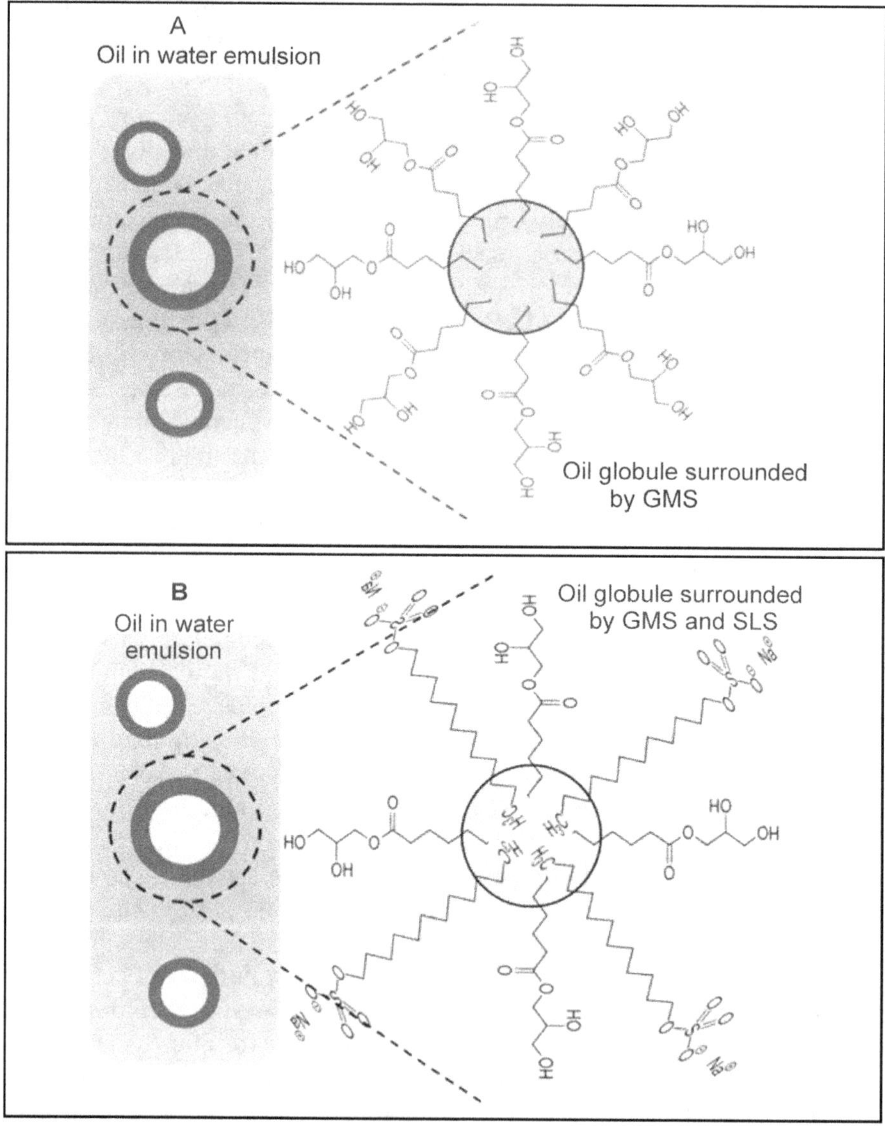

FIGURE 2.1 Diagrammatic representation of emulsified oil globules in an oil in water emulsion (A) oil globule surrounded by solo surfactant (GMS; HLB-5.5) molecules forming a soft monolayer leading to a comparatively unstable emulsion, (B) oil globule surrounded by combination of surfactants (GMS and

SLS; HLB-40) leading to a comparatively stable emulsion because of the rigid architecture provided by combination of surfactant molecules. It is also observed that the combination of surfactant having considerably different HLB values lead to stable emulsion than with surfactants of similar HLB values.

2.2.3 Co-solvents/Co-surfactants

As the name signifies these substances used to help solvation or emulsification in a bi-/multi-phasic system. It is discussed in the above section that a combination of surfactants is used in order to get better stability of emulsion, hence employment of a co-surfactant is justified in this case. Co-surfactants help in the formation of strong barrier membrane around the oil globules and inhibit the coalescence of oil droplets in the emulsion. Thermodynamically it reduces the interfacial tension as well as provide a better mechanical barrier function. It has also been observed to develop a repulsive layer around the dispersed globules which experiences an electrical repulsive force, making the emulsified droplets apart from each other. This electrical repulsive force is due to the surface charge on the oil globules, which might be owing to the molecular orientation of the surfactant. Similar to that of co-surfactant, the co-solvents also work as a supportive ingredients in the stability of emulsion. Co-solvents increase the solubility of the drug particle in the oil and help in formation of a stable biphasic system. Although SEDDS as such are not emulsion, rather these are isotropic mixture but finally SEDDS has to convert into emulsion and hence the role of co-solvent/-surfactant is very much crucial in the formulation of SEDDS.

Co-solvents that are commonly used in pharmaceutical field are alcohols but in SEDDS these are not preferred. The reason might be the volatility of these co-solvents, which might cause problems (degradation of capsule, precipitation of drug due to loss in alcohol content) while these SEDDS are delivered as a capsule dosage form. Other co-solvents may be polyethylene glycol, propylene glycol, glycerol etc., whereas any of the surfactants (Span, Tween, glyceryl stearate, cetyl alcohol, steryl alcohol, cetosteryl alcohol or even some polymers such as hydrophilic colloids) used in less quantity may act as co-surfactant. SEDDS is supposed to form emulsion *in situ* (less force for emulsification) so the role of co-solvents is very much important in facilitating the emulsification process. Compatibility of each co-surfactant/-solvent must be analyzed before formulation and development (Gursoy and Benita, 2004; Tang et al., 2008).

2.2.4 Pharmaceutical Additives

Oils, surfactants and co-solvents are the building blocks of SEDDS. These ingredients can form a stable SEDDS but none of these can assure stability for a long period. In such cases other additives are required to be incorporated in the SEDDS in order to assure the stability. It is very well known that oils are susceptible to oxidation to a great extent and any physical or chemical instability can be observed during the life time of the formulation. The oxidation products alter the molecular as well as thermodynamic balance in the SEDDS and also behave like a toxic ingredients. Employment of a suitable antioxidant is useful in this regard. Butylated hydroxy toluene (BHT) and butylated hydroxy anisole (BHA) are the most common antioxidants used in pharmaceutical preparations. It is worth mentioning that as like emulsion we are not free to use any types of antioxidants, rather in SEDDS lipophilic antioxidants are preferred due to their easy miscibility with oils. Lipids/oils are also inclined to degradation and it is usually initiated with a change in the pH of the SEDDS. In order to prevent such phenomena, edible buffers such as citrate, phosphate, cacodylate, borate, and bicarbonate buffers are used in the formulations. Other additives may be some polymers such as HPMC, but it is especially used to develop supersaturatable SEDDS (Gursoy and Benita, 2004; Rowe et al., 2009).

2.3   Formulation and Development

Formulation of the SEDDS is a multi-step process. There are four basic steps in the formulation of SEDDS comprising

  (i)   preformulation studies
  (ii) development of ternary phase diagram
  (iii) formulation of SEDDS by incorporating drug in to the isotropic mixture of oils, surfactants and co-solvents and
  (iv) development of a suitable dosage form incorporating the formulated SEDDS (Kohli et al., 2010; Pouton, 1997).

Fig. 2.2 gives the detailed formulation development scheme of SEDDS.

Preformulation studies include the investigation of the physicochemical properties of drug such as solubility, partition co-efficient, pKa and compatibility with other excipients. These studies suggest the suitable excipients that can be used for a specific drug molecules. It is notable that there are only few excipients available which could cause self-emulsification. Solubility studies are the prime area of interest in the SEDDS, as the selection of the oil phase solely depends on the solubility of drug molecule in that oil phase. The extent of solubility is also important as it will decide the amount of drug that can be accommodated in the SEDDS. The dose of the drug for the targeted diseases is to be taken into consideration during selecting the oil phase (Adeyeye and Brittain, 2008; Steele, 2004).

Phase behavior of three-component systems comprising water, oil and surfactant/co-surfactant mixture are generally characterized by isothermal triangular phase diagrams. Pseudo-ternary phase diagram is one of the competent methods for selection of best SEDDS formulation. A compromise of desired parameters including particle size, charge, drug entrapment, emulsification time and stability can be analyzed by this phase diagram. Different optimization techniques are also employed to investigate the best possible composition of SEDDS. Response surface methodologies (RSM) and factorial designs are used in the studies. The Central Composite and Box-Behnken designs are very popular among these as an optimization tool in SEDDS formulations. However these approaches are focused only for the selection of the suitable oil and surfactant in SEDDS but not for the whole emulsion formulation (Pouton, 1997). The next step in the formulation development is the preparation of the isotropic mixture of the selected excipients and the drug. The first step in this process is the solubilization of the required quantity of the drug in the oil/co-solvent which can be achieved by simply mixing the drug in the oil phase and if required an additional heat or mechanical force may be provided. The isotropic mixture should yield a clear solution of the excipients and the drug (Shao et al., 2010; Tang et al., 2008). This is the usual texture/consistency of the SEDDS, as majority of the excipients used in the formulation are liquid at room temperature. At the same time SEDDS may also be in semisolid form if the excipients used are very highly viscous/waxy in nature. In recent years solid SEDDS (S-SEDDS) is gaining popularity. Spray drying, solid dispersion, melt extrusion, nano-/micro-particle formulations are some of the strategies which are used to develop S-SEDDS in dry emulsion, nanoparticle, microspheres, pallets, and solid dispersion forms (Tang et al., 2008). Schematic flowcharts are shown in Fig. 2.3 and Fig. 2.4 exhibiting the steps in formulation of liquid/semi-solid and solid SEDDS.

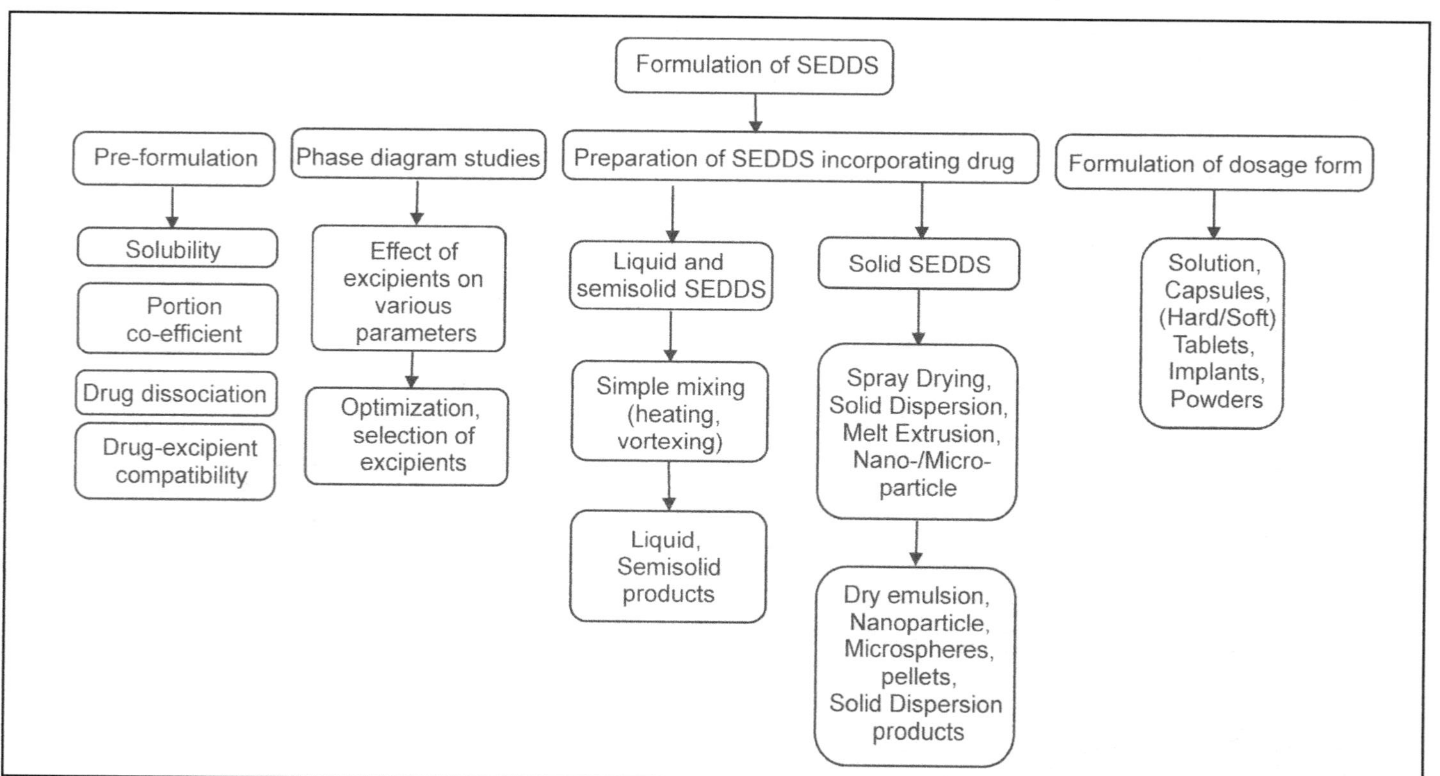

FIGURE 2.2 Scheme showing the formulation-development steps involved in SEDDS preparation.

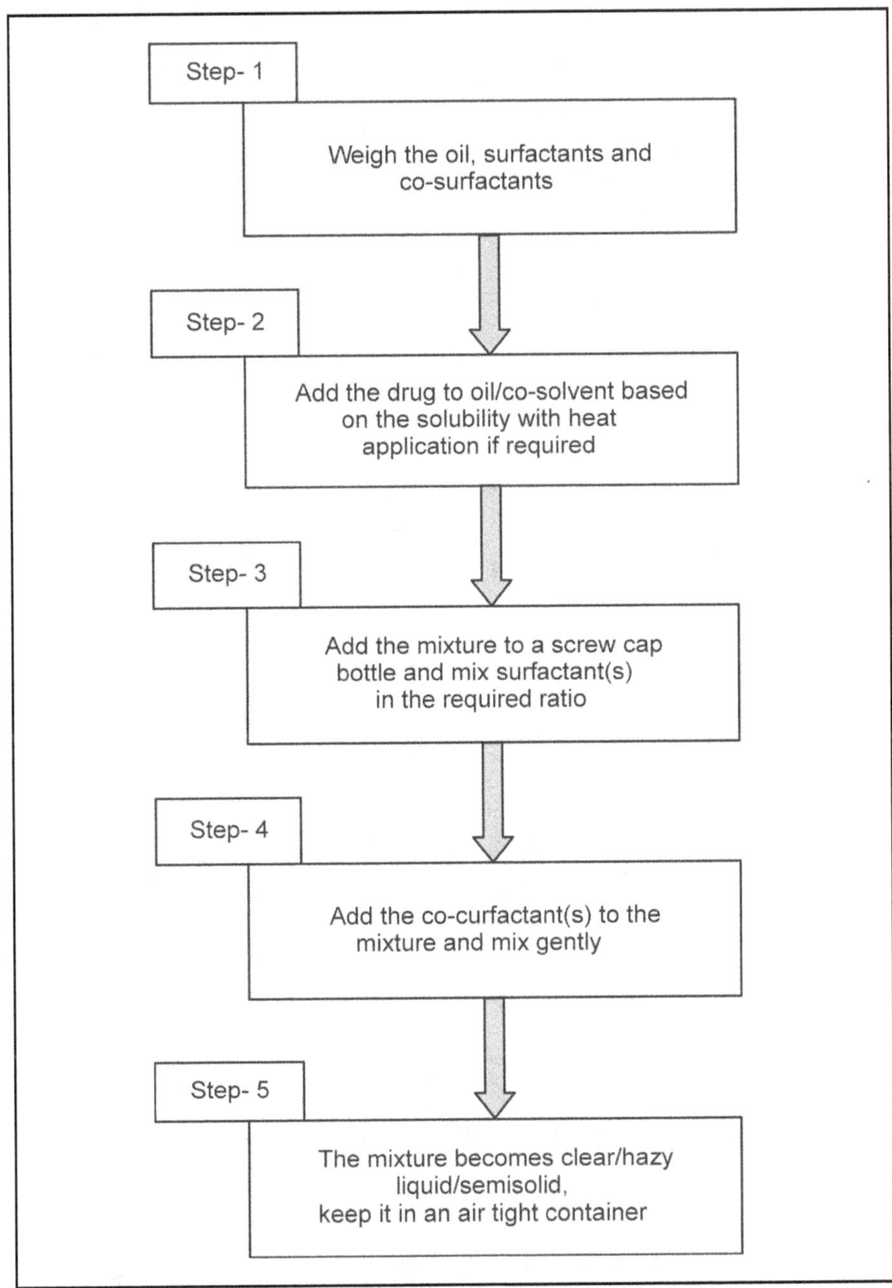

FIGURE 2.3 Steps involved in liquid/semisolid SEDDS formulation.

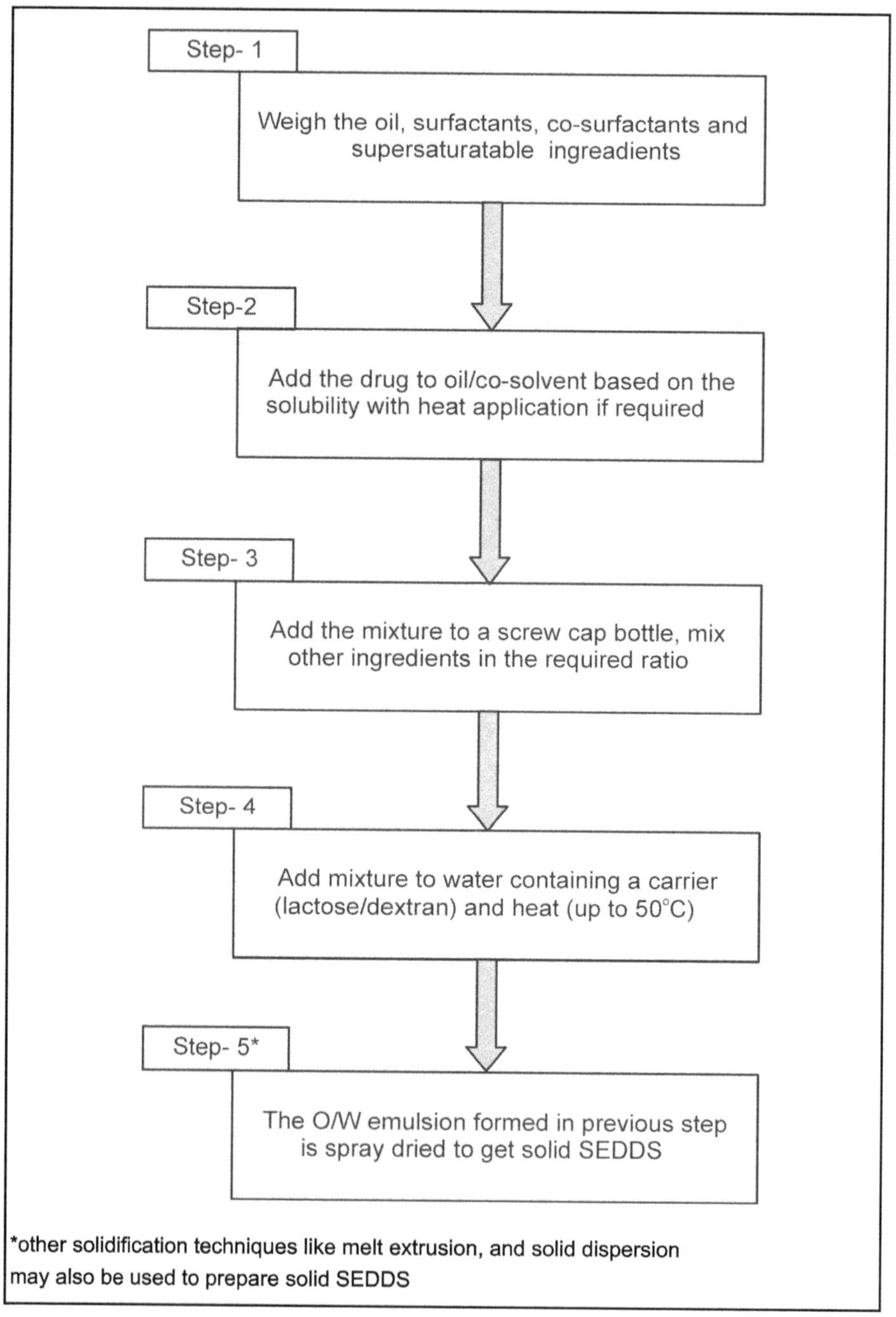

FIGURE 2.4 Steps involved in solid SEDDS formulation.

The last step in the formulation-development program is to give the formulated SEDDS a final shape in the form of a dosage form. If the SEDDS is in liquid or semisolid form then, it can be filled in to either a soft/hard gelatin capsule. Capsule filling and sealing is a routine tool which can be practiced in laboratory, pilot, and industrial scale. The capsule shell and SEDDS must have compatibility and it is the role of formulation scientist to resolve these issues well in advance. In case of S-SEDDS, different solid dosage forms viz. tablet, capsule, implants, powders and many other conventional and novel drug delivery systems can be developed (Breitkreitz et al., 2013; Park et al., 2013). Fig. 2.5 illustrates a diagrammatic representation of the soft/hard gelatin capsule containing the SEDDS and its formation as nano-/micro-emulsions in aqueous environment.

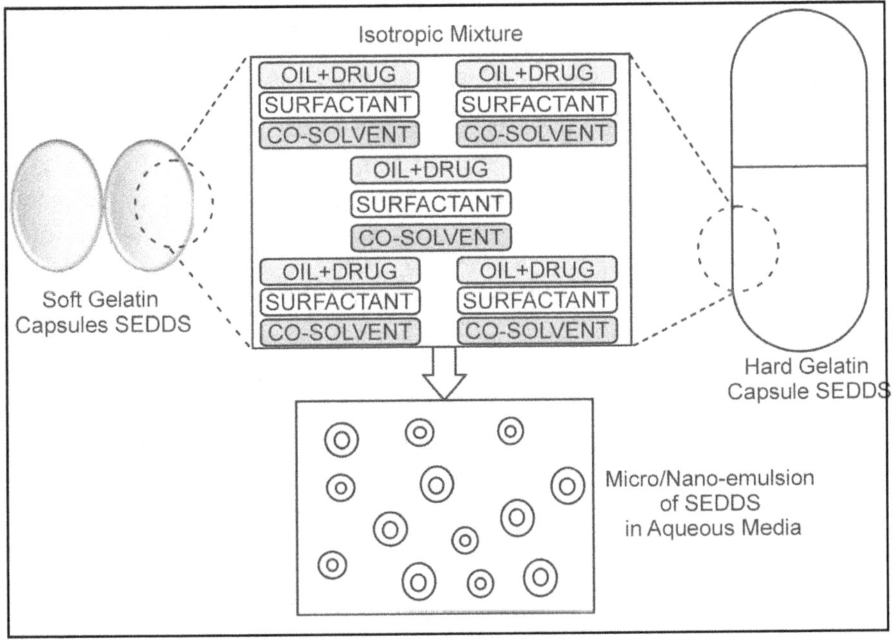

FIGURE 2.5 A diagrammatic representation of SEDDS in form of soft and hard gelatin capsule and formation of nano/microemulsion upon contact with aqueous media.

Now let us take a move to the mechanistic insight to the formation of SEDDS. Till date there is no concrete elucidated mechanism of formulation of SEDDS. To understand it in a better and simpler way let us take the example of conventional emulsification and then correlate with SEDDS. Now let us predict, what will happen a very less quantity of oil is added to water in a drop wise manner? Within a very short span of time, the oil droplets coalesce to form a bigger oil droplet. In other case, a complete dispersion of tiny oil droplets in water is achieved if the mixture is shaken vigorously with some mechanical means. Why is this happening? The reason lies in the fact that both the phases have diverse differences in polarity generating high interfacial tension and consequently system exhibits high free energy. In order to reduce the free energy of the system the oil droplets tend to coalesce forming bigger droplets. The free energy of the system is reduced by the addition of surfactants. The surfactant forms a layer around the dispersed oil droplets and minimizes the interfacial tension, which the oil droplets were trying to accomplish by coalescing in absence of surfactant. In a nutshell the surfactant provides comfort to the oil droplet and let it remains dispersed in the aqueous phase by reducing and dragging the free energy of the system in a comfort zone. Point to be noted is that in conventional system, it is achieved by application of heat or mechanical agitation.

Now let us consider the case of SEDDS, here we want the same phenomena to happen, but we are bit handicapped. In case of *in vivo* administration, we cannot provide heat or additional agitation, what we have maximum is $37\pm1°C$ as heat and gastric motility as agitation force that too vary from person to person. SEDDS should be developed composing such ingredients that a very little efforts will be required by water to get into the oil-surfactant surface with very less surface tension. This will lead to the development of a very fine emulsion. The oil-surfactant interface with water should behave very gently showing no or very less resistance to the entry of water. The initial process involved here is penetration of water to the oil-surfactant binary mixture forming a gel like structure. This will happen till the solubilization/saturation of water in the oil-surfactant surface. As and when the limit of water solubilization/saturation is reached, the water molecule will start breaking the oil-surfactant binary mixture and as an intermediate step, smaller oil-surfactant-water gel structure will be formed. Upon a gentle agitation these oil-surfactant-water gel structures get disrupted and form a fine emulsified system. Depending upon the employment of surfactant the self-emulsification may take place in few seconds or even in hours (Gursoy et al., 2003; Hong et al., 2006). Although these above discussed mechanism seems to be the most appropriate description of the sequential happening in the SEDDS but a deeper insight in to the self-emulsification phenomenon is needed.

2.4   Factors Affecting Formulation and Performance of SEDDS

Several factors may come in to play as far as the formulation-development and performance evaluation of SEDDS is concerned. The factors may be dependent on the API, excipients, manufacturing methods and volume of production, as well as the dosage form in which the SEDDS is intended to be delivered. The variation in these parameters are very much sensitive and unique for different formulations. However, a generalization can be made for those factors that significantly influence the formulation as well as the performance of SEDDS. These generalized parameters are almost common in all SEDDS formulations irrespective of their physico-chemical state. In the following section the major factors *viz.* excipients and physicochemical state of SEDDS and intended dosage form are discussed, how they affect the formulation and performance of SEDDS.

2.4.1 Excipients

SEDDS is kind of novel formulation where performance depends on the excipients, as self-emulsification can only be achieved by the combination of specific excipients in specific concentration. A minor variation may lead to alteration in the emulsification time, particle size, stability, bioavailability as well as therapeutic efficacy of the SEDDS formulation. Oil/lipid is the main ingredient in the SEDDS as it is usually chosen to solubilize the drug. After coming in contact with water, this oil phase is emulsified leading to formation of lipid emulsified globules containing drug which is entrapped with an aim to increase its bioavailability. The chain length of the oil/lipid affects the emulsifying capacity of SEDDS with various surfactants. Medium chain fatty acids are found to be effectively emulsified and absorbed from the intestine. Further the required HLB of these oils/lipids determines the selection of surfactant. It is already mentioned, that a combination of surfactants is always preferable for better stability. Oil with very low required HLB may lead to use of surfactants in HLB range of 4-6, which may interfere in the formation of O/W micro-/nano-emulsion. Use of oils with unsaturation is risk-full as it may lead to degradation during formulation or storage exemplifying the importance of selection of oil/lipid in the formulation of SEDDS.

Precipitation of drug after coming in contact with the aqueous media is an undesired but common phenomena in SEDDS, which leads to failure of formulation in terms of achieving its intended goal. The nature of oil/lipid significantly influences the precipitation of drug. Prasad and co-workers have investigated the effect of lipid chain length on the precipitation of a poorly water soluble drug contained in self-emulsifying drug delivery system (Prasad et al., 2013). In their study they employed two medium chain lipids Lauroglycol and Capryol, as well as two long chain lipids Labrafil and castor oil, where they observed that no precipitate was seen with long chain lipids SEDDS, whereas medium chain lipids SEDDS showed precipitation within 30 min of drug release from formulations. Such report clearly shows that oils/lipids have very crucial impact on the formulation of SEDDS. Lipids/oils in combination with surfactants have substantial effects on performance of SEDDS by assisting with the drug absorption in the GI tract. They put forth their effects by several complex mechanisms that lead to alteration in the biopharmaceutical properties of the drug, for instance

(i)   increased dissolution rate of the drug and solubility in the intestinal fluid,

(ii)   protection of the drug from chemical as well as enzymatic degradation in the oil droplets, and

(iii)   promoting the lymphatic transport of highly lipophilic drugs.

These mechanisms act simultaneously and are specific to lipids/oils of different nature.

The next ingredients in SEDDS are surfactants and the co-surfactants which determine the success of the formulation. The required HLB of the oil phase in the isotropic mixture of SEDDS may be achieved by the combination of surfactants and at the same time the amount of the same must be in sufficient quantity so that self-emulsification can be achieved. The optimization of interfacial tension and droplet size are formulation art which result in the formation of stable micro/nanoemulsion. Inadequate quantity of surfactants may not be able to form self-emulsion whereas higher concentration may lead to unwanted side effects. Surfactants with desired HLB may result in formation of SEDDS with different particle size and emulsification time. This is attributed to the fact that molecular arrangement of solo surfactant and combination of surfactants in developing emulsified globules are quite different. Hence there is variation in the formulation of SEDDS when prepared with various types of surfactants. As far as performance of SEDDS is concerned surfactants play a very significant role. Surfactants interfere with the rate of gastric emptying and also cause retarded movement of drug to the absorption site by increasing the viscosity of the formulation. Surfactants cause improvement in absorption of drug which is considered to be due to the allosteric rearrangement of the membrane protein. The membrane alteration effects of surfactants can be explained by

(i)   membrane-surfactant binding,

(ii) disruption of membranes through solubilization into lipoproteins, proteins, and mixed micelles,

(iii) protein-protein interactions, and

(iv) selective solubilization of some membrane components by the surfactant.

Researchers have demonstrated the impact of emulsion-based drug delivery systems on intestinal permeability and drug release kinetics (Buyukozturk et al., 2010).

Other ingredients such as supersaturatable substances affect the formulation by inhibiting the precipitation of drug present in the formulation. Xiao and group, have employed HPMC as a supersaturatable excipient and also demonstrated the mechanism of HPMC in preventing precipitation of drug in SEDDS (Xiao and Yi, 2013). They have shown that HPMC inhibited drug precipitation during the dispersion of SEDDS under gastric conditions by inhibiting the formation of crystal nucleus and the growth of crystals. HPMC was found to interfere with the rate of SEDDS lipolysis and benefited the distribution of drug molecules across the aqueous phase, at the same time it also decreased the sedimentation of drug by forming a viscous network.

2.4.2 Physicochemical State of SEDDS and Intended Dosage Form

The physicochemical state of the SEDDS has also important contribution in the formulation and performance of SEDDS. From stability aspects solid SEDDS are very much stable than liquid-/semisolid-SEDDS because of its less reactive features, whereas from manufacturing aspects the latter is simple involving easy unit operations like mixing, blending and heating than solid SEDDS which has complex unit operations like spray drying, solid dispersion, and melt extrusion. Solid SEDDS are not feasible to all drug molecules owing to its feature associated with application of hot air, at the same time agglomeration is a major problem in this method. Use of excipients like mannitol may solve such problems but it may increase the production cost of the SEDDS. Liquid SEDDS are finally delivered as solution or filled in soft gelatin capsules. In the solution state rate of reaction among the components of SEDDS is high and risk of stability with reference to environmental factor is elevated. Interaction of the surfactant with the container in case of liquid SEDDS and capsule shell with liquid-/semisolid-SEDDS cannot be ruled out and caution must be taken in this regard. Solid SEDDS formulation can be administered in form of powder, tablet, or capsule dosage forms. In case of tablet formulation, compressibility (hardness) and self-emulsification are two contradictory parameters. Inadequate harness will lead to higher friability whereas higher hardness will cause delay in self-emulsification. Other factors related to tablet compression such as generation of heat (mechanical action) and adhesion of materials to die-punch (due to lipids/oils, surfactants) may also interfere with the formulation as well as function of SEDDS. In an integrative study Gumaste and his team investigated the effect of adsorbed lipid and surfactant on tableting properties and surface structures of different silicates (Gumaste et al., 2013). Among the six different silicates, Neusilin(R) US2 was the only silicate able to produce tablets with acceptable tensile strength in presence of a lipid component at 1:1 W/W ratio due to the fact that the liquid was mostly adsorbed into the pores of the silicate rather than at the surface.

Flow-ability of the solid SEDDS is a point of concern in developing solid dosage forms. Agrawal et al, have examined the dissolution and dynamics of powder flow characteristics of griseofulvin solid SEDDS in combination with silica and silicates (Agarwal et al., 2009). Dissolution of drug from adsorbed-SEDDS was found to be dependent on pore length and nucleation at the lipid/adsorbent interface. Increase in dissolution rate was observed with an increase in surface area and was independent of the chemical nature of the adsorbents. They concluded that in order to manufacture free flowing powder containing liquid SEDDS, special attention should be given to particle size, specific surface area, type and amount of adsorbent (excipients). The degree of dispersion of SEDDS have momentous effect on the bioavailability of drug by decreasing the particle size and altering the surface area available for lipid digestion. Liquid/semisolid SEDDS is fast and better in this prospects whereas additional effect of disintegration and dissolution are seen in solid SEDDS.

2.5   Characterization

SEDDS is the to-be emulsion formulation incorporated in a suitable pharmaceutical dosage form. So the evaluation of this system is categorized in to two stages, first is characterization of the SEDDS and the second is evaluation of the pharmaceutical dosage form. Here in this section we will focus on the characterization of the SEDDS as the evaluation of pharmaceutical dosage forms *viz.* tablets, capsules etc. is very common and can be referred from text books dealing with pharmaceutical formulations. SEDDS is characterized for different parameters viz. self-emulsification efficiency, zeta potential, size-shape of droplets and their distribution, morphology of dispersed phase, stability of the SEDDS, toxicological issues and the therapeutic efficacy evaluation (Agarwal et al., 2009; Gursoy et al., 2003; Tang et al., 2008). The toxicological issues will be discussed as a separate section and the following section will describe the *in vitro* and *in vivo* evaluation of SEDDS.

2.5.1 Self-emulsification Efficiency

The first and very basic evaluation of SEDDS is the self-emulsifying efficacy. It can be done with visual observation by examining that upon mixing with aqueous media, the SEDDS is converting into a fine nano-/ micro-emulsion or not? The time required for self-emulsification may be noted and also the appearance of the developed emulsions must be observed. Usually the SEDDS should give rise to a clear homogeneous appearance to the naked eyes and in some instances it may give a bit hazy appearance depending on the size of droplets formed in the emulsion. Caution must be taken in evaluating the formation of any precipitate in the self-emulsification process. Formation of precipitate may occur due to higher partitioning of the hydrophobic drug molecule to the aqueous environment than the oil-surfactant mixture. Such observation indicates poor formulation and it may lead to poor bioavailability. After visual inspection the self-emulsification may also be examined by the sophisticated techniques by investigating the charge and droplet size and also the turbidity of emulsion developed by SEDDS (Shao et al., 2010; Xiao et al., 2013).

2.5.2 Zeta Potential

The charge of the colloidal particles/droplets is a major point of concern in any particulate, colloidal or vesicular systems. SEDDS is a colloidal system where the oil droplets are expected to be in the micro-/nano-meter size ranges and because of the presence of lipid as well as surfactants there is charge on the oil droplets. The charge always depends on the nature of surfactants and can be quantified by various instrumental techniques. Micro-electrophoretic techniques are most common in measuring zeta potential where the movement of oil droplets is measured under the influence of a known electric field. Electrophoretic light scattering techniques are used as an alternative for measuring the zeta potential. Usually the zeta potential of conventional SEDDS is found to be negative but employment of various surfactants and co-solvents may alter the zetapotential. Zeta potential is also a measure of kinetic stability of the SEDDS and a stable formulation may lead to better absorption *in vivo*. Some researchers claim the formulation of cationic SEDDS, as it has been found to interact preferably with the negatively charged cells in human body and increases bioavailability of drug molecules (Araya et al., 2005; Kohli et al., 2010).

2.5.3 Size and Size Distribution

SEDDS is intended to form micro-/nano-emulsion *in situ*/*in vivo* and the droplet size of the oil globules containing the hydrophobic drug molecule is in the nanometer range. To the naked eyes these micro-/nano-emulsions look clear or bit hazy but microscopically these are heterogeneous system containing a distribution of droplets of different size. The size and size distribution can be measured by automated laser diffraction technology. Techniques employed in size determination are photon correlation spectroscopy and coulter counter techniques which determine mean particle size and poly-dispersity index. Employment of suitable surfactants, co-surfactants and co-solvent sat appropriate concentration leads to the formation of emulsion with desired droplet size and distribution. The size and poly-dispersity index should be studied with regular interval of time to ensure the intactness and stability of the emulsion (Abdalla et al., 2008).

2.5.4 Morphology

The morphology of the micro-/nano-droplets formed by the SEDDS can be evaluated by the sophisticated transmission electron microscopy (TEM). The more advanced high resolution (HR) TEM and cryo-TEM are now-a-days preferred because of their high quality result. The emulsified droplets, coating on the droplets as well as their distribution can be studied by these techniques. The surface morphologies of the emulsified globules may be studied which is helpful in reviewing the aggregation and/or coalescence of the oil globules in the emulsion. Other powerful microscopic techniques such as atomic force microscopy (AFM), confocal microscopy and fluorescent microscopy may also be engaged in the morphological investigation of these colloidal systems (Abdalla et al., 2008; Karewicz et al., 2010).

2.5.5 Drug Content

Although most of the SEDDS undergo simple mixing of drug molecules in the oil/surfactant phase but still there are chances of loss of drug during various unit operations. Amount of drug incorporated into the SEDDS must be quantified in order to assure the does accuracy. The SEDDS is subjected to dilution with a suitable solvent system. The placebo formulation may be used as a blank control and the quantification may be done by any sophisticated analytical techniques such as HPLC, LCMS etc. The analytical method should be developed prior to the formulation and development process. The limit of drug content depends on the nature (therapeutic index) of the drug and may vary accordingly. The protocols for drug content may vary depending upon the type of SEDDS such as solution, dry emulsion, pellets, microspheres, solid dispersed powder and nanoparticles (Wang et al., 2010).

2.5.6 *In vitro* Drug Dissolution and *Ex Vivo* Drug Permeation

In vitro drug dissolution is one of the vital evaluation parameters as it examines the successful development of SEDDS. It can be done with the basket type USP/IP dissolution apparatus or by dialysis method. In either cases the SEDDS formulation may be kept inside the dialysis tube and placed in the dissolution medium. Some researchers suggest to directly add the SEDDS in the dissolution medium and run the experiments. Although the SEDDS may be dispersed in the aqueous media in few seconds/minutes but the drug being lipophilic in nature must not go into the aqueous media very soon. Early release of large amount of drug may cause precipitation which is undesirable in SEDDS. The amount of drug released in the medium may be quantified as discussed in the drug content evaluation section. As dissolution of drug around the biological membrane is the rate limiting step in absorption of drug from SEDDS formulation, the *in vitro* dissolution studies may be much helpful in predicting the behavior of SEDDS in *in vivo* conditions. Similar to the *in vitro* dissolution studies, the *ex vivo* permeation is also an important evaluation parameters. Franz diffusion cell may be used for this purpose and intestinal layer of animals like rat, rabbit, goat or pig can be used as the biological barrier. In order to mimic the biological environment in a more accurate way, the intestinal content may be added to the dissolution medium. The amount of drug permeated with respect to time can be analyzed by determining the amount of drug in the dissolution medium. The *ex vivo* drug permeation gives an indication of the permeability efficiency of the SEDDS which can be further examined by *in vivo* experimentation (Mercuri et al., 2011; Shao et al., 2010).

2.5.7 *In vivo* Bio-Distribution

The *in vivo* bio-distribution can be analyzed by administrating the SEDDS to animals preferably mice, rat or rabbit in the pre-clinical investigation. Permission of the animal ethical committee must be obtained prior to any animal experiments and regulatory protocols regarding animal handling must be followed. In a preplanned exercise the amount of drug in the blood/urine may be analyzed and the biopharmaceutical parameters viz. C_{max}, t_{max}, AUC, onset time, duration of action etc., can be evaluated and extrapolated for the entire therapeutic efficacy of the SEDDS. For the comparison purpose any commercially available formulation may be taken and subjected to the same set of experiments (Yan et al., 2012). A comparative oral bioavailability study of Tocotrienols (vitamin E isoforms) as SEDDS in comparison to commercially available UNIQUE E(R) Tocotrienols capsules has been investigated *in vivo* (Alqahtani et al., 2013). Results revealed that SEDDS formulation significantly increased the absorption and bioavailability of Tocotrienols. However, it was also observed that this effect was self-limiting because treatment with increasing doses of SEDDS led increase in free surfactants levels that negatively influenced tocotrienol transport protein function. This phenomena resulted in nonlinear absorption kinetics and a progressive decrease in Tocotrienols absorption and bioavailability.

2.5.8 Stability

The SEDDS is subjected to stability evaluation and the purpose of stability testing is to ensure the quality of drug product over a period of time under the influence of a variety of environmental factors such as temperature, humidity and light. SEDDS is a complex mixture system containing lipid and surfactants which are very much susceptible to the environmental degradation by any physical or chemical stimuli. ICH provides the worldwide accepted protocols for stability evaluation of drug products. In the stability evaluation, the SEDDS are subjected to the different accelerated and real time testing conditions. The first step in the stability testing is the selection of batches which must be performed in a random manner. The storage conditions should be

(i) $25 \pm 2°C/60 \pm 5$ % RH for 12 months in long term testing and

(ii) $40 \pm 2°C/75 \pm 5$ % RH for 6 months in accelerated testing conditions.

Certain parameters such as size, shape, charge, drug content, surface morphology etc., are studied in the stability analysis. Any physicochemical changes observed in the accelerated stability testing of SEDDS are further subjected to an intermediate condition e.g., $30 \pm 2°C/60 \pm 5\%$ RH. Any observable change during accelerated conditions as per ICH guidelines is defined as loss of potency from the initial assay value, any specified degradant exceeding its regulatory limit, alteration in pH, dissolution exceeding the specification limits as well as failure to meet specifications for appearance and physical properties e.g., color, phase separation, caking, hardness, etc. Based on the obtained results and data the SEDDS may qualify or fail the stability test. Apart from these, stability testing brings forward the degradation products over storage which might be a potent toxic product (Bhattacharyya and Bajpai, 2013; Wasan et al., 2009).

2.6   Fate of SEDDS *In vivo*

Before getting into the mechanistic insight of fate of SEDDS *in vivo*, let us ask a simple question ourselves that how very highly lipophilic dietary substances get absorbed from our body? Let us take the example of cholesterol (log *p*- 12, aqueous solubility approximately 10 ng/mL), being highly lipophilic it gets absorbed through the GIT. This becomes possible due to the bile acid mixed micelles. Oil soluble vitamins are also exposed to such conditions for absorption (Araya et al., 2006). As our SEDDS consists of lipids, what should be the mechanism for its enhanced uptake? Let us see in the section below.

SEDDS are composed of the drug, lipids/oils, surfactants as well as co-solvents and these ingredients especially lipids and surfactants determine the fate of SEDDS *in vivo*. Before being absorbed into blood or lymphatic system, lipids undergo certain chemical and physical alteration within the GIT. The emulsified SEDDS are digested by enzymes such as lipase and co-lipase both in stomach and intestine. During the digestion (bio-transformation) process the lipids of SEDDS get converted to comparatively more polar diglycerides, monoglycerides, and fatty acids. This is all about the chemical fate of the SEDDS in GIT which further undergoes certain physical process as a part of the pharmacokinetics. The moderately digested diglycerides, monoglycerides, and fatty acids in stomach are swept to the duodenum and further get emulsified due to the emulsifying nature of above digested molecules and shear force during gastric emptying (Gursoy et al., 2003; Gursoy and Benita, 2004).

The partly digested emulsion reaches the small intestine and causes secretion of bile salts and biliary lipids from the gallbladder. These biological components further emulsify the partially digested emulsion and reduce its particle size. Availability of the adequate bile salts allow these digested SEDDS products to be solubilized and incorporated into bile salt micelles forming an intestinal mixed micellar phase (Fig. 2.6). The solubilization of SEDDS digestion products in intestinal mixed micelles augments their dissolution. Monomolecular lipid is dissociated from the mixed micelles and get available to the enterocyte surface for absorption. Dissociation of the monomolecular lipid containing the drug molecule is hypothesized to be due to the acidic environment around the enterocyte. The concentration gradient in the intestinal lumen and enterocytes causes passive diffusion of these monomolecular lipids. The small and medium chain lipids get absorbed through enterocytes to reach the portal blood circulation (Fig. 2.7). As these lipids reach the liver they get digested in the hepatocytes' mitochondria releasing CO_2, H_2O, and energy whereas the drug finds its own way to elicit therapeutic effect.

The same thing does not happen to the long chain lipids, because of higher lipophilicity they instead of getting transported through enterocytes get trafficked through the endoplasmic reticulum, re-esterified and secreted into the intestinal lymph. Further through the central lymphatic system, these lipids enter into the systemic circulation. This is one of the mechanisms by which the drug molecule is protected from the hepatic first pass metabolism by bypassing the liver. From the lymphatic system the lipid containing drug gets in to the systemic circulation and further get associated with some lipophilic carriers and reach the target site to exhibit therapeutic action (Kohli et al., 2010; Tang et al., 2008). The above mentioned fate of SEDDS *in vivo* is based on some experimental findings and assumption too. Research is continuing to investigate more in this field which might show a different path to the SEDDS.

2.7   Safety and Toxicological Issues

SEDDS uses a large quantity of surfactant at around 30-60%. Such a high quantity of the surfactants, particularly if indicated for any chronic therapy, may lead to severe toxicological complications. It is well known that high concentrations of surfactant disrupts the biological membrane. Many surfactant molecules alter the membrane permeability and in some instances interfere with the enzyme system of the membrane. Much of such alterations are reversible but a long term exposure may lead to irreversible changes causing damage to the bio-membrane.

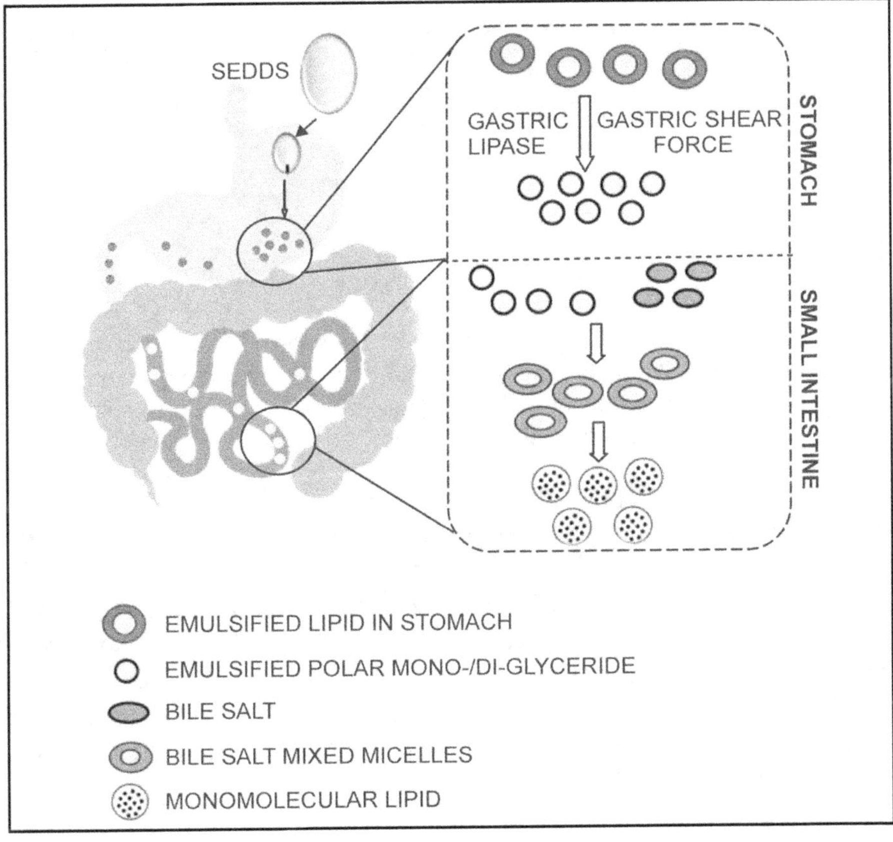

FIGURE 2.6 Diagrammatic representation of *in vivo* fate of SEDDS where after getting into stomach the SEDDS becomes fine emulsion and after coming in contact with lipase these emulsified globules degrades into mono-/di-glyceride. In intestine these glycerides come in contact with bile salt forming micellar complex and further in the micro-acidic environment of enterocytes these micellar complex dissociate into monomolecular lipids containing drug (this phenomena is specific to small and medium chain fatty acids).

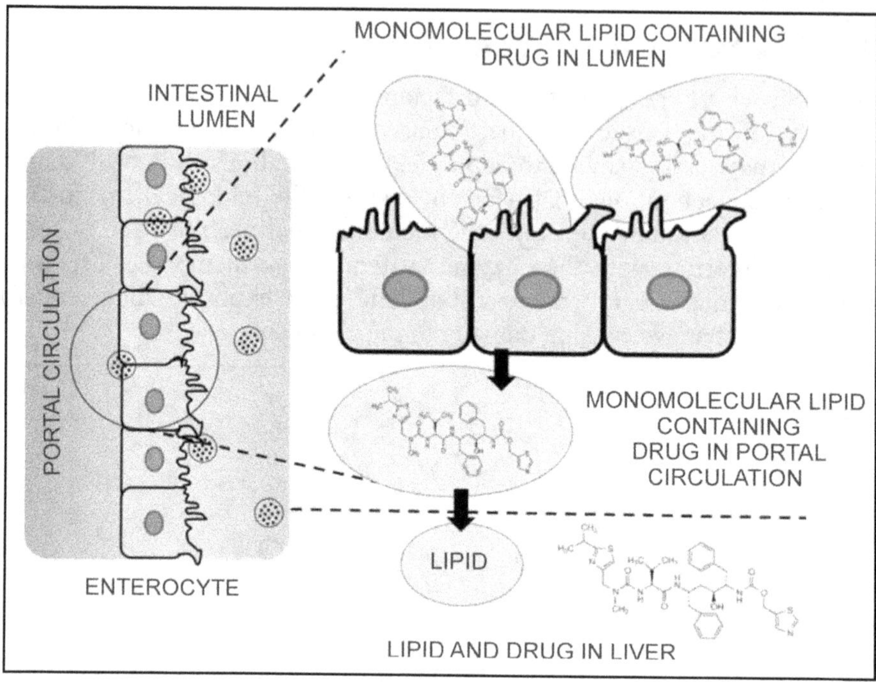

FIGURE 2.7 Diagrammatic representation of transport of monomolecular lipid containing drug (ritonavir) through enterocyte to portal circulation, where lipid is digested and drug gets transported to systemic circulation drug (this phenomena is specific to small and medium chain fatty acids).

Certain surfactants are also found to initiate adverse drug reactions. Some oils/lipids may have good properties with reference to formulation aspects owing to their high solubility and emulsifying properties but these may be allergic upon internal administration, and hence such ingredients should be avoided. As discussed in the stability section possible degraded products on storage must be analyzed for their toxic effects. Replacement of high content of synthetic surfactants with the natural surfactant can be studied in order to minimize the surfactant related adverse effect (Fischl et al., 1997; Palamakula and Khan, 2004).

2.8   Applications of SEDDS

Various drug molecules have been developed as SEDDS and as evident from commercially available products many chemotherapeutic molecules are successfully used via this delivery system. Apart from these, many drug molecules are reported for better therapeutic effect as SEDDS in comparison to the conventional dosage forms. Some of the reports from leading scientific journals showing wide applications of SEDDS in various diseases and disorders are discussed in Table 2.2. The prime objective of SEDDS is to develop oral formulation of such drugs which are failed via this route in conventional formulation as well as to increase the bioavailability of poorly bioavailable drugs through oral route. Apart from that increase in stability whether physical, or chemical and improvement in physicochemical activity in terms of taste, photo-stability etc. are also goals of formulation of SEDDS.

The first commercially successful SEDDS product was Neoral® containing Cyclosporine A as API which was developed by Sandoz (Novartis) in form of both as soft gelatin capsule and oral solution. The excipients incorporated in soft gelatin capsule were propylene glycol, corn oil-mono-ditriglycerides, polyoxyl 40 hydrogenated castor oil, DL-α-Tocopherol and alcohol (USP dehydrated, 9.5% W/V). The clue of better absorption of this drug with lipid solution was the turning point in the development of SEDDS of the same. Anticancer drugs like paclitaxel, docetaxel are yet to get success as oral formulation and SEDDS is expected to be the suitable delivery system.

TABLE 2.2

A brief account of applications of SEDDS

Drug candidate	Delivery system	Description	References
Bifendate (Chinese medicine for chronic hepatitis)	Solid SEDDS	A self-emulsifying pellet was developed by extrusion/ spheronization technology. SEDDS was composed of Miglycol (R) 840, a mixture of Cremorphor (R) EL and Solutol HS(R) 15, and Transcutol HP as the oil phase. Mixture of MCC, lactose, and mannitol (45:45:10, w/w/w) was taken as solid adsorbents. A 2.36-fold increase in oral bioavailability was observed in comparison to conventional formulation.	(Xiao et al., 2013)

TABLE 2.2 Contd...

Drug candidate	Delivery system	Description	References
Celecoxib (COX-2 inhibitor)	Supersaturatable SEDDS	Formulation is composed of Soluplus (precipitation inhibitor), Capryol 90 (oil), Tween 20 (surfactant), and Tetra-glycol (co-surfactant) in 1:4.5: 4.5 (volume) ratio. Results revealed highest Cmax and the smallest Tmax of SEDDS indicating rapid and enhanced absorption in comparison to conventional suspension.	(Song et al., 2013)
Phenobarbital (Antiepileptic)	Liquid SEDDS	SEEDS containing phenolbarbital were developed to improve its chemical stability, solubilizing capacity and taste-masking property. Optimized formulation with Cremophor RH40 20%, Capmul MCM L 4%, PEG 400 35% and sucralose 2% (w/w) was chosen in order to optimize taste-masking using an electronic tongue. A 5-fold increase in the efficacy with no sign of physical or chemical instability along with improved taste was observed.	(Monteagudo et al., 2013)
Itraconazole (Antifungal)	Liquid SEDDS	SEDDS based on PEGylated bile acids were prepared, where the number and length of PEG arms were varied to optimize the loading of itraconazole in the formulation. SEDDS showed good cyto-compatibility as revealed by MTT assays of SEDDS with Caco-2 and RAW 264.2 cells, and a low degree of hemolysis of human erythrocytes. Pharmacokinetic studies exhibited improved bio-availability of drug.	(Le Devedec et al., 2013)

TABLE 2.2 *Contd...*

Drug candidate	Delivery system	Description	References
Fenofibrate (Lipid regulating drug)	Solid SEDDS	Solid SEDDS containing fenofibrate was prepared by taking Labrafac WL1349 as oily phase, Cremophor EL as surfactant and Gelucire 44/14 as co-surfactant. The prepared pre-concentrate was solidified with PEG 6000. The dissolution of drug was enhanced by approximately 20-fold in simulated gastric fluid.	(Kanaujia et al., 2013)
Meloxicam (NSAID)	Powder SEDDS	A powdered SEDDS formulation of meloxicam was prepared and compared for oral bioavailability against commercial Mobic (R) tablets. The SEDDS formulation was prepared by *in situ* salt formation of meloxicam in a blend of lipid and was adsorbed on silica powder. Oral bioavailability of the formulation was evaluated in beagle dogs where powdered meloxicam SEDDS formulation showed a 1.3-fold increase in AUC in comparison to commercial Mobic (R) tablets.	(Agarwal et al., 2013)
beta-Arteether (Antimalarial)	Liquid SEDDS	SEDDS of groundnut/ sesame oil, Maisine 35-1, Tween 80/ Cremophor EL, and absolute ethanol containing beta-arteether were formulated. No toxicity against Caco-2 intestinal cells was observed. Using a mouse model, the efficacy of these arteether lipid formulations against *Plasmodium berghei* was evaluated. A daily dose of 24 mg/kg for 4 days led to complete cure for more than 45 days in 100% of treated mice and had an antimalarial efficacy comparable to that of an intramuscular oily solution	(Memvanga and Preat, 2012)

TABLE 2.2 *Contd...*

Drug candidate	Delivery system	Description	References
		of arteether and significantly higher than that of an oily solution of beta-arteether given orally at the same dose	
Tetrahydro-curcumin	Floating SEDDS pallets	Floating SEDDS were prepared to improve solubility, dissolution, and controlled release of the poorly water-soluble tetrahydrocurcumin. The formulation contains Labrasol, Cremophor EL, Capryol 90 andLabrafac PG. The liquid SEDDS was mixed with adsorbent (silicon dioxide), glycerylbehenate, pregelatinized starch, sodium starch glycolate, and micro-crystalline cellulose and transformed into pellets by the extrusion/spheronization technique. The optimum formulation had a floating efficiency of 93% at 6 h and provided a controlled release of THC over an 8 h period.	(Setthacheewakul et al., 2011)
Ibuprofen (NSAID)	Immediate-SEDDS tablets	Immediate-release self-emul-sifying tablets of ibuprofen was prepared with solidified SEDDS. The liquid SEDDS consisted of Capryol 90, Cremophor EL, Labrasol, and IBU at a ratio of 3:4:3:3, and was solidified with various adsorbents. The powder SEDDS was punched by a direct compression to prepare tablet. SEDDS tablets revealed remarkably higher dissolution rate of drug. This can be promising as a fast-releasing SEDDS tablet for quick onset of action.	(Kang et al., 2011)

TABLE 2.2 *Contd...*

Drug candidate	Delivery system	Description	References
Torcetrapib (Cholesteryl ester transfer protein inhibitor used in treatment of atherosclerosis)	Softgel SEDDS capsule	SEDDS formulations have been developed using MCT softgels in order to reduce the food effect observed in early clinical trials and to increase the dose per capsule. MCT/ Triacetin/ Polysorbate 80/ Capmul MCM (20/30/ 20/30) increased fasted exposure and thus reduced the food effect from 5- to 3-fold in dogs at a dose of 90 mg. Use of the lipophilic, GRAS cosolvent triacetin allowed a 2-fold increase in the dose per capsule.	(Perlman et al., 2008)
Cyclosporine (immune-suppressant)	Liquid SEDDS	Galactolipids, polar lipids commonly found in the chloroplast membranes of green plants, and a natural part of the human diet were employed as main surfactants in SEDDS containing Cyclosporine. The clinical trials were performed in healthy volunteers. It was found that fractionated oat oil and medium chain mono-glycerides (60:30:10 mono-, di- and tri-glycerides) promoted absorption, and resulted in a formulation with absorption characteristics nearly equal to the commercial formulation of cyclosporine, Sandimmun-Neoral.	(Odeberg et al., 2003)

2.9   Commercial SEDDS

As already narrated in the previous section SEDDS has got tremendous scope for industrial level production and commercialization. The success story of cyclosporine as a SEDDS formulation opened the way towards delivery of poorly soluble drugs via SEDDS. Many other drug molecules were experimented to be developed in to SEDDS but few among them could reach to the market. Again the reason for failure of many projects on this venture is either due to no significant difference in the conventional and developed SEDDS in therapeutic response or scale up complications. However, SEDDS is being actively researched and many possibilities are under exploration such as

(i)   formulation of solid SEDDS,

(ii) development of supersaturable SEDDS,

(iii) development of functional excipient/surfactant to minimize excipient based side effect, and

(iv) exploration of g-glycoprotein inhibition potential of excipients for multipurpose use etc.

It is expected that these attempts will bring a new boom in the commercialization potential of SEDDS. Table 2.3 gives a brief account of commercially available SEDDS and their characteristics (Kohli et al., 2010; Tang et al., 2008).

2.10 Future Prospects and Challenges

The future prospects of SEDDS can be categorized into two different facets viz. prospects and challenges in formulation and development (purely pharmaceutical issue) and prospects and challenges in successfully delivering the water insoluble drug molecules (pharmaceutical and biological issues). It has been evident from the literature that HLB values are utilized in the development of SEDDS as a qualitative measure. Many research papers describe that matching the HLB of oil phase and surfactant leads to the formation of stable emulsion. But surprisingly, the lucid science of HLB and its application is yet to be worked out in formulation and development of SEDDS. Almost all formulations of SEDDS reported till date are based on trial and error method of selecting surfactants. Challenges must be taken to find out the quantitative and qualitative relation of HLB of different surfactants on SEDDS and its performance. The second challenge in the development of SEDDS is the employment of this delivery system for target specific drug delivery. It is evident that the lymphatic system contains large numbers of lymphocytes, and thus offers attractive targets for cytokines. Lymphatic system is the site for many microorganisms/parasites such as leishmania parasites, tuberculi etc., and also channel for spreading of many tumor metastases. So the lymphatic uptake of SEDDS may be effective in treating many diseases. Inhibition of the reflux action of p-glycoprotein and pre-systemic metabolism of lipid/drug will also remain as future challenges in SEDDS.

TABLE 2.3

A brief account of commercially available SEDDS

Drug/ Characteristics (log P, solubility)	Brand name	Manufacturer	Indication	Formulation details
Cyclosporine [2.92, 9 µg/mL (water)]	Neoral®	Sandoz (Novartis Pharmaceuticals Corporation)	Immuno-suppressant used in organ transplantation	**Softgelatin capsule:** **API**-100 mg **Excipients**-propylene glycol, corn oil-mono-ditriglycerides, polyoxyl 40 hydrogenated castor oil, DL-α –tocopherol, Alcohol (USP dehydrated,9.5% wt/vol) **Oral solution:** **API**-100 mg/mL **Excipient**-same to softgel
Cyclosporine [2.92, 9 µg/mL (water)]	Sandimmune®	Novartis Pharmaceuticals Corporation	Immuno-suppressant used in organ transplantation	**Soft gelatin capsule:** **API**-25-100 mg **Excipient**-corn oil,Labrafil M 2125 CS, gelatin, glycerol, ethanol **Oral solution:** **API**-100 mg/mL in 12.5% ethanol **Excipient**-olive oil,Labrafil M 1944 **Injection:** **API**-50 mg **Excipient-** Cremophor® EL (polyoxyethylated castor oil), alcohol, nitrogen. Injection is diluted with 0.9% NaCl or 5% dextrose solution before administration

TABLE 2.3 *Contd...*

Drug/ Characteristics (log P, solubility)	Brand name	Manufacturer	Indication	Formulation details
Cyclosporine [2.92, 9 µg/mL (water)]	Panimun Bioral™	Panacea Biotech	Immuno-suppressant used in organ transplantation	**Available as** 25, 50 and 100, mg soft gelatin capsules 100 mg/ml oral solution Name of excipients are not disclosed
Cyclosporine [2.92, 9 µg/mL (water)]	Gengraf®	Abbott Laboratories	Immuno-suppressant used in organ transplantation	**Capsule:** **API**-25/100 mg in alcohol, USP, absolute, 12.8% v/v (10.1% wt/vol) **Excipients-** FD&C Blue No. 2, gelatin, polyethylene glycol, polyoxyl 35 castor oil, polysorbate 80, propylene glycol, sorbitanmonooleate, titanium dioxide **Oral solution:** **API-** 100 mg/mL **Excipient-** Propylene glycol Sorbitanmonooleate
Saquinavir [4.40, 5 µg/mL at pH 7 buffer]	Fortavase®	Hoffmann La Roche Incorporation	HIV protease inhibitor used in AIDS	**Softgelatin capsule:** **API**-200 mg **Excipient**-medium chain mono- and di-glycerides, povidone
Tipranavir [7.2, 5 µg/mL at pH 6 buffer]	Aptivus®	BoehringerIngelheim		**Softgelatin capsule:** **API**-250 mg **Excipient**-Polyoxyl 35 castor oil, propylene glycol, mono-/di-glycerides of caprylic/capric acid, 7% dehydrated alcohol

TABLE 2.3 Contd...

Drug/ Characteristics (log P, solubility)	Brand name	Manufacturer	Indication	Formulation details
Ritonavir [5.28, 0.37 µg/mL at pH 6 buffer]	Norvir®	AbbVie (Abbott Laboratories)		**Softgelatin capsule:** **API**-100 mg **Excipient**-polyoxyl 35castor oil, oleic acid, BHT, ethanol **Oral Solution:** **API**-80 mg/ml in ethanol (43% w/v) **Excipient**-polyoxyl 35 castor oil, propylene glycol, citric acid

References

Abdalla, A., Klein, S., and Mader, K. (2008). A new self-emulsifying drug delivery system (SEDDS) for poorly soluble drugs: characterization, dissolution, *in vitro* digestion and incorporation into solid pellets. *European journal of pharmaceutical sciences:* official journal of the European Federation for Pharmaceutical Sciences **35**, 457-464.

Adeyeye, M.C., and Brittain, H.G. (2008). Preformulation in solid dosage form development (Informa Healthcare New York).

Agarwal, V., Alayoubi, A., Siddiqui, A., and Nazzal, S. (2013). Powdered self-emulsified lipid formulations of meloxicam as solid dosage forms for oral administration. *Drug development and industrial pharmacy* **39**, 1681-1689.

Agarwal, V., Siddiqui, A., Ali, H., and Nazzal, S. (2009). Dissolution and powder flow characterization of solid self-emulsified drug delivery system (SEDDS). *Int J Pharm* **366**, 44-52.

Alqahtani, S., Alayoubi, A., Nazzal, S., Sylvester, P.W., and Kaddoumi, A. (2013). Nonlinear absorption kinetics of self-emulsifying drug delivery systems (SEDDS) containing tocotrienols as lipophilic molecules: *in vivo* and *in vitro* studies. *The AAPS journal* **15**, 684-695.

Araya, H., Nagao, S., Tomita, M., and Hayashi, M. (2005). The novel formulation design of self-emulsifying drug delivery systems (SEDDS) type O/W microemulsion I: enhancing effects on oral bioavailability of poorly water soluble compounds in rats and beagle dogs. *Drug metabolism and pharmacokinetics* **20**, 244-256.

Araya, H., Tomita, M., and Hayashi, M. (2006). The novel formulation design of self-emulsifying drug delivery systems (SEDDS) type O/W microemulsion III: the permeation mechanism of a poorly water soluble drug entrapped O/W microemulsion in rat isolated intestinal membrane by the Ussing chamber method. *Drug metabolism and pharmacokinetics* **21**, 45-53.

Bhattacharyya, A., and Bajpai, M. (2013). Oral bioavailability and stability study of a self-emulsifying drug delivery system (SEDDS) of amphotericin B. *Current drug delivery* **10**, 542-547.

Breitkreitz, M.C., Sabin, G.P., Polla, G., and Poppi, R.J. (2013). Characterization of semi-solid Self-Emulsifying Drug Delivery Systems (SEDDS) of atorvastatin calcium by Raman image spectroscopy and chemometrics. *Journal of pharmaceutical and biomedical analysis* **73**, 3-12.

Buyukozturk, F., Benneyan, J.C., and Carrier, R.L. (2010). Impact of emulsion-based drug delivery systems on intestinal permeability and drug release kinetics. *Journal of controlled release*: official journal of the Controlled Release Society **142**, 22-30.

Faisal, W., Ruane-O'Hora, T., O'Driscoll, C.M., and Griffin, B.T. (2013). A novel lipid-based solid dispersion for enhancing oral bioavailability of Lycopene – *in vivo* evaluation using a pig model. *Int J Pharm* **453**, 307-314.

Fischl, M.A., Richman, D.D., Flexner, C., Para, M.F., Haubrich, R., Karim, A., Yeramian, P., Holden-Wiltse, J., and Meehan, P.M. (1997). Phase I/II study of the toxicity, pharmacokinetics, and activity of the HIV protease inhibitor SC-52151. *Journal of acquired immune deficiency syndromes and human retrovirology*: official publication of the International Retrovirology Association **15**, 28-34.

Gao, P., Akrami, A., Alvarez, F., Hu, J., Li, L., Ma, C., and Surapaneni, S. (2009). Characterization and optimization of AMG 517 supersaturatable self-emulsifying drug delivery system (S-SEDDS) for improved oral absorption. *Journal of pharmaceutical sciences* **98**, 516-528.

Gumaste, S.G., Pawlak, S.A., Dalrymple, D.M., Nider, C.J., Trombetta, L.D., and Serajuddin, A.T. (2013). Development of Solid SEDDS, IV: Effect of Adsorbed Lipid and Surfactant on Tableting Properties and Surface Structures of Different Silicates. *Pharmaceutical research*.

Gursoy, N., Garrigue, J.S., Razafindratsita, A., Lambert, G., and Benita, S. (2003). Excipient effects on *in vitro* cytotoxicity of a novel paclitaxel self-emulsifying drug delivery system. *Journal of pharmaceutical sciences* **92**, 2411-2418.

Gursoy, R.N., and Benita, S. (2004). Self-emulsifying drug delivery systems (SEDDS) for improved oral delivery of lipophilic drugs. *Biomedecine & pharmacotherapie* **58**, 173-182.

Holmberg, K., Jönsson, B., Kronberg, B., and Lindman, B. (2003). Surfactants and polymers in aqueous solution, Vol 2 (John Wiley & Sons Chichester).

Hong, J.Y., Kim, J.K., Song, Y.K., Park, J.S., and Kim, C.K. (2006). A new self-emulsifying formulation of itraconazole with improved dissolution and oral absorption. *Journal of controlled release*: official journal of the Controlled Release Society **110,** 332-338.

Kanaujia, P., Ng, W.K., and Tan, R.B. (2013). Solid self-emulsifying drug delivery system (S-SEDDS) for improved dissolution rate of fenofibrate. *Journal of microencapsulation.*

Kang, M.J., Jung, S.Y., Song, W.H., Park, J.S., Choi, S.U., Oh, K.T., Choi, H.K., Choi, Y.W., Lee, J., Lee, B.J., et al,. (2011). Immediate release of ibuprofen from Fujicalin(R)-based fast-dissolving self-emulsifying tablets. *Drug development and industrial pharmacy* **37,** 1298-1305.

Karewicz, A., Zasada, K., Szczubialka, K., Zapotoczny, S., Lach, R., and Nowakowska, M. (2010). "Smart" alginate-hydroxypropylcellulose microbeads for controlled release of heparin. *Int J Pharm* **385,** 163-169.

Kohli, K., Chopra, S., Dhar, D., Arora, S., and Khar, R.K. (2010). Self-emulsifying drug delivery systems: an approach to enhance oral bioavailability. *Drug Discov Today* **15,** 958-965.

Lachman L., Libermen H., and J., K. (1990). The Theory and practice of industrial Pharmacy. In (Varghese publishing house), p. 366.

Le Devedec, F., Strandman, S., Hildgen, P., Leclair, G., and Zhu, X.X. (2013). PEGylated bile acids for use in drug delivery systems: enhanced solubility and bioavailability of itraconazole. *Molecular pharmaceutics* **10,** 3057-3066.

Lukyanov, A.N., and Torchilin, V.P. (2004). Micelles from lipid derivatives of water-soluble polymers as delivery systems for poorly soluble drugs. *Advanced drug delivery reviews* **56,** 1273-1289.

Memvanga, P.B., and Preat, V. (2012). Formulation design and *in vivo* antimalarial evaluation of lipid-based drug delivery systems for oral delivery of beta-arteether. *European journal of pharmaceutics and biopharmaceutics*: official journal of Arbeitsgemeinschaft fur Pharmazeutische Verfahrenstechnik eV **82,** 112-119.

Mercuri, A., Passalacqua, A., Wickham, M.S., Faulks, R.M., Craig, D.Q., and Barker, S.A. (2011). The effect of composition and gastric conditions on the self-emulsification process of ibuprofen-loaded self-emulsifying drug delivery systems: a microscopic and dynamic gastric model study. *Pharmaceutical research* **28,** 1540-1551.

Monteagudo, E., Langenheim, M., Salerno, C., Buontempo, F., Bregni, C., and Carlucci, A. (2013). Pharmaceutical optimization of lipid-based dosage forms for the improvement of taste-masking, chemical stability and solubilizing capacity of phenobarbital. *Drug development and industrial pharmacy.*

Odeberg, J.M., Kaufmann, P., Kroon, K.G., and Hoglund, P. (2003). Lipid drug delivery and rational formulation design for lipophilic drugs with low oral bioavailability, applied to cyclosporine. *European journal of pharmaceutical sciences*: official journal of the European Federation for Pharmaceutical Sciences **20**, 375-382.

Palamakula, A., and Khan, M.A. (2004). Evaluation of cytotoxicity of oils used in coenzyme Q10 Self-emulsifying Drug Delivery Systems (SEDDS). *Int J Pharm* **273**, 63-73.

Park, M.J., Balakrishnan, P., and Yang, S.G. (2013). Polymeric nanocapsules with SEDDS oil-core for the controlled and enhanced oral absorption of cyclosporine. *Int J Pharm* **441**, 757-764.

Perlman, M.E., Murdande, S.B., Gumkowski, M.J., Shah, T.S., Rodricks, C.M., Thornton-Manning, J., Freel, D., and Erhart, L.C. (2008). Development of a self-emulsifying formulation that reduces the food effect for torcetrapib. *Int J Pharm* **351**, 15-22.

Pouton, C.W. (1997). Formulation of self-emulsifying drug delivery systems. *Advanced Drug Delivery Reviews* **25**, 47-58.

Prasad, D., Chauhan, H., and Atef, E. (2013). Studying the effect of lipid chain length on the precipitation of a poorly water soluble drug from self-emulsifying drug delivery system on dispersion into aqueous medium. *The Journal of pharmacy and pharmacology* **65**, 1134-1144.

Rosen, M.J., and Kunjappu, J.T. (2012). Surfactants and interfacial phenomena (John Wiley & Sons).

Rowe, R.C., Sheskey, P.J., Quinn, M.E., and Press, P. (2009). Handbook of pharmaceutical excipients, Vol 6 (Pharmaceutical press London).

Setthacheewakul, S., Kedjinda, W., Maneenuan, D., and Wiwattanapatapee, R. (2011). Controlled release of oral tetrahydrocurcumin from a novel self-emulsifying floating drug delivery system (SEFDDS). *AAPS Pharm Sci Tech* **12**, 152-164.

Shao, B., Tang, J., Ji, H., Liu, H., Liu, Y., Zhu, D., and Wu, L. (2010). Enhanced oral bioavailability of Wurenchun (Fructus Schisandrae Chinensis extracts) by self-emulsifying drug delivery systems. *Drug development and industrial pharmacy* **36**, 1356-1363.

Singh, A., Worku, Z.A., and Van den Mooter, G. (2011). Oral formulation strategies to improve solubility of poorly water-soluble drugs. *Expert opinion on drug delivery* **8**, 1361-1378.

Song, W.H., Yeom, D.W., Lee, D.H., Lee, K.M., Yoo, H.J., Chae, B.R., Song, S.H., and Choi, Y.W. (2013). *In situ* intestinal permeability and *in vivo* oral bioavailability of celecoxib in supersaturating self-emulsifying drug delivery system. *Archives of pharmacal research*.

Steele, G. (2004). Preformulation as an Aid to Product Design in Early Drug Development.

Tang, B., Cheng, G., Gu, J.C., and Xu, C.H. (2008). Development of solid self-emulsifying drug delivery systems: preparation techniques and dosage forms. *Drug Discov Today* **13,** 606-612.

Wang, Z., Sun, J., Wang, Y., Liu, X., Liu, Y., Fu, Q., Meng, P., and He, Z. (2010). Solid self-emulsifying nitrendipine pellets: preparation and *in vitro/in vivo* evaluation. *Int J Pharm* **383,** 1-6.

Wasan, E.K., Bartlett, K., Gershkovich, P., Sivak, O., Banno, B., Wong, Z., Gagnon, J., Gates, B., Leon, C.G., and Wasan, K.M. (2009). Development and characterization of oral lipid-based amphotericin B formulations with enhanced drug solubility, stability and antifungal activity in rats infected with Aspergillus fumigatus or Candida albicans. *Int J Pharm* **372,** 76-84.

Xiao, L., and Yi, T. (2013). [Mechanisms of hydroxypropyl methylcellulose for the precipitation inhibitor of supersaturatable self-emulsifying drug delivery systems]. Yao xue xue bao = *Acta pharmaceutica Sinica* **48,** 767-772.

Xiao, Y., Wang, S., Chen, Y., and Ping, Q. (2013). Self-emulsifying bifendate pellets: preparation, characterization and oral bioavailability in rats. *Drug development and industrial pharmacy* **39,** 724-732.

Yan, Y.D., Marasini, N., Choi, Y.K., Kim, J.O., Woo, J.S., Yong, C.S., and Choi, H.G. (2012). Effect of dose and dosage interval on the oral bioavailability of docetaxel in combination with a curcumin self-emulsifying drug delivery system (SEDDS). *European journal of drug metabolism and pharmacokinetics* **37,** 217-224.

3   Colon Specific Drug Delivery Systems

Arvind Gulbake[1], Pramod Kumar[2], Prashant Khare[3] and Nitin K. Jain[4]

[1]Centre for Interdisciplinary Research, D.Y. Patil University, Kolhapur-416 003, Maharashtra, India.

[2]School of Life Sciences, The University of Nottingham, Nottingham, U.K. NG7 2RD.

[3]Baylor Institute for Immunology Research, Dallas, TX-75204, USA.

[4]Department of Biotechnology, Ministry of Science & Technology, New Delhi-400 003, India.

3.1   Introduction

The oral route is most preferred and widely acceptable route for drug administration to the patients. It has received maximum attention for sustained and controlled release drug delivery systems because of greater flexibility in dosage form design compared to parentral preparations. Patient acceptance for oral drug administration is very high as it is relatively safe route of drug administration, and the constraints pertaining to sterility and plausible damage at the site of administration are minimal. Spatially oral drug delivery can be broken down into two major zones: intestinal and colon. Colon targeted drug delivery systems offer vital therapeutic advantages in a number of colonic diseases such as Crohn's disease, amobiasis, spastic colon and colorectal cancer. Infact colon specific delivery of many therapeutics has been found to be more effective than routine systemic delivery of the same agents (Filipe, 1979). Conversely, colon can also be accessed via rectum for the purpose of drug drelilvery; suppositories are effective due to the confined spread and enema solutions are applied to treat sigmoid diseases of the descending colon. However, the common disadvantage of rectal dosage forms (suppositories and enemas) is high variability in distribution of administered drugs. Keeping in mind these limitations, the oral route is preferred but absorption and degradation of the active ingredient in hostile environment of upper gastrointestinal tract (GI tract) is a major obstacle and must be overcome for successful colonic drug delivery. The current chapter focused on rationale behind colon drug delivery employing oral route, their advantages, limitations and various updates on colonic drug delivery carriers. We need to study the structure and functioning of various parts of GI trat to understand the need of colonic drug delivery, thus these subject are also explained in brief.

3.2 Anatomy and Physiology of Gastro Intesitinal Tract

Physiolgic/pathophysiologic conditions prevailing in gastro intesitinal tract (GI tract) can have considerable influence on drug delivery by oral route. The human GI tract is divided mainly into stomach, small intestine and large intestine (Karasov and Hume, 2010; Sekirov et al., 2010). Each part is assigned to have different functions, essential for vital processes of body.

3.2.1 The Stomach

The stomach is the first part of human GI tract and lies between esophagus and small intestine. Food material or dosage form enters into stomach via esophagus. In the same manner microorganisms from mouth and saliva get entry into stomach. The bacterial count of saliva is around 107 CFU/ml with aerobic and anaerobic bacteria in same number. There is drastic reduction in the number of microorganisms due to strong acidic pH that prevails in the stomach and it may vary from 104-108 CFU/ml in presence of food that causes the elevation of pH to 4.0. As food mixes with gastric juice only the acid-resistant bacteria survive in this acidic environment. Gram-positive and aerobic microfloras are predominantly present in stomach.

3.2.2 The Small Intestine

Duodenum, jejunum and ileum are three parts of small intestine. The duodenum is first short sessile section, followed by the jejunum, a long greatly coiled part forming the two-fifth portion and the distal three-fifth part forms the ileum. The small intestine contains huge bacterial population compared to stomach due to presence of favourable environment. The microflora of the duodenum resembles that of the stomach whereas ileum resembles the colonic microflora. The bacterial concentration of the duodenum is in the order of 103-104 CFU/ml with bacterial species predominantly gram positive and aerobic in nature that include Streptococci, Staphylococci, Lactobacilli and anaerobic Veillonella. The bacterial growth is reduced due to bile juice, lysozyme and peristaltic movements. In the jejunum and the upper ileum very few microorganisms are present including Lactobacilli and Enterococci (Thadepalli et al., 1979). In the distal ileum, gram-negative bacteria begin to outnumber the gram-positive organism and bacterial concentration becomes high.

3.2.3 The Large Intestine

The large intestine extends from the ileocaecal junction to the anus and is divided into three main parts: the colon, the rectum and the anal canal. In terms of size and complexity, the human colon falls between that of carnivores such as the ferret, which has no identifiable junction between ileum and colon, and herbivores, which have a voluminous caecum. The cecum, colon ascendens, colon transversale, colon descendens, and rectosigmoid colon are the different parts of the colon which is approximately 1.5 m long. Unlike the small intestine, the colon does not have any villi. However, the surface of the colon is increased to approximately 1300 cm^2 due to presence of plicae semilunares, which are crescentic folds (Mrsny, 1992). The physiology of the proximal and distal colon differs in several aspects related to their functions (Fig. 3.1) and may affect drug absorption. The physical properties of the luminal contents of the colon also change, from liquid contents in the caecum to semisolid contents in the distal colon. The absorption of drugs from the colon depends on rate of blood flow to and from the absorptive epithelium. The superior mesenteric artery provides arterial blood supply to the proximal colon and the inferior mesenteric artery to the distal colon. Venous drainage is via the superior (proximal colon) and inferior (distal colon) veins. The proximal colon receives a greater share of the blood flow than more distal parts, although total colonic blood flow is less than that of the small intestine.

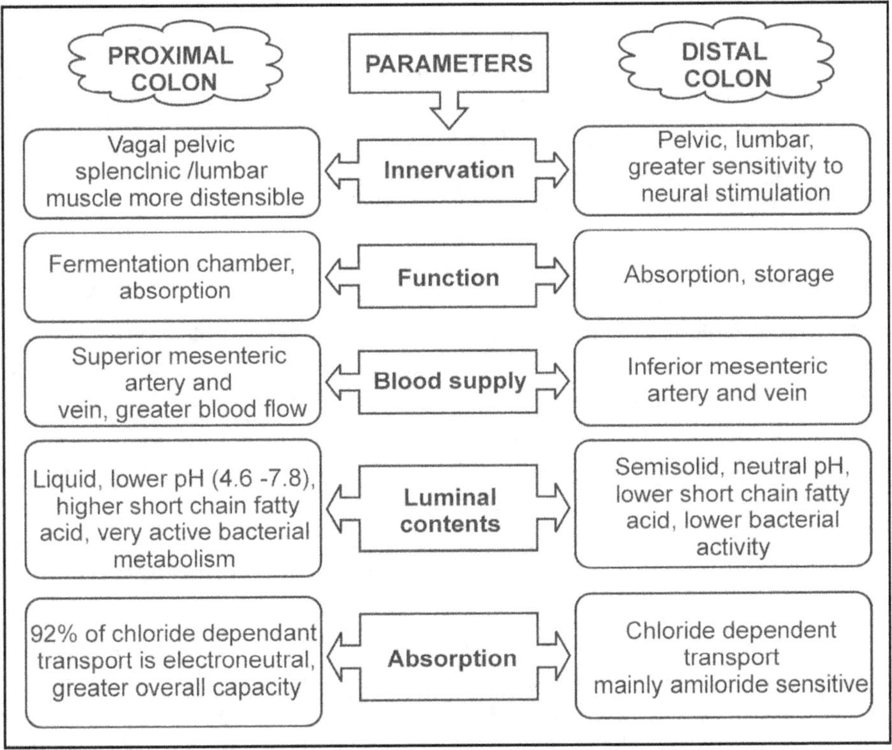

FIGURE 3.1 Characteristic features of proximal and distal colon.

3.3 Important Factors Considered for Colonic Drug Delivery

The absorption of drugs from colon is greatly hampered by small area available, higher viscosity of colonic contents, less exposure of the molecules to the epithelium and unusual binding of drug with dietary or metabolites of colonic bacteria in the lumen. The other barriers of colonic absorption are lipid bilayer of the individual epithelial colonocytes, the occluding junction complex (OJC) and mucus layer at the epithelial surface. Still the colon, as a site for drug delivery, offers several distinct advantages on account of a near neutral pH, longer transit time, relatively low proteolytic enzyme activity, and greater responsiveness to absorption enhancers. All these criteria favor colon as a site for the delivery of various bioactive, including proteins and peptides (Haupt and Rubinstein, 2002). The pharmaceutical formulations available for this site are slow release oral formulations or enemas and foams. The adverse effects appear to be more frequent after administration of oral formulations compared with rectal formulations due to the large degree of systemic absorption from the upper GI tract. The delivery systems targeted to colon should remain intact in the hostile environment of upper GI tract. The major variables, which have influence on the performance of colon specific drug delivery systems, are discussed below:

3.3.1 Gastric Emptying

The arrival of an oral dosage form at the colon is determined by the rate of gastric emptying. Particle size, physicochemical charecteristic and feeding state which strongly affect the residence time of particles in the stomach. An increase in level of acidity, osmolarity and caloric value slows down gastric emptying. Various emotional factors like; stress increases gastric emptying rate, whereas depression slows it down. Fasted and fed conditions also affect gastric empting of dosage forms. Liquid dosage form and small pellets (2-7 mm in size) were shown to be emptied from the stomach quite rapidly (Meyer et al., 1985) and were not greatly affected by the digestive state of the individual, while large singly unit systems i.e., tablet were retained for long periods of time, depending on the size of the meal. Under fasting condition, capsules and tablets generally clear the stomach within 1 hour, while dosing after a meal results in gastric retention times in excess of 10 hours (Davis et al., 1986).

3.3.2 Small Intestinal Transit

The mean transit time of dosage form in the small intestine is about 3-4 hours to reach the ileocaecal valve. It has been shown that transit through the small intestine in healthy subjects is consistent as compared to gastric emptying and no or little influenced by the physical state and size of the dosage form. The dosage form is exposed to enzymes such as esterase, lipase, amylase, protease, nuclease and brush border enzymes present in the small intestine. Higher bacterial levels in the ileum can affect the release of drugs from the prodrug-based systems and also the stability of peptides and proteins.

3.3.3 Colonic Transit

The transit through the large intestine show considerable variability as compared to the small intestine. Gender can also influence the transit, shorter transit time in men in comparision to women. There is no or very small variations in dietary fiber transit and age do not significantly alter the transit time of the colon. Adults show a colonic transit time of capsules and tablets for 20-35 hours. The longer transit time improve the residence time and the contact of the dosage form with the microflora in the colon, which is important for release of drug from the dosage form completely. In addition, colonic transit rate does not discriminate between solids and small volumes of liquid and is also independent of dosage form size.

3.3.4 Gastrointestinal pH

The pH of the stomach is 1.5-2 or 2-6 in fasted and non non-fasted conditions, respectively. This condition is responsible for degradation of acid/pH sensitive drugs and enteric coating may prevent the pH-related degradation problem of drug delivery systems. The pH gradient in the GI tract is not exactly in increasing order. Passing from the jejunum through the mid small bowel and the ileum, pH increases slightly from 6.6-7.5, further decreases to 6.4 in the right colon. The mid and left colon has pH values of 6.6 and 7.0, respectively. Because of minimal pH gradients between the ileum and the colon, the use of pH-dependent polymers alone in colon targeted drug delivery systems does not appear to selectively release the drug in the colon. However, it is still possible to exploit the pH variations in the GI tract to formulate colonic delivery dosage forms (Chourasia and Jain, 2003).

3.3.5 Colonic Microflora

The bacterial population in the human colon is 1011-1012 CFU/ml, which produce enzymes and secretory products important to carry out several metabolic reactions. Several of these enzyme systems are currently being used to deliver drugs selectively to the colon and others part of GI tract and have great potential in the design of specific colon targeted delivery systems. The composition and population of intestinal microflora remain constant under normal conditions, but pathological conditions or the disease state of the colon may significantly modify the colonic microflora. Obvious alternations in the colonic microflora following oral administration of antibiotics during infectious diseases significantly affect the colonic delivery of drug formulations dependent on the bacterial degradation for release. It is also possible that some of the metabolic products of the microflora can inactive drugs or potentiates their side effects (Cleusix et al., 2008).

3.3.6 Disease State of Large Intestine

In general, the absorption of a number of drugs have been affected by intestinal diseases such as inflammatory bowel disease (IBD), Cohn's disease, diarrhea, constipation, and gastroenteritis. Many of these disorders are also often associated with increased nausea and vomiting reflexes, which may expel drug content. The release and absorption characteristics of colon specific drug delivery systems may be affected by disease states of the large intestine (Table 3.1). Antibiotic-induced depression of intestinal motility, particularly the muscaris mucosae, may facilitate antibiotic-resistant bacterial overgrowth leading to colitis. These compounds also initiate or exaggerate diarrhea by altering control of epithelial function of the distal colon (Goldhill et al., 1996).

Enzymes produced by colonic microflora have been proposed for triggering local delivery of anti-inflammatory azo bond drugs and prodrugs to the colon. This approach relies on the metabolic activity of digestive flora, which may be affected by the disease sates of the patients. Bacterial enzymes used for colon targeted drug delivery are found to be decreased or become inactive in active Crohn's disease (Carrette et al., 1995). In the case of pouchitis, azoreductase and nitroreductase activity of bacteria were higher after recovery than during attacks of pouchitis. These factors should be taken into consideration for the therapeutic usefulness of steroid glycosides and azo bond drugs for colonic delivery.

TABLE 3.1

Pathophysiological conditions affecting colon specific drug delivery systems

Pathological conditions	Colonic absorption of drugs affected by pathophysiological alteration
Diarrhea	Increased motility and the frequent passage of hypertonic liquid feces in diarrhea significantly affect the performance of colonic drug delivery systems.
Crohn's disease	The inflammatory response is confined to the mucosa and submucosa of the colon. The thickening of the submucosa and mucosa may reduce surface area and impede diffusion.
IBD	Diarrhea, fever, steatorrhea and anemia, obstruction of lymphatic drainage and hyperplasia of lymphoid tissue, may markedly affect the performance of colon delivery system.
Antibiotic associated colitis	This is related to the overgrowth of *Clostridium difficile* and its subsequent toxin production. The falsified mucosal surface may reduce drug absorption from colon.
Constipation	Weakened peristaltic movement of bowel reduces diffusion and availability of drug at colonic absorption sites

TABLE 3.1 *Contd...*

Pathological conditions	Colonic absorption of drugs affected by pathophysiological alteration
Gastroenteritis	Because of viral or bacterial infection, the toxins produced may increase mucosal secretions and increase the intestinal motility leading to diarrhea. This may markedly influence the drug residence time in colon and drug absorption
GI tract infections	Colonic bacterial infections and protozoal infestations are characterized by extensive diarrhea. Extremely low transit time and increased mucus production often disturb the localization and absorption of drug. Toxins produced may damage transport processes, thereby impairing drug absorption processes.
Hirchsprung's disorder	A severe form of constipation in which bowel movement occurs only once or twice a week. This tremendously impedes the movement of colonic dug formulation and consequently its absorption.

3.4 Drug Candidates for Colon Specific Drug Delivery

The colon is utilized as a specific site for the purpose of increasing the bioavailability, absorption and stability or for achieving the local release of the drugs. The bioavailability of poorly absorbable drugs such as nifedipine, diclofenac, ibuprofen, theophylline and isosorbide can be improved by using this approach. Drugs which cause irritation to the gastric mucosa are suitable candidate to increase the bioavailability by fabrication in the form of colon specific delivery systems. Proteins and peptide drugs are digested in the hostile environment of upper GIT and the bioavailability of such drugs can also be considerably increased by using colon specific delivery systems (kumar et al., 2013). In case of several diseases associated particularly with the colonic site such as amebiasis (metronidazole, secnidazole), colon cancer (5-flurouracil, doxorubicin, bleomycin), ulcerative colitis (sulfasalazine, mesalamine, balsalazide) and Crohn's disease (5-aminosalicylic acid, prednisolone, hydrocotisone) demand the drugs in intact form at the pathological site.

3.5 Formulation Approaches for Colon Specific Drug Delivery

Formulations for colonic drug delivery are, in general, delayed-release dosage forms which may be designed either to provide a 'burst release' or a sustained/prolonged release at the colonic site. The proper selection of a formulation approach is dependent upon several important factors including:

(a) pathology and pattern of the disease, especially the affected parts of the lower GI tract or pathophysiological changes in the colon

(b) physicochemical and biopharmaceutical properties of the drug such as solubility, stability and permeability at the intended site of delivery, and

(c) the desired release profile of the active ingredient.

The formulation of colon specific drug delivery systems have been categorized in four basic approches:

1. temporal control of delivery (depends on passage of time),

2. pH-based delivery (triggered by a change in local pH as the formulation passes down the GIT),

3. enzyme-based delivery (the enzymes found locally in a region of the gut breakdown a prodrug or a formulation to release the active therapeutic moiety, and

4. pressure-based systems (variations in pressure along the lumen of the GI tract is used to trigger the drug release).

Some other mechanism used for colon specific delivery are; osmotic controlled drug delivery, prodrug based systems, microbial triggered approach, commensal bacteria and hydrogels based systems.

3.5.1 Timed Release/Delayed Release Dosage Forms

Timed release or delayed release approach is based on the principle of delaying the drug release from formulation until it enters into the colon. The strategy in designing timed-release systems is to resist the acidic environment of the stomach and to undergo a lag phase of predetermined span of time, after which release of drug takes place. The lag time in this case is the time required by the dosage form to transit from the mouth to colon. However, such systems suffer from following disadvantages:

1. Gastric emptying time varies markedly between subjects or in a manner dependent on type and amount of food intake.

2. Gastrointestinal movement, especially peristalsis or contraction in the stomach would result in change in transit of the drug.

3. Accelerated transit through different regions of the colon has been observed in pathophysiological conditions i.e., IBD, the carcinoid syndrome, diarrhea and ulcerative colitis.

The Pulsincap® was first formulation introduced based on this principle to overcome above metioned limitations (MacNeil ME, 1990). It is very similar in appearance to hard gelatin capsule; the water insoluble main body is developed by exposing the body to formaldehyde vapour which may be produced by the addition of trioxymethylene tablets or potassium permanganate to formalin or any other method. The body contains bioactive agent and pluged by a hydrogel, which is covered by a water-soluble cap. The whole system is coated with an enteric polymer to avoid the problem of variable gastric emptying. After entering the capsule in small intestine the enteric coating dissolves and the hydrogel plug starts to swell. The amount of hydrogel is such adjusted that it pops out only after the stipulated period of time to release the bioactive agent (Fig. 3.2).

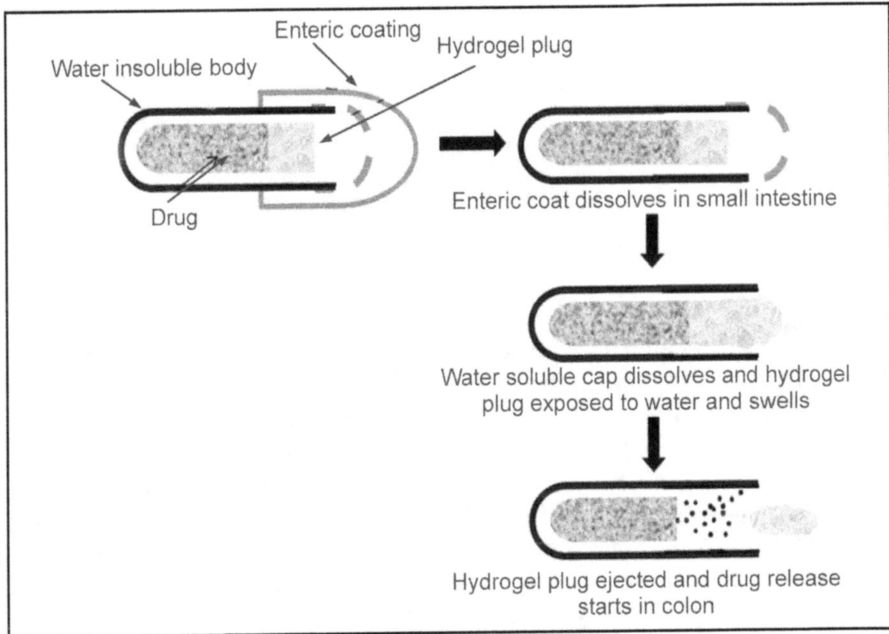

FIGURE 3.2 Drug release mechanism from Pulsincap®.

3.5.2 Osmotic Controlled Drug Delivery

A novel colon drug delivery system was introduced by Alza Corporation, to target the drug locally to the colon, which is known as OROS-CT. The

OROS-CT is timed release or delayed release osmotic dosage form for drug delivery to the colon (Fig. 3.3) (Theeuwes F, 1990). The OROS-CT osmotic therapeutic system can be a single osmotic unit or can compromise as many as 5-6 small push-pull units, 4 mm in diameter contained within a hard gelatin capsule (Swanson et al., 1987). A bilayer push pull unit comprises of osmotic push layer and a drug layer, both surrounded by a semipermeable membrane. An orifice is drilled through the membrane next to the drug layer. The gelatin capsule containing the push-pull units dissolves immediately after the OROS-CT is swallowed. The individual units are enteric coated to prevent release in the stomach, and the release process is triggered by the change in pH of the intestinal fluid upon gastric emptying. Following triggering, a delay period has been built in to the system to concide with the normal small intestinal residence time i.e., 3 hours.

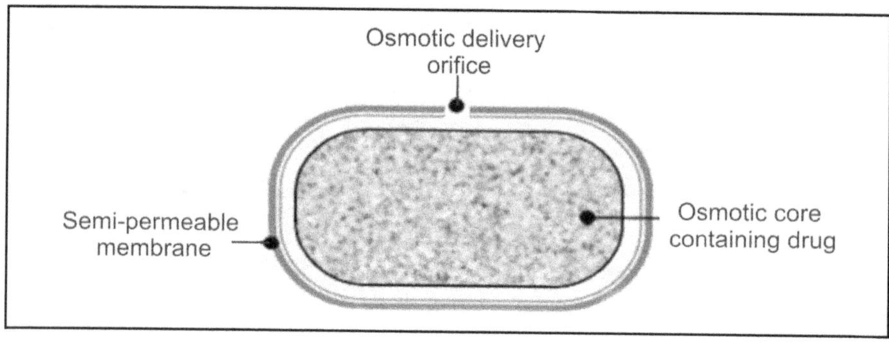

FIGURE 3.3 OROS Capsule.

A multiple coated oral dosage form consisting of core coated with three polymeric layers has been developed (Gazzaniga et al., 1994). The inventor described a novel oral time based drug release system for colon-specific delivery. The system designed to exploit the relatively constant small intestinal transit time of dosage forms consists of drug-containing cores coated with three polymeric layers. The outer layer dissolves at pH above 5, followed by the intermediate swellable layer, made of an enteric material. The system provides the expected delayed release pattern, as also indicated by the preliminary *in vivo* studies on rats. Several other drug delivery systems have developed that rely upon the relatively constant transit time of small intestine (Fukui et al., 2000).

The enteric coated timed-release press-coated tablets (ETP tablets) were developed by coating enteric polymer on timed-release press-coated tablets composed of an outer shell of hydroxypropyl cellulose and core tablet containing diltiazem hydrochloride as a model drug (Fig. 3.4). To evaluate whether ETP tablets could have been of use in the gastrointestinal tract, ETP tablets with a layer of phenylpropanolamine hydrochloride (PPA) (a marker of gastric emptying) between the enteric coating layer and outer shell were prepared, and administered to beagle dogs. The gastric emptying time and lag time after gastric emptying was evaluated by determining the times at which PPA and diltiazem hydrochloride first appeared in the plasma (Ishibashi et al., 1998). To develop a new colon targeting formulation, which can suppress drug release completely during early 2 hours in the stomach and release the drug rapidly after a lag time of 3 ± 1 hours in the small intestine, the use of press-coated tablets with hydroxypropylmethylcellulose acetate succinate (HPMCAS) in the outer shell has been investigated.

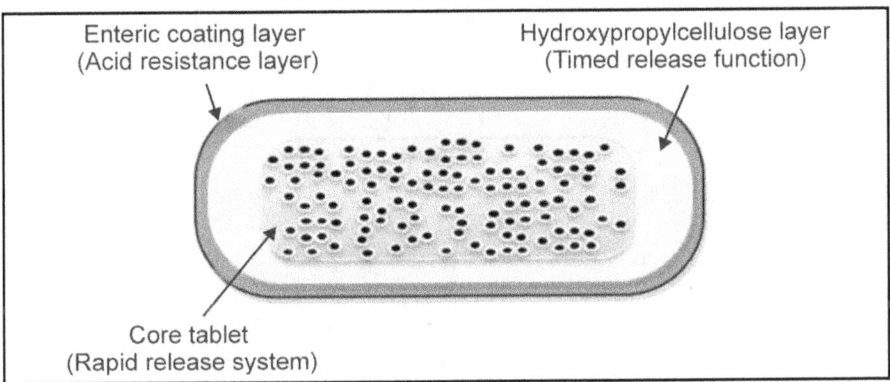

FIGURE 3.4 Enteric coated timed- release press-coated tablet.

3.5.3 pH Dependent Systems: Enteric Coating

Several therapeutic agents can be delivered selectively to the colon by utilizing the pH difference of the different regions of the GIT. Enteric coatings have been used for drug substances that are destroyed by acid or gastric enzymes or cause gastric irritation or produce nausea if released in the stomach.

The pH difference in gastric acid and intestinal fluid determines the salvation of enteric coated polymers used in such systems. To ensure gastric resistance, a coating material should be impermeable until reaching a pH of at least 5-6. The polymers that dissolve at relatively high pH values (pH 8), raises concern as to whether the coating will dissolve promptly at the colonic site and provide opportunity for drug absorption or other intended effects. The first reported use of enteric coating is credited to Unna in 1884, who introduced a medication based on keratin coated pills (Hollander, 1986). The enteric polymers are long chain molecules characteristically display acidic or acidic ester groups, which provide the pH sensitivity necessary for enteric coating activity. Apparently, it is highly desirable for pH-dependent colonic formulations to maintain their physical and chemical integrity during passage through the stomach and small intestine and reach the large intestine where the coating should disintegrate to release the drug locally (Fig. 3.5). It should be however noted that GI fluids might pass through the coat while the dosage form transits through the small intestine. This could lead to premature drug release in the upper parts of GI tract with consequent loss of therapeutic efficacy.

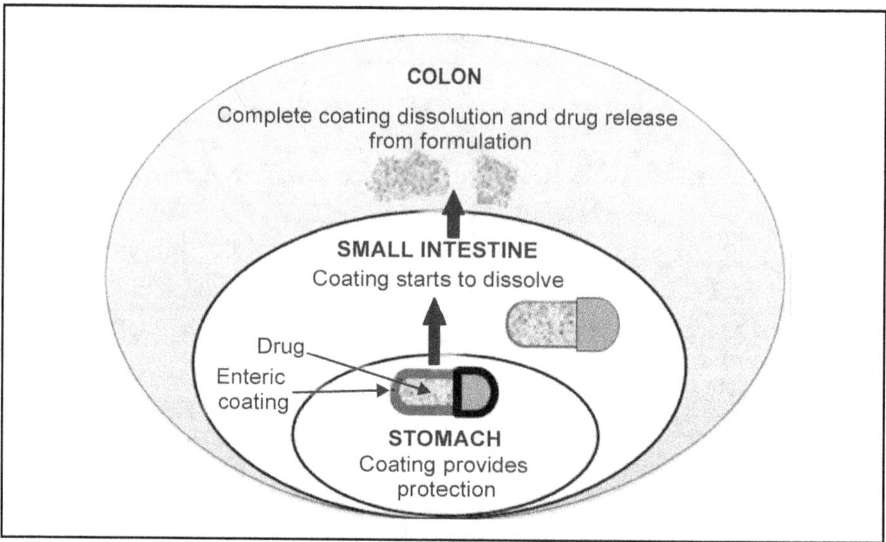

FIGURE 3.5 Schematic representation of pH sensitive polymer coated colon specific capsule.

One approach to overcome this problem is to apply higher coating levels of enteric polymers; however, this also allows influx of GI fluids through the coat, and the thicker coats often rupture under the influence of contractile activity in the stomach. In general, the amount of coating required depends upon the solubility characteristics (solubility, dose/solubility ratio) of the drug, desired release profile, surface area of the formulation, and composition of the coating solution/dispersion. Coating approach is one of the simplest formulation technologies available for colon-specific delivery. The enteric polymers commonly used are derivatives of acrylic acid and cellulose. These polymers have ability to withstand an environment ranging from low pH (~1.2) to neutral pH (~7.5) for several hours. A detail list of various enteric polymers with there respective pH based solubility is given in Table 3.2.

TABLE 3.2

Enteric polymers utilized in development of modified-release formulations for colonic delivery

Enteric polymers	Optimum pH for dissolution
Polyvinyl acetate phthalate (PVAP) (Coateric®**)	5.0
Cellulose acetate trimellitate (CAT)	5.5
Hydroxypropyl methylcellulose phthalate (HPMCP)	----
HP-50	5.0
HP-55 and HP-55S	5.5
Hydroxypropylmethylcellulose acetate succinate (HPMCAS)	----
*LF Grade	5.5
*MF Grade	6.0
*HF Grade	6.8
Methacrylic acid copolymer, Type C (Eudragit® L100-55*)	5.5
Methacrylic acid copolymer dispersion (Eudragit® L30D-55**)	
Methacrylic acid copolymer, Type A	6.0
(Eudragit® L-100* and Eudragit® L12,5)	
Cellulose acetate phthalate (CAP) (Aquateric®**)	6.0
Methacrylic acid copolymer, Type B	7.0
(EudragitÒS-100* and Eudragit® S12, 5)	
EudragitÒ FS30D**	7.0
Shellac (MarCoat 125*** & 125N***)	7.0

*suitable for aqueous dispersion; **available as aqueous dispersion;

***available as aqueous solution

The enteric coating can be applied to a wide variety of solid core formulations such as tablets, capsules, mini tablets, pellets or granules. The tablets or capsules containing coated pellets or granules can be further coated with a suitable enteric polymer which may be same or different polymer than that used for coating of pellets or granules. The enteric coating of orally administered dosage forms is an effective method for modifying and obtaining control drug delivery to small intestine. In some studies it is concluded that the change in luminal pH may not be used reliably and routinely as a mechanism to deliver drugs specifically in the colon (Ashford et al., 1993). Nevertheless, a number of colonic delivery systems have been designed to exploit such a pH-triggered release.

3.5.3.1 CODES™

CODES™ is a combinational approach based on of microbially triggered and pH dependent colon drug delivery system. This technology avoids influence by pH variation in the vicinity of the cecum with individuals or by diet and is designed to release a drug specifically in the colon without relying on time control. It has been developed for the colon site specific release utilizatlizing a unique triggered mechanism involving lactulose. CODES™ comprising a composition containing a drug coated with an organic-acid-soluble macromolecular substance (Eudragit E) and a saccharide (lactulose) which rapidly generates an organic acid by the action of enteric bacteria in a lower gastrointestinal tract and then subsequently overcoated with an enteric material (Eudragit L). Outermost coat of Eudragit L protect the system in gastric fluids and former Eudragit E protects the core from alkaline pH of the small intestine (Fig. 3.6). At the colonic site microbial content triggers the degradation of lactulose. While polysaccharide (lactulose) is dissociated into monosaccharides (organic acids) and the pH surrounding the system comes down favoring dissolution of the acid soluble coating and subsequent drug release (Patel, 2011).

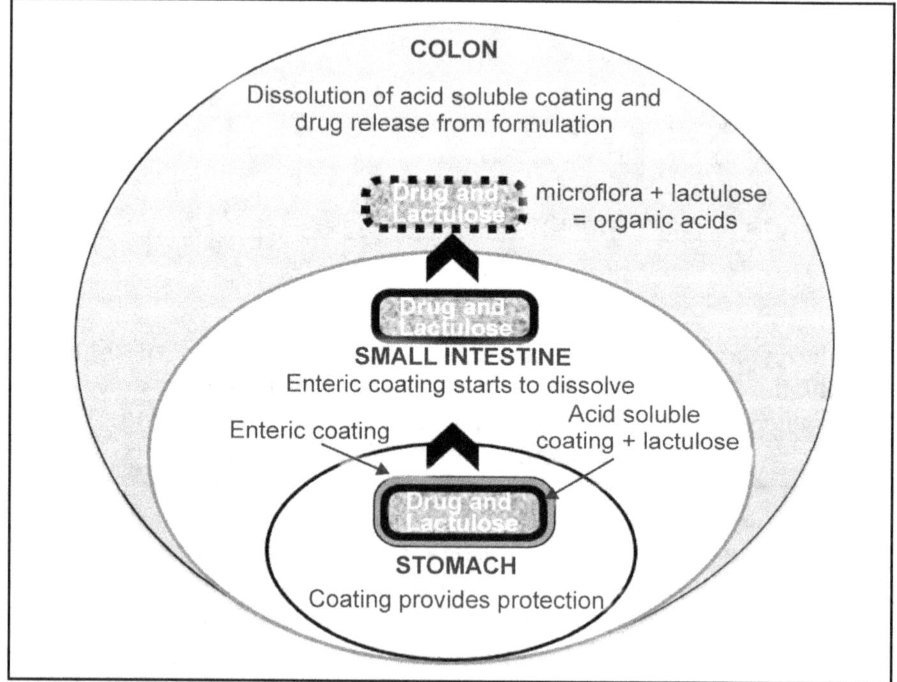

FIGURE 3.6 Schematic representation of CODES™.

3.5.4 Prodrug Based Systems

The pharmacologically inactive moity of a parent bioactive molecule that requires *in vivo* biotransformation to release the active form of bioactive is called prodrug. Prodrug approach involves the formation of a covalent linkage between bioactive and carrier in such a manner that after oral administration it maintains the integrity of the dosage forms in the hostile environment of upper GIT and converted into parent drug/active molecule in the colon. Site specific drug delivery through produrg could be achived by utilizing some specific properties of the target site, i.e., altered pH or high activity of certain enzymes relative to the non-target tissues for the prodrug-drug conversion. Vast variety of enzymes, such as azoreductase, glycosidase, polysaccharidases, cyclodextrinase etc., are produced by bacterial flora and are successfully exploited for site specific colon drug delivery with prodrugs. A number of prodrugs have been developed in the past that are capable of targeting non steroidal anti-inflammatory drugs to the larger bowel. The colonic bacteria produce a wide array of glucosidases and polysaccharidases that are capable of hydrolyzing glycosides and polysaccharides, respectively. Different approaches of prodrugs such as azo bond prodrug, glycoside conjugate, glucoronide conjugate, cyclodextrin conjugate, dextran conjugate, amino acid conjugates have been utilized by different scientists around the globe (Minami et al., 1998). The unique glycosidase activity of the colonic microflora for steroid glycosides form the basis of a new colon targeted drug delivery system. Drug glycosides are hydrophilic and thus, poorly absorbed from the small intestine. Once such a glycoside reaches the colon it can be cleaved by bacterial glycosidases, releasing the free drug to be absorbed by the colonic mucosa. Prodrugs utilizing azo linkages are sulfasalazine, ipsalazine, balsalazine, and olsalazine and have been developed for the delivery of 5-amino salicylic acid to the colon for localized treatment of IBD (Fig. 3.7).

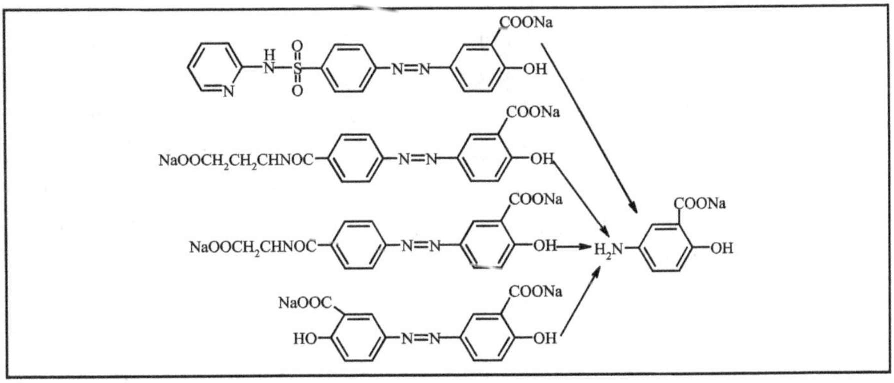

FIGURE 3.7 Derivatives of 5-amino salicylic acid bearing azo bond.

3.5.5 Pressure Based Drug Delivery Systems

The colon encounters higher pressure than small intestine due to peristalsis movements. Peristaltic movements of intestines along with gastric contractile activity are responsible for the propulsion of intestinal contents. The design of pressure controlled drug delivery system is based upon above mechanism. Intensity and duration of this pressure varies with the muscular contractions in the visceral organs (Aggarwal et al., 2011; Challa et al., 2011). Takaya and others developed pressure controlled colon drug delivery capsules using water insoluble polymer Eudragit S (Takaya et al., 1998). The drug release depends on the disintegration of a water-insoluble polymeric capsule due to pressure in the lumen of the colon. The thickness of the ethylcellulose membrane is the most important factor for the disintegration of the formulation. The system also appeared to depend on capsule size and density. Because of reabsorption of water from the colon, the viscosity of luminal content is higher in the colon than in the small intestine. It has therefore been concluded that drug dissolution in the colon could present a problem in relation to colon-specific oral drug delivery systems.

3.5.6 Microbial Triggered Approach

The basic principle involved in this method is degradation of polymers by microflora present in colon and release of drug. Polysaccharides offer an alternative substrate for the bacterial enzymes present in the colon. In this approach we take the advantage of interior flora microbes while in probiotic principle we have to deliver the microflora from external source.

A large number of polysaccharides have already been studied for their potential as colon-specific drug carrier systems (Table 3.3), such as chitosan, pectin, guar gum, chondroitin sulphate, dextrans, cyclodextrin, inulin, amylose, sodium alginate and locust bean gum. Many of these polymers are already used as excipients in drug formulations or are constituents of the human diet and are therefore generally regarded as safe.

TABLE 3.3

Characteristics of various biodegradable polysaccharides for colon targeted drug delivery

Polysaccharide	Chemical name	General properties	Bacterial species
Amylose	α-1,4 D-glucose	Unbranched, constituents of starch, used as excipient in tablet formulation	Bacteroids, Bifidobacterium
Arabinogalactan	β-1,4 and β-1,3 D-galactose β-1,6 and β-1,3 D-arabinose and D-galactose	Natural pectin, hemicellulose, used as thickening agent	Bifidobacterium
Chitosan	Deacetylated β-1,4 N-acetyl-D-glucosamine	Deacetylated chitin, used as absorption enhancing agent	Bacteroids
Chondroitin sulfate	β-1,3, D-glucuronic acid and N-acetyl-D-glucosamine	Mucopolysaccharide, contains various amounts of sulfate ester groups at the 4- or 6- position	Bacteroids
Cyclodextrin	α-1,4 D-glucose	Cyclic structures of 6,7 or 8 units, high stability against amylase, used as drug solublizing agent and absorption enhancer	Bacteroids
Dextran	α-1,6 D-glucose, α-1,3 D-glucose	Plasma expanders	Bacteroids
Guar gum	α-1,4 D-mannose, α-1,6 D-galactose	Galactomannan, used as thickening agent	Bacteroids, Ruminococcus
Pectin	α-1,4 D-galacturonic acid and 1,2 D-rhamnose with D-galactose and D-arabinose side chains	Partial methyl ester, commonly used as thickening agent	Bacteroids Bifidobacterium, Eubacterium
Xylan	β-1,4 D-xylose with β-1,3 L-arabinose side chains	Abundant hemmicellulose of plant cell walls	Bacteroids Bifidobacterium

3.5.7 Commensal Bacteria

The human body supports the growth of variety of bacteria and fungi, which are collectively called the normal flora or "normal microbiota". These microbes are harmless, and for the most part they do not cause disease and are even beneficial. The normal flora can be commensal, if they benefit from the association with the host; whereas the host is not affected i.e., they enjoy symbiotic relationship. The normal micro flora comprises of a permanent population of organisms that vary in both number and kind from one site to another. The commensal bacteria offer the means and opportunities for protein delivery through GI Tract mucosa by site specific drug delivery systems. They have been evolved to colonize a specific niche such as oral cavity, the gut, the urogenital tract or the rectum. L. sporogenes are normal resident of mouth, colon, vagina and intestine. Genetically engineered live vector system such as recombinant commensal bacteria, L. sporogenes producing or releasing an enzyme, packed as granules and coated with polymers may be used as model which may be helpful in lowering blood substrate level. After disintegration of granules, the recombinant strain expresses heterologous proteins on their surface or secrete into the colon. These engineered bacteria are conserved pathway to express and anchor their surface proteins to colon and provide prolonged delivery of enzyme. This approach can be used to deliver a recombinant commensal at a specific location where it can colonize, grow and subsequently secrete a biologically active protein to produce a therapeutic effect at desired site. These systems would minimize or eliminate the problems associated with other conventional or novel dosage forms and get success in achieving continuous and prolonged delivery of proteins in colon. Jain et al., developed and characterized engineered commensal bacteria for site-specific targeting of galactokinase and glutamate dehydrogenase (Jain et al., 2003).

3.5.8 Hydrogel

The potential of hydrogel for oral colon drug delivery has been studied by various research groups (Table 3.4). The three basic types of hydrogels named as azo cross-linked, alcohol cross-linked and aldehyde cross-linked hydrogels are used for colon specifically drug delivery. The hydrogels are developed by different synthetic approaches. They can be obtained by cross-linking polymerization of N-substituted (meth) acrylamides, N-tert-butylacrylamide and acrylic acid with 4,4'-di(methacryloylamino) azobenzene, 4,4'-di(N-methacryloyl-6-aminohexanoylamino) or 3,3',5,5'-tetrabromo-4,4, 4',4'-tetrakis (methacryloylamino) azobenzene as the crosslinking agents (Brondsted and Kopecek, 1992). An alternative approach is cross-linking polymeric precursors. In this case, a reactive linear polymeric precursor was first prepared by copolymerization of N, N-dimethacrylamide, N-tertbutylacrylaminde, acrylic acid, and N-methacryloylglycylglycine p-nitrophenyl ester. The precursors were then cross-linked with N, N' (aminocaproyl)-4, 4'-diaminoazobenzene on the nitrophenyl ester to form the hydrogel structure. The hydrogels were also prepared by polymer–polymer reaction using the same polymeric precursor with the corresponding copolymer containing side chains terminating in NH$_2$ groups. Glutaraldehyde was found to be model candidate from aldehyde family to be used as cross-linker for various polymers. Guar gum hydrogel discs of ibuprofen were delveloped by Das et al in 2006 using glutaraldehyde as a cross-linking agent (Das et al., 2006). Poly vinyl alcohol is another molecule which has its own cross-linking property which was used to cross link succinyl, adipoyl and sebacoyl chloride to get hydrogel foaming polymers (Yang et al., 2002).

TABLE 3.4

Hydrogels for colon specific drug delivery

Type of hydrogel	Materials	Description	Reference
Azoaromatic hydrogels	Acidic comonomers	The gel structure remains intact in the stomach and liberates the drug upon arrival in the colon due to degradation of crosslinks	(Kopeček et al., 1992)
	Methacryloyloxy azobenzene and HEMA	Faster *in vitro* release of 5-flurouracil in presence of azo reductase in the culture of intestinal flora	(Shantha et al., 1995)
	N,N-dimethylacrylamide, N-t-butylacrylamide, and acrylic acid	*In vitro* and *in vivo* degradability depends on the degree of swelling of the gels	(Brondsted and Kopecek, 1992)
Inulin hydrogels	Methacrylated inulin, copolymerized with the aromatic azo agent BMAAB and HEMA or MA	Uptake of the water in the gels inversely proportional to the methacrylated inulin feed concentration, the degree of substitution of the inulin backbone and concentration of BMAAB.	(Maris et al., 2001)
	Inulin reacted with glycidylmethacrylate in N,N-dimethyl formamide in the presence of 4-dimethylaminopyridine	Inulin hydrogels formed by free radical polymerization of aqueous solutions of methacrylated inulin.	(Vervoort et al., 1997)
	Methacrylated inulin or Methacrylated dextran and BMAAB	More pronounce degradation of azo-dextran gels than azo-inulin gels by dextranase	(Stubbe et al., 2001)

TABLE 3.4 Contd...

Type of hydrogel	Materials	Description	Reference
Dextran Hydrogels	Dextran crosslinked with diisocyanate	Degradation of the hydrogels in human colonic fermentation model.	(Hovgaard and Brøndsted, 1996)
	Activated dextran (T-70) conjugated with 4-aminobutyric acid and crosslinked with 1,10-diaminodecane	Enhanced release of bovine serum albumin from the hydrogels by addition of dextranase in buffer solution.	(Chiu et al., 1999)

3.5.9 Redox-Sensitive Polymers

Biodegradation of azo polymers has been extensively studied in the literature (Gingell, 1973). The analogues of these polymers are cleaved by intestinal enzymes via azo bonds. There are many such novel polymers that are hydrolyzed nonenzymatically by enzymatically generated flavins for colon targeting. These reactions used the NADPH as its electron source. As NADPH is oxidized, the electron mediator (reduced flavins) acts as an electron shuttle from the NADPH dependent flavoprotein to the azo compound. Bragger et al., demonstrated its azo reducing activity, which could enlighten some factors affecting the bacterial reduction (cleavage) of azo compounds. A common colonic bacterium, Bacteroides fragilis was used as test organism and the reduction of azo dyes amaranth, Orange II, tartrazine and a model azo compound, 4,4'-dihydroxyazobenzene were studied (Bragger et al., 1997). It was found that the azo compounds were reduced at different rates and the rate of reduction could be correlated with the redox potential of the azo compounds. Similar observations were made with another colonic bacterium Eubacterium limosum. Disulphide compounds can also undergo degradation due to the influence of redox potential in the colon. Noncrosslinked redox-sensitive polymers containing an azo and/or a disulfide linkage in the backbone have also been synthesised (Schacht et al., 1996).

3.6 Colon Specific Polymeric Carrier Systems

Carrier is one of the most important entities essentially required for successful transportation of the loaded drug(s). Carrier systems can do so either through an inherent characteristics or acquired (through structural modification), to interact selectively with biological targets, or otherwise they are engineered to release the drug in the proximity of target cell lines demanding optimal pharmacological action.

3.6.1 Biodegradable Polysaccharide Carriers

Polysaccharides are long carbohydrate molecules of repeated monomer units joined together by glycosidic bonds. The use of GI microflora as a mechanism of drug release via polysaccharides carriers in the colonic region has been of great interest to researchers in recent times. They are digested by the colonic microflora and broken down to simple saccharide units. The polysaccharide based delivery systems protect the bioactive from the hostile conditions of the upper GI tract and bioactive is released in the colon through hydrolysis of the glycosidic linkages (Fig. 3.8). The main saccharolytic species responsible for this biodegradation are Bacteroides and Bifidobacteria.

The majority of bacteria are present in the distal gut although they are distributed throughout the GI tract. Endogenous and exogenous substrates, such as carbohydrates and proteins escape digestion in the upper GI tract but are metabolized by the enzymes secreted by colonic bacteria. Sulphasalazine, a prodrug consisting of the active ingredient mesalazine, was the first bacteria-sensitive delivery system designed for the successful delivery of the drug to the colon (Schacht et al., 1996). Most of these polymers are used in pharmaceutical compositions and are considered generally regarded as safe (GRAS) excipients. A coating composition of a mixture of pectin, chitosan and hydroxypropyl methylcellulose was proven to be very efficient as the tablets coated with this composition passed intact through the stomach and small intestine and broken down in the colon for the release of active agents.

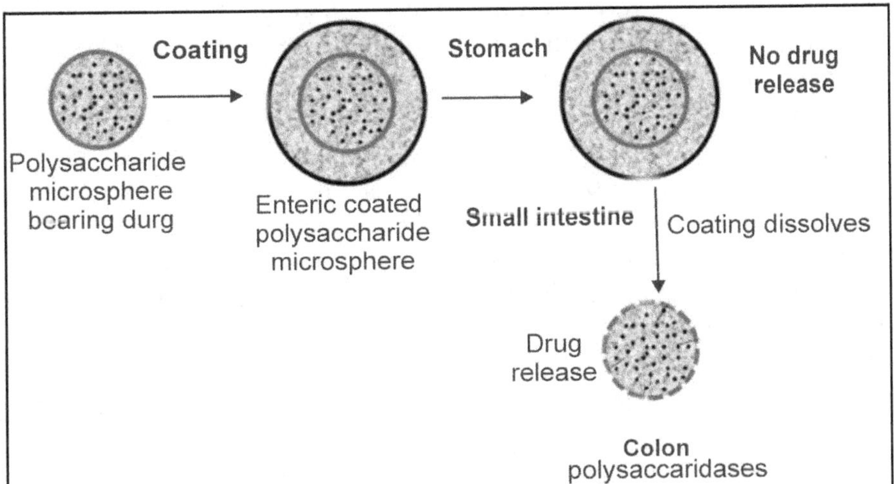

FIGURE 3.8 Drug release mechanism from polysaccharide based colon specific particulate systems.

3.6.2 Microspheres Based Systems

In case of IBD, sustained release devices like pellets, capsules or tablets have less efficiency due to diarrhea which induces their elimination and reduces the total residence time requeired for drug release. It has also been shown that drug carrier systems with a size larger than 200 μm would be subjected to fast bowel evacuation due to diarrhea, resulting in a decreased GI transit time and reduced efficiency. Therefore, a multiparticulate system in the micron size range could be a useful option in the design of a suitable dosage form for IBD. In the study performed by Lamprecht and coauthors, Eudragit P-4135 F, a new pH-sensitive polymer was used to prepare microparticles of 5-fluorouracil for the treatment of colorectal cancer (Lamprecht et al., 2003). The pH-sensitive eudragit group of polyacrylates (Eudragit P-4135 F) possesses a dissolution threshold slightly above pH 7.2. This was found to be very useful in ulcerative colitis mainly affects the distal part of the colon and an early drug loss towards the non-inflamed tissue was also reduced. The multiparticulate system bearing metronidazole for successful colon specific delivery has been developed by us (Chourasia and Jain, 2004). Studies suggest the involvement of macrophages and dendritic cells in active IBD (Seldenrijk et al., 1989). Since these immune cells have an important pathophysiological role, they should be considered in the therapeutic strategy for patients with IBD. It was reported that biodegradable microspheres could be efficiently taken up by macrophages. Therefore, the direct uptake of anti-inflammatory agents by macrophages achieved with the use of microspheres has better response as immunosuppressive effect and more useful for treatment of patients with IBD. In a study by Nakase et al., dexamethasone was incorporated into poly (DL-lactic acid) microspheres and administered to mice induced with experimental colitis. It was observed that serum dexamethasone levels were not increased after oral administration of dexamethasone microspheres but at the same time the microspheres facilitated mucosal repair of experimental colitis (Nakase et al., 2000). The colon has always attracted as a potential site for the systemic absorption of peptide drugs due to low proteolytic enzyme activity and hence several insulin delivery system based on microsphers have been reported in literature. This strategy could be ideal strategy for the treatment of IBD where local action in colon is needed without systemic drug burden.

3.6.3 Nanoparticle Based Systems

Nanotechnologies have the potential to revolutionize the drug development process and changing the landscape of the pharmaceutical industry. The approval of more than two-dozen products based on therapeutic nanoparticles for clinical use has generated great enthusiasm in both academia and industry, although the first generation nanoparticles therapeutics are relatively simple and only provide clinical benefits across a narrow range of clinically validated drugs. Nano sized colloidal drug carriers composed of natural or synthetic polymers have also been investigated for colon specific drug delivery. Orally administered nanoparticles serve as carriers for different types of drugs and have shown to enhance their solubility, permeability and bioavailability to the colon. Various polymeric nanoparticles have also been investigated for the delivery of protein and various peptide drugs. It was shown that nanoparticles tend to accumulate at the site of inflammation in IBD because a strong cellular immune response occurs in the inflamed regions due to increased presence of neutrophils, natural killer cells, macrophages and so on in the case of colitis. It has been reported that microspheres and nanoparticles could be efficiently taken up by these macrophages. This results in accumulation of the particulate carrier system resulting in prolonged residence time in the desired area. A study by Lamprecht group has demonstrated an increased nanoparticles deposition in the inflamed tissue of the colon compared with the healthy control organ. These biodegradable nanoparticles were developed using the polymer poly(lactic-coglycolic acid). However, an important area of concern is to prevent loss of nanoparticles in the early transit through GI tract. Moreover, particle uptake by Payer's patches and/or enzymatic degradation may cause the release of entrapped drug leading to systemic drug absorption and undesired effects. In order to overcome this problem, in a study, drug loaded nanoparticles were entrapped into pH sensitive microspheres, which serve to deliver the incorporated nanoparticle to their site of action, thereby preventing an early drug leakage. The use of eudragit P-4135F prevents drug release in the upper GI tract during intestinal passage and permits selective drug delivery in the colon.

Nanoparticles have a large specific surface, which is indicative of high interactive potential with biological membrane. The bioadhesive nature of nanoparticles has also been investigated for site specific delivery. Since the interaction is of non-specific nature, bioadhesion can be induced by binding nanoparticles with different molecules. For covalent attachment, the nanoparticle surface has to show free functional groups, such as carboxylic or amine residues. The gliadin (protein isolated from wheat gluten) nanoparticles were conjugated with lectins (glycoproteins of non-immune origin which provide specific bioadhesion), fluorescently labeled and evaluated for bioadhesive potential on isolated intestinal segments. It was shown that gliadin nanoparticles have a high capacity of non-specific interaction with intestine and the binding of lectin provided greater specificity for colonic mucosa.

3.6.4 Ligand Anchored Polymeric Nanoparticles

The application of nanoparticle technologies to drug delivery has demonstrated significant impact on many areas of medicine. The strategy is useful for systemic delivery of drugs like proteins and peptides in addition to the local colonic pathologies. It provides the means for various diseases sensitive to the circadian rhythms such as asthma, angina and arthritis. Thus there is need of more research in this area specific for drug uptake at the colon site is necessary. The bioactive targeting specific to molecular and cellular levels has emerged as a convincing paradigm with immense potential for therapeutic and diagnosis purpose. However, such targeting poses enormous challenges and needs to overcome physiological, biochemical, and pharmaceutical barriers. Passive and active targeting approaches have been used to guide drug bearing carrier to specific cells or tissues. Passive targeting implies accumulation of a drug at a particular site due to various physicochemical, anatomical, pathophysiological, and chemical attributes, whereas active targeting deals with surface modification of a drug/carrier with site-specific ligands. Surface modification of polymeric nanoparticles by receptor-specific ligands and surface protein-specific antibodies are essential for targeting them to specific disease and allowing them to selectively interact with cells or receptors for active delivery. Surface modification could be achieved by coupling these site-specific moieties by various physical and chemical means. The physical means involves adsorption of ligand and antibodies to the surfaces of nanoparticles by hydrophobic and ionic interaction, whereas chemical means comprise covalently or noncovalently conjugating the target-specific ligands to nanoparticle surfaces. Surface functionalization of nanoparticles for active delivery is either based on direct coupling or coupling the ligands on stealth particles. This modulates spatial placement of nanoparticles to specifically defined targets. The ligand mediated carrier system can effectively used to deliver anticancer drug to colorectal cancer. Jain and co-workers have developed HA anchored polysaccharide nanoparticles for site specific delivery of encapsulated anticancer drug to the colorectal cancer (Jain et al., 2010). The general mechanism of drug targeting through ligand anchored polymeric nanoparticles to the colorectal cancer cells is represented in Fig. 3.9.

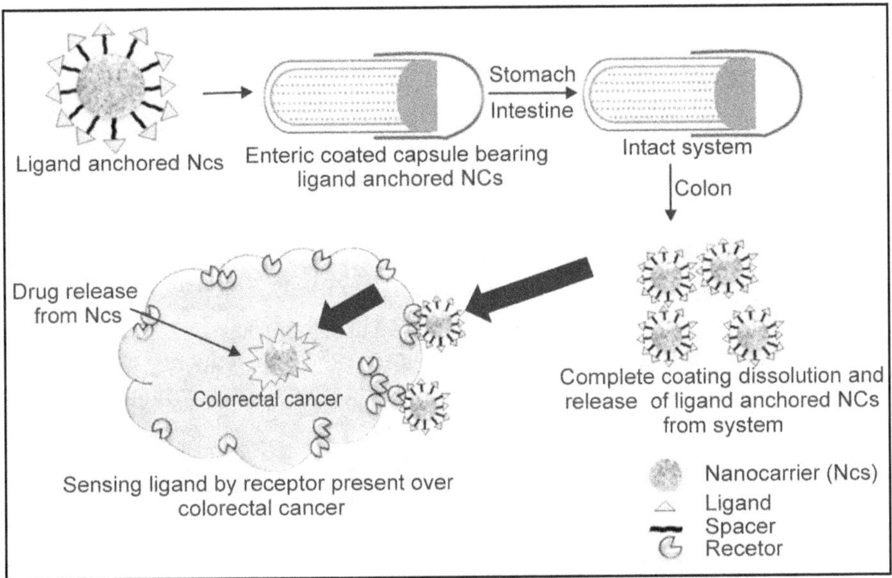

FIGURE 3.9 Effective drug targeting through ligand anchored polymeric nanoparticles.

3.7 Conslusion

From above discussion, we can be familiar with the development of colon specific drug delivery system. Colon specific drug delivery has attained great popularity for the delivery of drugs for the treatment of local diseases as well as potential site for the systemic delivery of therapeutic peptide and proteins. Colon as a site for drug delivery, offers number of favorable factors e.g., near neutral pH, reduced digestive enzymes activity, a long transit time, as well as an increased responsiveness to the absorption enhancers. There are number of other issue to be addressed while formulation of colon specific drug delivery systems. The colon targeting is complicated, with reliability and delivery efficiency depends on person to person response. Another limitation associated with colon specific delivery is with poorly soluble drug because the fluid content in colon is much lower and more viscous. Thus successful delivery through this site requires being in solution form before it reaches colon and/or should dissolve in luminal fluid of colon easily. The resident colonic microflora also affects the drug performance via metabolic degradation and need to be addressed before such formulations. The surface area of colon is lower and numerous tight junctions are present in colonic area that restricts the drug transport to the systemic circulation.

References

Aggarwal, S., Sharma, S., Lal, S., and Choudhary, N. (2011). Recent trends in colon targeted drug delivery system. *Research Journal of Pharmaceutical, Biological and Chemical Sciences* **2,** 406-415.

Ashford, M., Fell, J.T., Attwood, D., Sharma, H., and Woodhead, P.J. (1993). An *in vivo* investigation into the suitability of pH dependent polymers for colonic targeting. *International Journal of Pharmaceutics* **95,** 193-199.

Bragger, J.L., Lloyd, A.W., Soozandehfar, S.H., Bloomfield, S.F., Marriott, C., and Martin, G.P. (1997). Investigations into the azo reducing activity of a common colonic microorganism. *International journal of pharmaceutics* **157,** 61-71.

Brondsted, H., and Kopecek, J. (1992). Hydrogels for site-specific drug delivery to the colon: *In vitro* and *in vivo* degradation. *Pharmaceutical Research* **9,** 1540-1545.

Carrette, O., Favier, C., Mizon, C., Neut, C., Cortot, A., Colombel, J.F., and Mizon, J. (1995). Bacterial enzymes used for colon-specific drug delivery are decreased in active Crohn's disease. *Digestive Diseases and Sciences* **40,** 2641-2646.

Challa, T., Vynala, V., and Allam, K.V. (2011). Colon specific drug delivery systems: A review on primary and novel approaches. *International Journal of Pharmaceutical Sciences Review and Research* **7,** 171-181.

Chiu, H.-C., Hsiue, G.-H., Lee, Y.-P., and Huang, L.-W. (1999). Synthesis and characterization of pH-sensitive dextran hydrogels as a potential colon-specific drug delivery system. *Journal of Biomaterials Science, Polymer Edition* **10,** 591-608.

Chourasia, M.K., and Jain, S.K. (2003). Pharmaceutical approaches to colon targeted drug delivery systems. *Journal of Pharmacy and Pharmaceutical Sciences* **6,** 33-66.

Chourasia, M.K., and Jain, S.K. (2004). Design and development of multiparticulate system for targeted drug delivery to colon. *Drug Delivery: Journal of Delivery and Targeting of Therapeutic Agents* **11,** 201-207.

Cleusix, V., Lacroix, C., Vollenweider, S., and Le Blay, G. (2008). Glycerol induces reuterin production and decreases Escherichia coli population in an *in vitro* model of colonic fermentation with immobilized human feces. *FEMS Microbiology Ecology* **63,** 56-64.

Das, A., Wadhwa, S., and Srivastava, A.K. (2006). Cross-linked guar gum hydrogel discs for colon-specific delivery of ibuprofen: Formulation and *in-vitro* evaluation. Drug Delivery: *Journal of Delivery and Targeting of Therapeutic Agents* **13**, 139-142.

Davis, S.S., Hardy, J.G., and Fara, J.W. (1986). Transit of pharmaceutical dosage forms through the small intestine. *Gut* **27**, 886-892.

Filipe, M.I. (1979). Mucins in the human gastrointestinal epithelium: a review. *Investigative & cell pathology* **2**, 195-216.

Fukui, E., Miyamura, N., Uemura, K., and Kobayashi, M. (2000). Preparation of enteric coated timed-release press-coated tablets and evaluation of their function by *in vitro* and *in vivo* tests for colon targeting. *International Journal of Pharmaceutics* **204**, 7-15.

Gazzaniga, A., Iamartino, P., Maffione, G., and Sangalli, M.E. (1994). Oral delayed-release system for colonic specific delivery. *International Journal of Pharmaceutics* **108**, 77-83.

Gingell, R. (1973). Substrate non-specificity of Streptococcus faecalis azoreductase. *Xenobiotica* **3**, 165-169.

Goldhill, J.M., Rose, K., and Percy, W.H. (1996). Effects of antibiotics on epithelial ion transport in the rabbit distal colon *in-vitro*. *Journal of Pharmacy and Pharmacology* **48**, 651-656.

Haupt, S., and Rubinstein, A. (2002). The colon as a possible target for orally administered peptide and protein drugs. *Critical Reviews in Therapeutic Drug Carrier Systems* **19**, 499-551.

Hollander, A.W. (1986). Development of dermatopathology and Paul Gerson Unna. *Journal of the American Academy of Dermatology* **15**, 727-734.

Hovgaard, L., and Brøndsted, H. (1996). Current applications of polysaccharides in colon targeting. *Critical Reviews in Therapeutic Drug Carrier Systems* **13**, 185-223.

Ishibashi, T., Hatano, H., Kobayashi, M., Mizobe, M., and Yoshino, H. (1998). Design and evaluation of a new capsule-type dosage form for colon- targeted delivery of drugs. *International Journal of Pharmaceutics* **168**, 31-40.

Jain, A., Jain, S.K., Ganesh, N., Barve, J., and Beg, A.M. (2010). Design and development of ligand-appended polysaccharidic nanoparticles for the delivery of oxaliplatin in colorectal cancer. *Nanomedicine: Nanotechnology, Biology, and Medicine* **6**, e179-e190.

Jain, N.K., Chourasia, M.K., Jain, S., and Jain, S.K. (2003). Development and characterization of engineered commensal bacteria for the delivery of enzymes. *Indian Journal of Pharmaceutical Sciences* **65**, 113-121.

Karasov, W.H., and Hume, I.D. (2010). Vertebrate Gastrointestinal System. In Comprehensive Physiology (John Wiley & Sons, Inc.).

Kopeček, J., Kopečková, P., Brøndsted, H., Rathi, R., Říhová, B., Yeh, P.Y., and Ikesue, K. (1992). Polymers for colon-specific drug delivery. *Journal of Controlled Release* **19**, 121-130.

kumar, J.R., Muralidharan, S., Dhanaraj, S.A., and Umadevi, S.K. (2013). A novel drug delivery systems of colon targeted: A review. *Journal of Pharmaceutical Sciences and Research* **5**, 42-47.

Lamprecht, A., Yamamoto, H., Takeuchi, H., and Kawashima, Y. (2003). Microsphere design for the colonic delivery of 5-fluorouracil. *Journal of Controlled Release* **90**, 313-322.

MacNeil ME, R.A., Stevens HN (1990). Dispensing device, WIPO, ed.

Maris, B., Verheyden, L., Van Reeth, K., Samyn, C., Augustijns, P., Kinget, R., and Van den Mooter, G. (2001). Synthesis and characterisation of inulin-azo hydrogels designed for colon targeting. *International journal of pharmaceutics* **213**, 143-152.

Meyer, J.H., Dressman, J., Fink, A., and Amidon, G. (1985). Effect of size and density on canine gastric emptying of nondigestible solids. *Gastroenterology* **89**, 805-813.

Minami, K., Hirayama, F., and Uekama, K. (1998). Colon-specific drug delivery based on a cyclodextrin prodrug: Release behavior of biphenylylacetic acid from its cyclodextrin conjugates in rat intestinal tracts after oral administration. *Journal of Pharmaceutical Sciences* **87**, 715-720.

Mrsny, R.J. (1992). The colon as a site for drug delivery. *Journal of Controlled Release* **22**, 15-34.

Nakase, H., Okazaki, K., Tabata, Y., Uose, S., Ohana, M., Uchida, K., Matsushima, Y., Kawanami, C., Oshima, C., Ikada, Y., et al. (2000). Development of an oral drug delivery system targeting immune-regulating cells in experimental inflammatory bowel disease: A new therapeutic strategy. *Journal of Pharmacology and Experimental Therapeutics* **292**, 15-21.

Patel, M.M. (2011). Cutting-edge technologies in colon-targeted drug delivery systems. *Expert Opinion on Drug Delivery* **8**, 1247-1258.

Schacht, E., Gevaert, A., Kenawy, E.R., Molly, K., Verstraete, W., Adriaensens, P., Carleer, R., and Gelan, J. (1996). Polymers for colon specific drug delivery. *Journal of Controlled Release* **39**, 327-338.

Sekirov, I., Russell, S.L., Antunes, L.C.M., and Finlay, B.B. (2010). Gut Microbiota in Health and Disease. *Physiological Reviews* **90**, 859-904.

Seldenrijk, C.A., Drexhage, H.A., Meuwissen, S.G.M., Pals, S.T., and Meijer, C.J.L.M. (1989). Dendritic cells and scavenger macrophages in chronic inflammatory bowel disease. *Gut* **30**, 484-491.

Shantha, K.L., Ravichandran, P., and Rao, K.P. (1995). Azo polymeric hydrogels for colon targeted drug delivery. *Biomaterials* **16**, 1313-1318.

Stubbe, B., Maris, B., Van den Mooter, G., De Smedt, S.C., and Demeester, J. (2001). The *in vitro* evaluation of 'azo containing polysaccharide gels' for colon delivery. *Journal of Controlled Release* **75**, 103-114.

Swanson, D.R., Barclay, B.L., Wong, P.S.L., and Theeuwes, F. (1987). Nifedipine gastrointestinal therapeutic system. *The American Journal of Medicine* **83**, 3-9.

Takaya, T., Niwa, K., Muraoka, M., Ogita, I., Nagai, N., Yano, R., Kimura, G., Yoshikawa, Y., Yoshikawa, H., and Takada, K. (1998). Importance of dissolution process on systemic availability of drugs delivered by colon delivery system. *Journal of Controlled Release* **50**, 111-122.

Thadepalli, H., Lou, S.M.A., Bach, V.T., Matsui, T.K., and Mandal, A.K. (1979). Microflora of the human small intestine. *The American Journal of Surgery* **138**, 845-850.

Theeuwes F, G.G., Wong PSL (1990). Delivery of drug to colon by oral dosage form, U.P. authority, ed.

Vervoort, L., Van Den Mooter, G., Augustijns, P., Busson, R., Toppet, S., and Kinget, R. (1997). Inulin hydrogels as carriers for colonic drug targeting: I. Synthesis and characterization of methacrylated inulin and hydrogel formation. *Pharmaceutical Research* **14**, 1730-1737.

Yang, L., Chu, J.S., and Fix, J.A. (2002). Colon-specific drug delivery: new approaches and *in vitro/in vivo* evaluation. *International journal of pharmaceutics* **235**, 1-15.

4 Targeting of Bioactives to Peyer's Patches

Piush Khare[1], Mohini Chaurasia[2], Prashant Khare[3], S. K. Paliwal[4], Nitin K. Jain[5] and Manish K. Chourasia[6]

[1]Eiman Pharma Pvt Limited, 1/1 Palm Road, Shipra Sun City (Gaziabad), National Capital Region, 201 014, India.

[2]Amity Institute of Pharmacy, Amity University, Lucknow-226 028, India.

[3]Baylor Institute for Immunology Research, Dallas, TX-75246, USA.

[4]Department of Pharmaceutical Sciences, Banasthali University, Banasthali-304 022, India.

[5]Department of Biotechnology, Ministry of Science & Technology, New Delhi-400 003, India.

[6]Pharmaceutics Division, CSIR-Central Drug Research Institute, Lucknow-226 031, India.

4.1 Introduction

Targeting is an advanced aspect of drug delivery; wherein the drug is delivered to a patient in a manner that increases the concentration of the drug in a specific part of the body relative to others. Targeted drug delivery seeks to concentrate the medication in the tissues of interest while reducing the relative concentration of the medication in the remaining tissues which in turn manifests the effect of drug in the targeted organ and no other parts of the body. This improves efficacy of the therapeutic agent while reducing side effects which may have been caused due to non specific distribution of the same. However, it is not easy for a drug molecule to specifically access its desired destination in the complex cellular network of an organism. Therefore any approach which facilitates the drug molecule in reaching preferably to its desired site comes under the purview of targeting. The inherent advantage of this technique has been the reduction in dose, dosing frequency and side effects of the drug. A huge amount of research is being carried out and implemented for the development of a targeted drug delivery and is being highly taken up industrially in form of various projects. In the same

"

sequence oral delivery of the drug is also now being coupled with the knowledge and tool of targeting to increase the therapeutic benefits of drug. It is common knowledge that oral delivery has always been and will always be the most convenient method of administration of the drugs to the patient since it does not require any expertise and professional competence. This contributes towards the ease of application as well as patient compliance. Moreover constraints such as maintenance of sterility as in case of parenteral dosage form do not apply to oral dosage form. May it be delivery of drugs or vaccines; oral route has been the most preferred route. But the delivery of therapeutics through oral route in some cases especially with respect to vaccines suffered a drawback viz. low bioavailability due to poor absorption/poor presentation. These bioactive agents mainly suffer from low bioavailability due to their instability within the harsh conditions of the gastrointestinal tract (GI tract) and low mucosal permeability (Salman et al., 2005). Approaches have been postulated for the delivery through carrier based system viz. liposomes/nanoparticles. Application of the targeting principles to the delivery of the drugs has opened new vistas in the field. This particularly has been possible through the targeting of the drugs and therapeutics to the Peyer's patches of the intestine whereby the active agent can be internalised across the epithelium through the M-cells mediated uptake. Strategies and application preceded by a brief discussion of the tissues involved in this phenomenon are being discussed in this chapter.

4.1.1 Small Intestine

The small intestine (small in diameter compared to the large intestine) is divided into three sections:

The duodenum, about 25 cm (10 inches) long, receives chyme from the stomach through the pyloric sphincter. Ducts that empty into the duodenum deliver pancreatic juice and bile from the pancreas and liver, respectively.

The jejunum, about 2.5 m (8 feet) long, is the middle section of the small intestine. The lining of the jejunum is specialized for the absorption of small nutrient particles by enterocytes, which have been previously digested by enzymes in the duodenum. Jejunum is involved in the passive transport of sugar fructose and the active transport of amino acids, small peptides, vitamins, and most glucose.

The ileum, about 3.6 m (12 feet) long, is the last section of the small intestine. It ends with the ileocecal valve (sphincter), which regulates the movement of chyme into the large intestine and prevents backward movement of material from the large intestine.

The functions of the small intestine include the following:

- *Mechanical digestion:* Segmentation mixes the chyme with enzymes from the small intestine and pancreas. Bile from the liver separates fat into smaller fat globules. Peristalsis moves the chyme through the small intestine.

- *Chemical digestion:* Enzymes from the small intestine and pancreas break down all four groups of molecules found in food (polysaccharides, proteins, fats, and nucleic acids) into their component molecules.

- *Absorption:* The small intestine is the primary location in the GI tract for absorption of nutrients.

The small intestine contains the same four standard layers that are generally present in most parts of the gastrointestinal tract: the mucosa, submucosa, muscularis and serosa. The mucosa and submucosa of small intestine hold some special features which facilitate variety of processes. The mucosa includes a columnar epithelium with glands called crypts of Lieberkuhn; absorptive cells; mucus-secreting goblet cells; Paneth cells, which secrete lysozymes; enteroendocrine cells, which secrete hormones. The mucosa is involved in the formation of series of fingerlike (leaflike) projections called villi, which increase its absorptive surface area several times; lamina propria (connective tissue); and muscularis mucosa.

The ileum has subepithelial aggregates of lymphoid tissue along the antimesenteric border; these are called Peyer's patches. Mucosa is much thicker in the jejunum than in the ileum and is arranged in spiral folds called plicae circulares, which appear as valvulae conniventes on plain abdominal radiographs. The submucosa contains the blood vessels and the Meissner nerve plexus; the muscularis propria contains inner circular and outer longitudinal muscles and myenteric (Auerbach) nerve plexus; and the serosa covering the organs of the peritoneal cavity is called the visceral peritoneum.

4.1.2 Peyer's Patches

Peyer's patches belong to a class of organized mucosal lymphoid tissues which are present in small intestine specifically in the illeal region of the small intestine. They are formed of or contain groups of lymphoid follicles that occur along the wall opposite the mesentric attachment of the small intestine (Ermak and Giannasca, 1998). The number of the follicles of which they are composed of as well as size and their distribution along the intestine vary from species to species (Griebel and Hein, 1996). These patches are evenly distributed in the rodents throughout the intestine with 5-10 follicles present within each Peyer's patch (Griebel and Hein, 1996) whereas in rabbits the Peyer's patches are 1 cm in diameter with 40-50 follicles in each patch (ABE, 1977) (Abe and Ito, 1978). On the other hand, the patch size in the humans increases distally, the largest being located generally in the terminal part of the ileum (Griebel and Hein, 1996). The largest population of the patches has also been reported to be present in the terminal ileum (Fasano, 1998). These patches represent one of the different gut associated lymphoid tissues or commonly cited as GALT which have been reported as inductive sites for the generation of the mucosal immune responses against the antigens. Also the Peyer's patches have been referred to as the most important structural units of the gut associated lymphoid tissue. The GALT has some features which are also characteristic of the Peyer's patches. These consist of an epithelial layer known as follicle associated epithelium (FAE) which is exposed to the lumen. The lymphoid tissues are characterized and the FAE can be distinguished from the normal epithelium by the presence of the M-cells that in particular lie over the lymphoid tissue and are specialized for the endocytosis and transport of the antigen/particulates to the intraepithelial space. Fig. 4.1 is a schematic representation of the Peyer's patches.

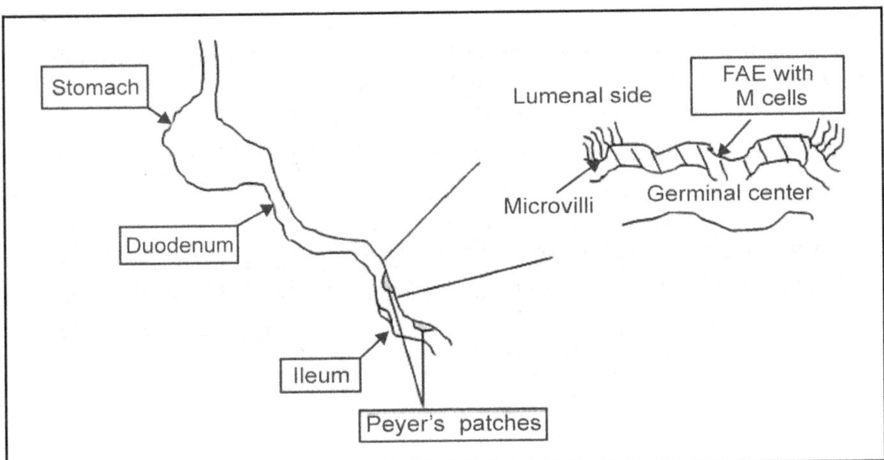

FIGURE 4.1 Diagramatic representation of Peyer's patches and their location.

4.1.3 M-Cells

Membranous epithelial cells (M-cells) are specialized epithelial cells overlying the subepithelial lymphoid follicles in the gastrointestinal and respiratory tracts. These are specialized for sampling viruses and bacteria and perform a critical role in immune surveillance in mucosal tissues. As it has already been mentioned these cells transport antigens from the lumen to the extracellular space, allowing access to lymphocytes, macrophages, and plasma cells. In suckling and adult animals they are involved in the transport of macromolecules. M-cells are generally found on the follicle-associated epithelium overlying Peyer's patches. The location of the Peyer's patches has already been discussed in the preceding section of this chapter. The epithelial lining overlying these patches possess a reduced number of goblet cells which successively results in reduction of the mucus secretion which in turn makes the M-cell's surface more conducive and feasible to antigen or particulate binding (Wolf and Bye, 1984). The M-cell apical surface is modified with less frequent shorter microvilli and a thinner glycocalyx so as to provide more contact of the antigen/particulates to the cells. The basolateral membrane is invaginated to form an intraepithelial pocket or space which houses the leukocytes. The alterations are favourable for and facilitate endocytosis and phagocytosis of microorganisms and their consecutive transport across the epithelium. The apical membrane possesses capability of rapidly responding to the bound bacteria or to the inert particles in form of phagocytosis. It has been shown that the apical membrane can also conduct endocytosis of the fluid phase molecules which is defined as pinocytosis (Bockman and Cooper, 1973). Pathogenic bacteria and viruses can recognize the M-cell surface and exploit its transcellular transport pathway to gain entry into host tissues. For the same reasons, M-cells also may be more easily accessible for nano-particles and microspheres. Due to their potential with regards to phagocytosis the M-cells sample and transport the synthetic microspheres exposed to their surface in a manner similar to microorganisms and thus can play an essential role in the delivery of vaccines and drugs to mucosal lymphoid tissues. In certain tissues, M-cell apical membranes exhibit distinct receptors which have been identified with monoclonal antibodies and lectins. Fig. 4.2 is an artistic portrayal of the location of M-cell and Fig. 4.3 represents the mechanism involved in the uptake of the particles or bacteria by the M-cells.

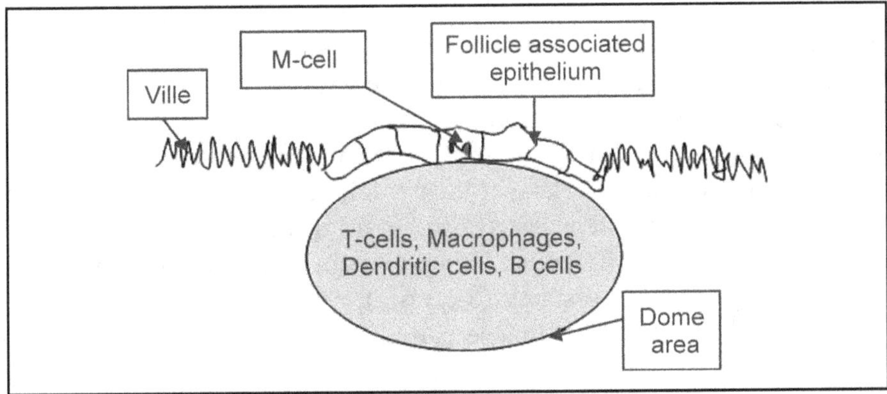

FIGURE 4.2 Diagrammatic representation of the location of the M-cells with adjoining structures.

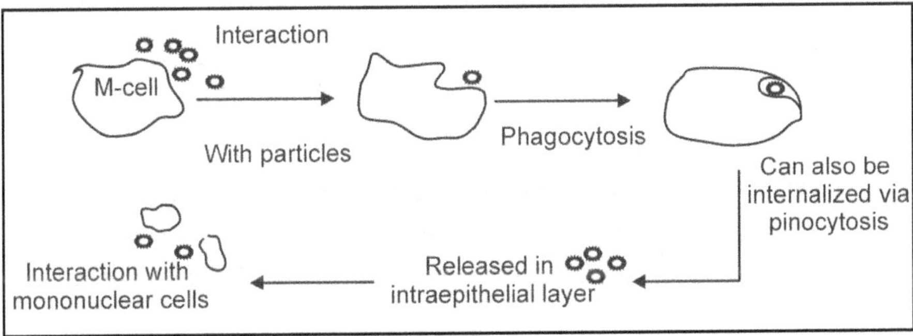

FIGURE 4.3 Mechanism of the uptake of the particles by M- cells.

4.2 Targeting of Therapeutics to Peyer's Patches

Use of Peyer's patch as target site for the delivery of the drugs and other therapeutics has evolved out recently with a number of research articles reporting existence of an absorptive mechanism for particulate matter at the intestinal site. The same had been a matter of controversy for many years and it was thought that such transport is very limited, unusual and to which a no clear scientific reason could be assigned. It is interesting to note that more than a century back it was thought that the normal intestine epithelial layer is impermeable unless and until it is wounded or inflamed and that only the inflamed mucosa allows the microorganism to pass, as per the study report of Basset and Carne in 1907. A review by (Florence, 1997) mentions study performed by Kumagai in 1923 which included the feeding of Indian ink to the rabbits. The study elucidated that the ink was found in large amounts in the epithelial lining of the lymph follicles as compared to the epithelial cells. The conclusion indicated towards the possibility of operational phagocytotic activity present at the site. This was succeeded by yet another study (Volkheimer, 1964) where extensive studies on the uptake of the particles through the intestine were performed on quantitative basis also. Investigations on variety of the materials present in different sizes, were performed which included corn starch (3-25 μm), potato starch (5-10 μm), rice starch (3-10 μm), PVC particles (5-100 μm) and cellulose particles. It was found that all of the particles could be traced out in the circulation and were able to find their way into the blood stream (Volkheimer, 1964). Before we proceed to the discussion related to the particle uptake one must know the possible routes of the absorption through the gastrointestinal tract. It has been suggested by some of the researchers (Florence, 1997; Kreuter, 1991) that the absorption through the gastrointestinal tract occurs via three mechanisms or three possible routes as mentioned below:

1. Through paracellular route/pathway
2. Through transcellular/intercellular pathway which involves the normal epithelial cells of the intestine
3. Through M-cell mediated transport/uptake in Peyer's patches

The last mode of uptake mentioned above i.e., M-cell mediated transport has been studied by many researchers and is a matter of discussion in the present context. It is well evident that the uptake of macromolecules through the M-cells acts as the source of immunity for the newborn. The bacteria and the reoviruses possess the ability to get absorbed and can target themselves to the cells of the gut (Florence, 1997). Florence has reviewed and laid emphasis on the fact that if we can trace out and decipher the mechanism underlying the uptake of the bacteriae or viruses which gain entry through the route naturally, the carrier or the particulates can be targeted to the lymphoid tissues in much better way. It has been postulated that the mechanism responsible for the uptake of the micro-nanoparticles resembles and is similar to that noticed for the bacteria (Ermak et al., 1995; Landsverk, 1988). This cellular basis for the uptake of the particles along with the transport of the bacteria and viruses has been reported by many scholars which needs a special mention in this section.

It has become evident through variety of studies and research done in this very field that the microorganisms find their way through Peyer's patches and gain entry into the circulation which results in the contraction of the disease spread by the particular pathogen. A number of pathogens have been reported which colonize on the epithelial surface of the intestine as well as invade into the underlying layers. These generally bind to the M-cell surface for gaining entry into the deeper layer/tissues of the intestine. It has been postulated that these microorganisms use adhesions to bind to the apical membrane components of the epithelial cells (Hultgren et al., 1993). Also the structure of the M-cell surface enhances and facilitates intimate contact of the microorganisms resulting in the high affinity interactions between the M-cell and microbial membranes. Reports indicate that the bacteria, yeast and protozoa are taken up by the cells through phagocytosis whereas the viruses are taken up by receptor mediated endocytosis (Marcial and Madara, 1986; Owen et al., 1986; Wolf and Bye, 1984). Poliovirus which is transmitted by oral route proliferates in the Peyer's patches and gains entry into the systemic circulation through Peyer's patch tissue (Bodian, 1955). Selective binding of the M-cells to wild type poliovirus type 1 as well as to attenuated sabin strain with subsequent endocytosis have been demonstrated when the same were incubated with the human Peyer's patch explants (Siciński et al., 1990). Bacteriae which are non invasive but colonize in the epithelial layer of intestinal lumen are also taken up by the M-cells. *Vibrio cholerae* is one of such bacteriae which when binds to the M-cell surface leads to assembling of the actin filaments and eventually leads to the phagocytosis and subsequent transport. There are different bacteriae which spread into the body and are translocated through M-cell mediated pathway to result in a local or systemic disease. *Campylobacter jejuni, Yersinia enterocolitica* and *Y. Pseudotuberculosis* bind to the M-cells, find their way into the mesentric lymph nodes and are translocated to liver and spleen. *Salmonella typhi* and *S. typhimurium* are known to cause typhoid fever and gastroenteritis respectively in humans. The bacteriae localize mainly in the Peyer's patches and they are known to attach and bind specifically to the M-cells after which they gain entry into the circulation. It has been reported that these pathogens possess selective binding to the M-cells which has been shown in mouse and rabbit ligated intestinal loop model (Ermak and Giannasca, 1998). It has been shown that *S. typhimurium* attachment to the Peyer's patch M-cell induces extrusion of the cytoplasm and apical surface of the M-cell into the lumen leading to the breach of the epithelial barrier of FAE (Jones et al., 1994).

Although the case with *Salmonella typhi* is a bit different since the bacteria is phagocytosed and can be transported without any such effects as resulting in the lysis of M-cells as in the case of the *S. typhimurium* even at higher doses (Pascopella et al., 1995). It has been elucidated that the *S. typhimurium* possess three fimbrial adhesion operons that mediate adherence of these pathogens to the epithelial cells (Bäumler et al., 1997). *Shigella flexneri* is also known to invade the intestinal mucosa through M-cell mediated translocation. It has been reported that the organism spreads in the follicle associated epithelium and infects the adjoining epithelial cells with subsequent intervention of the macrophages and ultimately resulting in the loss of follicle associated epithelial cells (Perdomo et al., 1994; Zychlinsky et al., 1992). There are various other kinds of pathogens which interact with the M-cells. They breach the epithelial layer and may gain entry into the circulation or to liver and spleen through the M-cell mediated uptake and precipitate the disease.

4.2.1 Uptake of Particles through Peyer's Patch

It is evident from the previous discussion that the bacteria and other pathogens can gain entry across the epithelial barrier into the circulation through the M-cell uptake. This technique has been studied and explored by many researchers with regards to particulate uptake. Several studies have been conducted in order to institute this phenomenon and many efforts have been levied to develop delivery of drug loaded particles through the similar approach by utilising and taking advantage of the M-cell mediated Peyer's patch uptake. It has been reported that the uptake of the microparticles by the M-cells is similar to that of the process responsible for bacterial uptake by the cells (Ermak et al., 1995; Landsverk, 1988). The particles after being exposed to the M-cells are phagocytosed by the cells (the number can vary for each case) and the contents are emptied into the intraepithelial pocket from where they are either engulfed or pass into the sub epithelial region. A schematic representation of the same has been given in Fig. 4.3. It has been reported that the smallest particles that can be transported include liposomes, nanoparticles which are 20-200 nm in size whereas the largest particles include microspheres of 10 μm diameter (Ermak et al., 1995; O'Hagan, 1994). Study related to polystyrene and poly (lactic-co-glycolic acid) microspheres contained within the ligated intestinal sac containing Peyer's patch showed that the microparticles were taken up by the M-cells. Electron microscopy of the samples revealed that the polystyrene microspheres between 200-650 nm diameter in bovine ileal patches whereas PLGA microspheres between 1-4 μm in rabbit Peyer's patches were translocated to the basolateral region through M-cells (Ermak et al., 1995; Landsverk, 1988). (Childers *et. al.,* 1989) also studied and observed the endosomal uptake of the liposomes by the Peyer's patch tissue in rat gut loop model (Childers et al., 1989). In a seperate study uptake of the ferritin containing liposomes by the Peyer's patch tissue has been observed (Chen and Langer, 1997). Chen *et. al.,* in their study reported that the Peyer's patches are the principal site where the polymerised liposomes are absorbed and gain entry across the gut after administration of the liposomes through oral gavage in mouse (Chen et al., 1996). Yoo and group performed study for targeting of the chitosan nanoparticles to Peyer's patches towards the delivery of a protein vaccine (Yoo et al., 2010). *In vitro* and *in vivo* studies indicated towards a fact that the localisation of chemically modified nanoparticles (coupled to a peptide) into the Peyer's patch tissue was enhanced. According to their view the modified delivery system could be advantageous for delivery of the vaccine.

From the above discussion one aspect should be taken into account which has also been described by many scholars that a size dependent mechanism also exists at the site of Peyer's patches. Eldridge et al., have reported this phenomenon and they found in their study that particles greater than 10 μm were not taken up by the Peyer's patch tissue (Eldridge et al., 1990). In an study conducted by jain and team the mice were fed with fluorescent polystyrol nanoparticles between 100 nm to 1 μm and the histological investigation revealed that particles less than 1 μm were translocated to mesentric lymph nodes (Jain et al., 1989). Higher uptake of smaller particles resulted as compared with that of the larger ones. They also found that the larger particles of 3 μm could not be detected. Gilley and co-workers in their experiment included microparticles of different polymers and of different size range (Gilley et al., 1988). They reported that particles between 1 μm to 10 μm are taken up by the Peyer's patch tissue whereas microspheres larger than 10 μm do not gain entry into the tissue. Furthermore the particles between 5 μm to 10 μm remain in the Peyer's patch tissue and may remain there for months. Also the microspheres were seen to penetrate the gut at Peyer's patch tissue specifically. A different study by Desai and his group elucidated the effect of the particles size on the uptake of the biodegradable PLGA microparticles of variable size (Desai et al., 1996). The authors formulated the microparticles of 100 nm, 500 nm, 1 μm and

10 µm. It was found that the microparticles of size range of 100 nm exhibited a 15 to 250 folds higher uptake than the particles of the larger sizes. The particles with smaller size diffused throughout the submucosal layer and were also present on the serosal side of the Peyer's patches. The microparticles of the higher size range i.e., 500 nm, 1 µm and 10 µm were taken up to a much lesser extent and these particles were localized in the epithelial lining of the Peyer's patch tissue. The results indicated potential toward the development of the microparticles for delivery of protein or therapeutics through the Peyer's patch route. Florence has reviewed this very phenomenon describing the uptake of particles (Florence, 1997). The review stressed over the fact that the particle size is a key factor which plays role in the uptake of the particles. The uptake has been reported as a natural process which does not involve any damage. The review holds a mention of research on the similar aspect which directs one to the fact that particle in the size range of 3-10 µm may get localised or are sequestered within the Peyer's patches. The same has been a matter of debate and research for last few decades. The author is of the view that the Peyer's patch targeting is a naturally occurring process and the same can be utilised for the development of the vaccines. A different study indicated that the microparticles between 50-500 nm were dispersed at approximately 10% efficiency rate but the rate of the particles between 1-3 µm was much lower (Desai et al., 1996). The review by Ermak and Giannasea postulates that in order to target the Peyer's patch tissue effectively the optimum particle size should be in the range of 0.5-2 µm whereas the enhanced access to systemic circulation could be brought about with smaller sizes less than 500 nm (Ermak and Giannasea, 1998). It is well evident from the above discussions that particle size of the delivery system exerts effect on the uptake of the micro/nanoparticles and is one of the important factors in designing of the targeted drug delivery system directed towards the Peyer's patch tissue. Some of the other factors which play a role in the development of the Peyer's pacth targeted drug delivery system are being described below:

4.2.1.1 Size of the Micro/Nanoparticles

The size of the delivery system plays a major role in the determination of the efficacy of targeting which has been discussed in detail in the previous section of this chapter. Fig. 4.4 is an illustrative representation of the size dependent uptake of the particles.

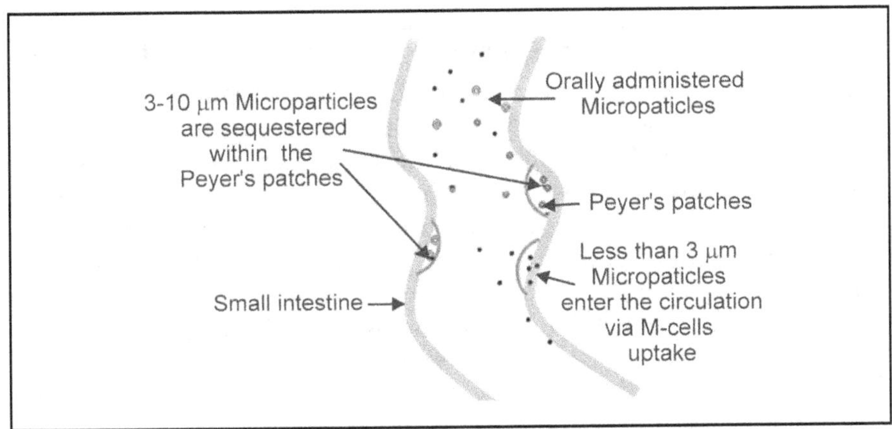

FIGURE 4.4 Size dependent uptake of the particles by the Peyer's patch tissue.

4.2.1.2 Species Difference and Number of Peyer's Patches

It has been observed that the translocation of the particles through the Peyer's patch tissue also depends on the number of the Peyer's patches which varies from species to species. The humans and mice possess similar number of the M-cells but the uptake is reduced in mice. This has been attributed to lower frequency of the M-cells as well as reduced transport activity in mice (Jepson et al., 1993; Pappo and Ermak, 1989). It has been reported that the rabbits have more number of Peyer's patches than rodents (Chen and Langer, 1998) as well as it has also been reported that they possess more density of Peyer's patches than humans (Gruber et al., 1987) and hence this creates difference in the magnitude of the uptake of the particles when both are compared. In a study the particles were inoculated in the rabbit intestinal loop containing Peyer's patches as well as in murine Peyer's patches. The results revealed that the uptake in case of rabbit was higher by a magnitude when compared to that of the murine patches (Pappo and Ermak, 1989). A different experiment which assessed the uptake of the 3 µm particles indicated the variation in the uptake of particles in different animals. It was found that the absorption was higher in rats as compared to hamsters whereas it was minimum for mice when compared to others. Apart from this variation between species a regional difference in the uptake of the particles has also been witnessed in murine follicle associated epithelium wherein the uptake from lateral sides of the structure was approximately two times more than when compared to the uptake from the apex (Porta et al., 1992).

4.2.1.3 Hydrophillic/Hydrophobic Nature of the Microparticles

The body has been reported to handle and respond the materials differently based upon their physicochemical properties. It has been noticed that the hydrophobic particles easily gain access through the Peyer's patch tissue rather than the hydrophilic ones. The surface characteristic of the particles and its absorption through the Peyer's patch tissue depends on the nature of the particles. It is reported that the particles with greater hydrophobicity are absorbed but the other one with low hydrophobicity such as cellulose and its derivatives are not taken up.

4.2.1.4 Type of Polymer

It is evident from the previous discussion that the properties and surface characteristics play role in the uptake of the particles from the Peyer's patches. The type of the polymer from which these particles or delivery systems are formulated do levy effect on the uptake of the particles. There are reports in support of the statement. In a study which compared the uptake of the polystyrene particles with that of the PLGA biodegradable microparticles showed that the biodegradable microparticles of PLGA were not taken up efficiently. Moreover the transported PLGA particles did not show selective binding to the M-cells (Jepson et al., 1993). Attempts have been made by the researchers to modify the polymer so as to target it efficiently to the tissue. A number of bioadhesives have been utilised for the same purpose. It has been reported that the gelatine modified PLGA was sampled efficiently in comparison to other modified polymer or PLGA taken alone (Trantolo D.J et al., 1996). In a different study it has been found that 0.5 µm polystyrene particles were efficiently endocytosed by the rabbit's Peyer's patches whereas the PLGA microparticles failed to target the M-cells (Jepson et al., 1993; Pappo and Ermak, 1989). Uptake of the non-ionized polystyrene nanoparticles was found to be greater than the uptake of the negatively charged carboxylated nanoparticles by the Peyer's patch tissue following oral gavage (Jani et al., 1989). Thus all the reports indicate toward the fact that the type of polymer has role in the particulate uptake by the Peyer's patches which definitely is due to the change of the surface characteristics with the change of the polymer.

4.2.1.5 Influence of Co-administered Agents

There are different factors which play role in the uptake of the nano/ microparticles. Another possible factor which can influence the uptake of the particulate drug delivery systems or particulate matter from the intestine is co-administered material which can be food, drink or drugs.

Few decades back volkheimer (Volkheimer, 1977) has demonstrated a similar phenomenon. It was found that the consumption of coffee increased uptake of the particles whereas the decaffeinated coffee did not have any effect on the uptake of the particles. It was also found that continuous smoking enhanced the uptake of the particles. Co administration of the drugs such as caffeine, papaverine, neostigmine increased the uptake of the microparticles whereas drugs such as atropine, polysorbate 20 decreased the uptake of the particles. This clearly shows that the dietary habits and oral administration of other agents such as drugs and drinks do have effect on the uptake of the particles through the Peyer's patch tissue.

4.2.1.6 Fluid Volume and Osmotic Parameters

It has been reported that the uptake of nanoparticles increased when administered with higher volume of water which has been suspected due to inefficient barrier function (Eyles et al., 1995). Moreover the uptake of the particles was higher when these were administered with hypotonic solutions as compared to isotonic solution indicating that osmotic parameters may also have role in the uptake of the particles.

4.3 Role of Peyer's Patches in Design and Development of Oral Vaccines

Peyer's patch tissue and M-cells have also been extensively explored for the design and development of the vaccine for a variety of diseases through the active targeting of the antigen to the Peyer's patches. The targeting leads to the presentation of the antigen(s) to the specific presentation cells resulting in the development of the immunity and also refinement of the immunization procedure which generally involves the parenteral route. A number of studies have been conducted with respect to the delivery of vaccines through the route being discussed in this chapter. Neutra and Kozlowski in 2006 have reviewed the challenges involved in development of the mucosal vaccines and discussed over the sites for the delivery of such vaccines. The same outlines various mucosal inductive sites for the delivery of the vaccines one of which is Peyer's patch tissue which holds T-cells, B-cells and dendritic cells which in turn have been stated to be specialized for the adaptive immune response. The review also mentions the role of M-cells that deliver the antigen through the transepithelial transport to intraepithelial lymphocytes as well as to the subepithelial lymphoid tissues. Development of the particulate vaccines for the delivery of the antigen can be advantageous since the micro/nano carrier systems have access to the M-cells which in turn transport them to the Peyer's patches depending upon the size of the carrier system already discussed earlier. These carrier systems enter the mucosal inductive sites i.e., Peyer's patches from where they can associate with that of the dendritic cells resulting in uptake and also gain access to the subepithelial lymphoid tissues. This can serve as one of the modes of delivery of antigen to the Peyer's patch tissue thereby contributing to the development of the mucosal vaccines. A study indicated that the antigens could be retained on the mucosal surfaces by the use of the polymers like chitosan which resulted in the enhancement of the antigen uptake thereby increasing the immune responses (McNeela et al., 2000). The potential of chitosan in the development of oral vaccines has been reviewed (Prego et al., 2005). Hence the use of micro/nanoparticulate systems fabricated out of these types of polymers which are biodegradable and biosafe can be of great advantage in the delivery of the vaccines through oral route which is conducive with more patient compliance (Kraehenbuhl and Neutra, 2000). Moreover the encapsulation of the antigens into such nano/micro drug delivery systems confers them with protection from degradation by lumenal factors limiting absorption and hostile environment of the gastrointestinal tract. Also slow degradation of the carrier system leads to a sustained release of the antigen which adds to the improvement of the vaccine delivery (Neutra and Kozlowski, 2006).

Here it is worth to mention that the delivery of the vaccines can also be brought about by modes other than the particulate delivery by the use of the attenuated strain of pathogen which associate directly to the M-cells and uses the M-cell mediated transport to enter the mucosal lymphoid tissues available in the intestine (Jones et al., 1994; Siciński et al., 1990). Such type of vaccines utilising the M-cell mediated transport include live attenuated poliovirus vaccine (Modlin, 2004) and live attenuated S. typhi vaccine (Levine, 2000). A number of reports have been published with respect to targeting of the vaccines to the Peyer's patch tissue. Yoo and team developed chitosan nanoparticles which were conjugated to a novel M-cell homing peptide which could target specifically the nanoparticles to the Peyer's patches resulting in the development of an efficient oral vaccine (Yoo et al., 2010). It was found that the peptide coupled nanaoparticles possessed enhanced efficiency in binding affinity and specific localization into the follicle associated epithelium of the Peyer's patch tissue. In a study by Channarong and co-workers oral DNA vaccine was developed which was targeted to the Peyer's patches (Channarong et al., 2011). Chitosan coated liposomes were prepared for the delivery of the DNA. The improvement and enhancement in the Peyer's patch targeting efficiency was brought about by the development of the polyplex loaded liposomes. Polyplex was formed by coacervation of DNA with chitosan which was followed by the loading of the polyplex into the liposomes which were then coated with the chitosan solution. The polyplex formation enhanced the positive charge. It was found that the chitosan coated polyplex liposomes had higher potential to deliver the DNA in comparison to the normal chitosan coated liposomes. This phenomenon has been attributed to the net positive charge and coating of the chitosan which enhanced the internalization of the DNA. A diagrammatic representation of the same has been given in Fig. 4.5. A very recent research by Tawade and his research team demonstrated the development of an oral vaccine against ovarian cancer. The vaccine was constituted of microparticles developed from polymers Eudragit FS30D and hydroxyl propyl methyl cellulose acetate succinate. The vaccine was targeted to the Peyer's patches specifically through the use of M-cell specific ligand. The results of the study indicated potential of the vaccine against the ovarian cancer as the vaccinated mice showed a significant retardation in the tumor volume which was up to six folds as compared to the non vaccinated mice after tumor challenge. Hunter et al., 2012 advocated the targeting of Peyer's patches with respect to delivery of vaccine/antigen where agents with higher potency but low volume are to be delivered. Vaccination through targeting of M-cells or Peyer's patch tissue can result in the elicitation of difference responses i.e., the particles which are sequestered within the Peyer's patches and target immune cells may elicit the IgA response whereas the particles which escape the patch region into the lymphoid region can be instrumental for generation of the systemic IgG responses (Ermak et al., 1995).

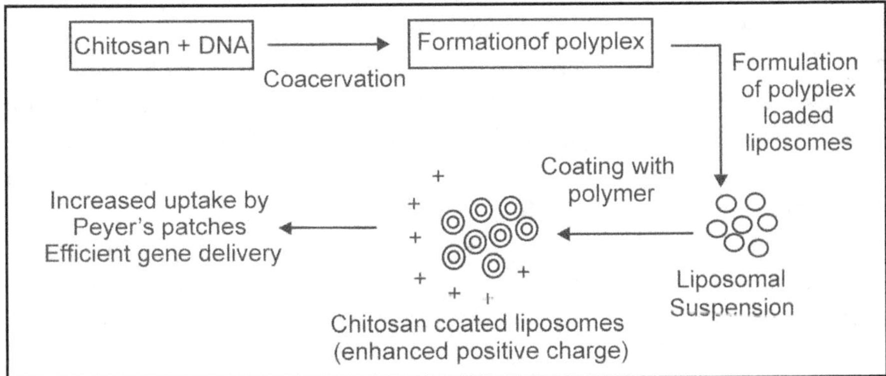

FIGURE 4.5 Schematic representation of gene delivery through Peyer's patches.

4.4　Targeting Strategies

Peyer's patch represents potential site for the delivery of bioactives and vaccines through drug delivery systems directed to these tissues for different anticipated effects. The same has been explored and different targeting strategies have been designed and approached to specifically achieve site specific delivery. Although size of the delivery system has been utilised as a tool to target the Peyer's patch tissue and the same has been discussed in detail in the preceding part of this chapter mentioning different research which indicate the fact that particles of larger size are sequestered within the patches whereas the smaller size particles gain entry through the M-cells into the circulation. Apart from these studies there are other strategies which have been designed to target the tissue or the M-cell directly. Some of these strategies are being mentioned as here under.

4.4.1　Lectin Mediated Targeting

The inherent ability of the M-cells to transcytose variety of the microbes and present them to the antigen presenting cells has been developed in the targeting of the oral vaccines to these cells in order to achieve a good immune response by many workers and the potential of the same have been elucidated in many reports. These cells have been utilized as the ideal target to which the vaccine can be delivered providing an access to the mucosal immune system. As a consequence the M-cells have been targeted and lectins in particular have been explored much in this regard. There have been a variety of studies and specifically the studies related to the lectin binding showed that the M-cells express a particular glycosylation pattern on their surface (Jang et al., 2004; Kozlowski et al., 2002). Moreover, it is also reported that the *Ulex europaeus* agglutinin-I selectively binds to the apical M-cell surface which in turn is a lectin possessing specificity for α-1-fucose residues (Lavelle et al., 2000; Wang et al., 2005). It has been shown in a study that the M-cell based targeting developed protective immunity against the infection caused by the gastrointestinal pathogens. It was found that the oral vaccination constituting killed whole *Helicobacter pylori* and Ulex europaeus agglutinin I (UEA-I)/*campylobacter jejuni* and UEA-I provided protective immune responses against the live challenge in a mouse model (Chionh et al., 2009). In a different study Gupta and his group developed PLGA nanoparticles loaded with HBSAg for oral immunization against hepatitis B (Gupta et al., 2007). The work included the targeting of the developed PLGA nanoparticles by anchoring them with *Ulex europaeus* agglutinin-I. Confocal laser scanning microscopy demonstrated that the lectinized nanoparticles (anchored with that of the UEA-I) were predominantly associated with that of the M-cells. Moreover the serum anti-HBsAg titre obtained after oral immunization with HBsAg loaded lectin anchored nanoparticles was comparable with that of the titre obtained after administration of the alum-HBsAg through the intramuscular route. Also the lectin anchored stabilized nanopartilces exhibited enhanced immune response as compared to stabilized non-lectinized nanoparticles. Similarly a study by Foster and co-researchers also utilised UEA-I wherein the polystyrene microspheres of the size range of 0.5 μm were covalently coated with that of the UEA-I and the microparticles were administered by injection into the ligated gut loops as well as through oral gavage (Foster et al., 1998). It was found that the particles coated with UEA-I were specifically directed to the M-cells and the lectin coated microparticles were rapidly endocytosed (Foster et al., 1998). Fig. 4.6 is a schematic representation of the process involved. M-cells targeting capability of UEA-I can also be achieved by anchoring or coating of UEA-I over other carrier systems including liposomes and solid lipid nanoparticles. Apart from UEA-I some other M-cell directed lectins have been used in order to target M-cells. The comparative efficacy of UEA-I and wheat germ agglutinin lectin in achieving M-cell specificity has been studied using liposomes. Both the lectins enhanced the uptake of the polymerised liposomes however the quantum of uptake was higher with UEA-I lectin (Chen et al., 1996). Another member from lectin family is tomato lectin which has also been used to target carrier system to the Peyer's patches/M-cells. Polystyrene microspheres having 0.5 μm size were prepared and coupled to tomato lectin with intention of targeting M-cells. It was observed that the bioadhesion of polystyrene microspheres to the rat intestinal tract was enhanced due to coupling with tomato lectin. The coupling resulted in a 50 fold increase in the translocation to the systemic circulation after the lectin conjugated microspheres were administered orally to the mouse (Hussain and Florence, 1998). The use of lectins enhances the targeting of the particulates to the M-cells although the efficiency may vary as mentioned earlier. Also the size plays an important role since the smaller particle size may have greater access to the lectin binding sites on the M-cell glycocalyx (Ermak and Giannasca, 1998).

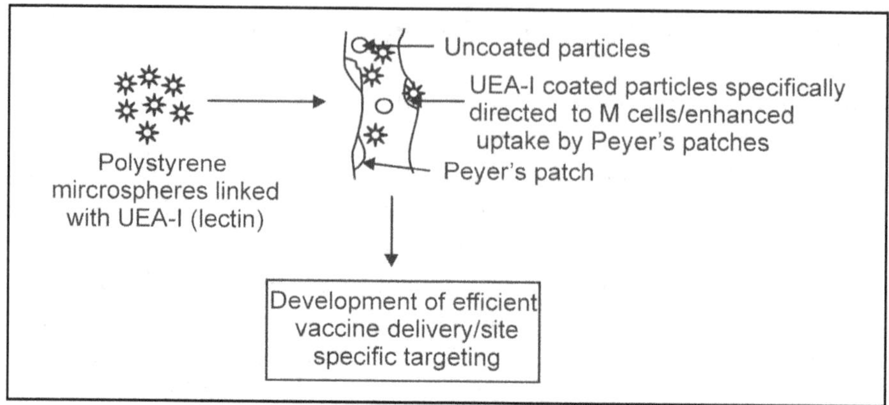

FIGURE 4.6 Diagrammatic representation of the potential of lectins in M-cell targeting.

4.4.2 Antibody Mediated Targeting

The approach considers the use of monoclonal antibody which are specific for the M-cells. These antibodies are tagged with that of the particle and is delivered *in vivo*. The particle by virtue of the selectivity of the antibody for the M-cells is directed to these cells and hence the targeting is accomplished whereby the antibody acts as a ligand. A monoclonal antibody mAb 5B11 has been tested *in vitro* in the presence of isolated Peyer's patch domes which contained lymphoid cells as well as follicle associated epithelium. It was found that antibody possessed more intimate contact with apical membrane of the M-cells in comparison to the adjoining cells (Ermak and Giannasca, 1998; Kabok et al., 1995). Similarly the targeting potential of the monoclonal antibody has been tested *in vivo*. The mAb 5B11 antibody and its isotype with non relevant specificity were coupled to the fluorescent polystyrene microparticles with different colors. These were than incubated in ligated intestinal loops. It was found that the uptake of the microspheres coupled with that of the M-cell specific mAb was three times more than when compared to that of the uncoupled microparticles or non specific antibody coupled microparticles (Pappo et al., 1991).

4.4.3 Other Targeting Ligands

Apart from lectins and M-cell specific antibody, immunoglobulins also find place among the ligands in the targeting of the M-cells. Secretory IgA possess a protective function and also prevents the adherence of the the microbes to the epithelial cell surface but the same has also been deployed to target the M-cells since it selectively bind to the M-cell surface. According to a report secretory IgA, monoclonal IgA and IgA antibody-antigen complex bind specifically to the M-cells and are transported by them (Weltzin et al., 1989). In a study the polystyrene microspheres coated with secretory IgA were delivered to the ligated intestinal loop in a murine model. It was found that the uptake of the microspheres was increased up to 4 folds in the case of IgA coated microspheres compared to the microspheres coated with BSA (Porta et al., 1992). In a different study IgA coupled liposomes were taken up to a greater extent with higher efficiency as compared to the uncoupled liposomes when both were delivered to the mouse Peyer's patches (Zhou et al., 1995). A different approach also exists in order to achieve immunoglobulin targeting with the use of antibody specific for the cell surface antigens. It has been reported that the uptake and internalization of polystyrene microspheres was enhanced by coating with a mouse monoclonal antibody i.e., IgM which specifically was directed against antigen expressed on the apical surface of M-cells (Pappo et al., 1991). It is well evident that microbes/ bacteriae such as *S. typhi, S. typhimurium* and polio virus target the M-cells. Following this it has been postulated that the microbial adhesion property of these microbes could be exploited to target the M-cells. Study by Hussain and Florence involved the delivery of polystyrene nanoparticles coated with invasion-C192 which is an amino acid fragment of the invasion protein. This strategy resulted in increased uptake of the nanoparticles by the intestinal epithelium (Hussain and Florence, 1998; Leong et al., 1990).

4.5 Evaluation of the Uptake of Particles

Numerous strategies and plans prevail to target the Peyer's patch tissue but in order to assess whether or not these are efficient and instrumental in the accomplishment of the goal for which they are designed, it is necessary to evaluate the same. There are different methods and models which have been developed for the evaluation of the intestinal uptake of the particulate systems and comprise of both qualitative as well as quantitative methodologies. Albeit all of the methods employed lead to the evaluation of the uptake but these differ in certain aspects viz. ease of evaluation of uptake of micro/nanoparticulate delivery systems and precision of the method. Some of the important methods and models are being discussed briefly in this section.

4.5.1 Microscopic Methods

Light microscopy, fluorescent microscopy and confocal laser scanning microscopy can be utilised for the evaluation of the particles uptake through the intestinal tissue. The particles can be observed through the light microscopy with respect to their size and shape however, more appropriate results can be obtained with the use fluorescent microscopy which is due to its better sensitivity and also fluorescence imparts better visualization (Lavelle et al., 2000; Wells et al., 1988). One can compare between the different particles via separate labelling of the particles with different flourochromes/fluorescent dyes. Confocal laser scanning microscopy is an advance technique which provides better results with respect to the localisation of the particles in a particular tissue. The particulate uptake can be observed in a more efficient way since the technique provides a three dimensional view by scanning of the sample in x-y-z planes and one can know the degree of penetration of the particles into the tissue. Uptake of the particles can be assessed either qualitatively or quantitatively. Qualitative assessment can be demonstrated through the histology of the tissue samples and the presence of the particles can be observed through direct visualization. On the other hand the quantitative assessment of the particles requires the measurement of the number of the particles or the extent of the particulate uptake wherein the tissue is treated to extract out the particles in form of suspension. The particulate suspensions can be further centrifuged to concentrate the suspension and the particles are counted with the help of the hemocytometer although it has been reported that it is accompanied by errors (Eyles et al., 1995). Hence the advanced techniques which make use of radioactivity or fluorescence can be advantageous measuring the uptake quantitatively. The techniques like fluorescent activated cell sorting and electron microscopy are being widely utilised.

4.5.2 Electron Microscopy

Electron microscopy can be utilized to assess the localization of the particles in a particular tissue sample. Scanning electron microscopy (SEM) and Transmission electron microscopy (TEM) both can be used for the detection of the particles. In TEM the aqueous dispersion (one drop) is placed over a 400-mesh carbon-coated copper grid followed by negative staining with phosphotungstic acid solution (3% w/v, adjusted to pH 4.7 with KOH) and the grid is placed at the accelerating voltage of 95 KV and photomicrographs are taken at suitable magnification. Transmission electron microscopy has also been utilized in the determination of the uptake of the nanoparticles by the macrophage cells (Pinto-Alphandary et al., 1994).

4.5.3 Fluorescent Activated Cell Sorter

This is another technique through which the uptake of the fluorescent labelled nano/microparticles by the macrophages/phagocytic cells can be measured. Jenkins et. al., used the technique to measure the particle absorption in the lymph samples (Jenkins et al., 1994). Delie reported that the technique requires only a small fraction of the sample for the assessment and the sensitivity of the measurement depends on the fluorescence of the particles rather than on the size of the particles as in case of the evaluation through histological screening (Delie, 1998).

4.5.4 Radioactivity and Fluorometry

The quantification of the uptake of the particles can also be done by the use of the radio labelled particles where the extent of the uptake can be measured through the radioactivity of the tissue sample which can be correlated directly to the degree/extent of particles localized in the tissue. Fluorometry can also be used to determine the number of the particles taken up by the tissue which is done by the measurement of the fluorescent emitted by the samples and correlating it with the number of the particles with the help of the standard curve of the fluorescent dye/material.

4.6   Models for Assessment of Uptake

There are various models which have been developed by different workers to assess the particulate uptake. The assessment can be made through *in vivo*, *ex vivo* or *in vitro* methods. In order to perform *in vivo* assessment a method of closed intestinal loop can be employed (Damge et al., 1996; Porta et al., 1992). The technique utilizes a methodology whereby a intestinal segment is ligated at a specific part of the intestine and the segment is not deprived of the blood supply to assess the uptake in a realistic way. Hence one can compare the uptake in segment containing Peyer's patches to one not possessing the patches. The methodology has been employed by Well's et. al., to measure the uptake of latex particles in different segment of the intestine. The results indicated phagocytosis of the particles occurs (Wells et al., 1988). An another technique make use of a special cage i.e., Bollman's cage in which the animal is confined and remains awake during the experiment as against the experiment in former case in which the flow of blood and lymph are reduced due to anaesthesia and hence realistic results can be obtained with the use of Bollman's cage. Similarly there are *ex-vivo* experiments for the assessment of the particulate uptake and permeability of the drugs across the tissue. In this method a piece of fresh intestine is placed in a chamber and certain amount of drug is placed in the donor compartment and it is taken out of the receiving chamber. Moreover different samples can be run and analyzed simultaneously. Scherer et al., 1993 observed the transport of the particles across the pig patch tissue and the results demonstrated the fact that the particles were not transported across the tissue devoid of Peyer's patches. *In-vitro* model include the incubation of the particles with the cell culture which may include different types of cells viz. Caco-2 cells. It has been reported that caco-2 cells when cultured with Peyer's patch lymphocytes transform into M-cell like cells and transport the particles more efficiently (Kernéis et al., 1997). Different models can be utilized to predict the uptake and the selection of model depends on the fact as to whether one wants to obtain an insight about the uptake or wishes to check the effect of the factors such as particle size, shape, charge etc., on the uptake of the particles.

4.7   Conclusion and Future Prospects

Peyer's patch targeting has been a lucrative field for the researchers especially those involved in oral delivery related to the development of the particulate systems for the delivery of the drugs and vaccines. It has been almost a century when the research on Peyer's patch uptake and M-cell mediated transport was supported with some published reports. Since then there have been many reports regarding the uptake of the particles. Albeit there were also some intermittent contradictory reports that lead to controversies about the uptake of the particles through the Peyer's patches but the recent research has indicated that such transport does exists. Majority of the reports indicate toward the fact that such uptake exists at the site of patches and that the M-cells are involved in the transport has been established. Published reports have shown different strategies to target delivery systems to the site i.e., peyer's patch and make them amenable for uptake or transport by the M-cells. The systems could be developed for either drug or vaccine targeting. Also one could find the use of different polymers in the development of such targeted delivery system bearing drug or vaccines. The variations in the data of the several published reports are observed which possibly could be due to factors such as inter species difference which is due to use of different animals in the study and the use of different models to assess the targeting. Hence more illustrative research is required to be instituted in order to circumvent such problems. The prospects are bright provided more stress is levied on the understanding of the M-cell biology and its characteristics for development of newer strategies. Efforts are also required to assess the potential of such approaches of delivery to Peyer's patch and M-cells with respect to the humans.

References

Abe, K. (1977). A qualitative and quantitative morphologic study of Peyer's patches of the mouse. *Arch Histol Jpn* **40,** 407.

Abe, K., and Ito, T. (1978). Qualitative and quantitative morphologic study of Peyer's patches of the mouse after neonatal thymectomy and hydrocortisone injection. *American Journal of Anatomy* **151,** 227-237.

Bäumler, A., Tsolis, R., and Heffron, F. (1997). Fimbrial adhesins of Salmonella typhimurium. In Mechanisms in the pathogenesis of enteric diseases (Springer), pp. 149-158.

Bockman, D.E., and Cooper, M.D. (1973). Pinocytosis by epithelium associated with lymphoid follicles in the bursa of Fabricius, appendix, and Peyer's patches. An electron microscopic study. *American Journal of Anatomy* **136,** 455-477.

Bodian, D. (1955). Emerging concept of poliomyelitis infection. *Science* **122,** 105-108.

Channarong, S., Chaicumpa, W., Sinchaipanid, N., and Mitrevej, A. (2011). Development and evaluation of chitosan-coated liposomes for oral DNA vaccine: the improvement of Peyer's patch targeting using a polyplex-loaded liposomes. *Aaps Pharmscitech* **12,** 192-200.

Chen, H., and Langer, R. (1997). Magnetically-responsive polymerized liposomes as potential oral delivery vehicles. *Pharmaceutical research* **14,** 537-540.

Chen, H., and Langer, R. (1998). Oral particulate delivery: status and future trends. *Advanced drug delivery reviews* **34,** 339-350.

Chen, H., Torchilin, V., and Langer, R. (1996). Lectin-bearing polymerized liposomes as potential oral vaccine carriers. *Pharmaceutical research* **13,** 1378-1383.

Childers, N., Denys, F., McGee, N., and Michalek, S. (1989). Ultrastructural study of liposome uptake by M-cells of rat Peyer's patch: an oral vaccine system for delivery of purified antigen. *Regional immunology* **3,** 8-16.

Chionh, Y.-T., Wee, J.L., Every, A.L., Ng, G.Z., and Sutton, P. (2009). M-cell targeting of whole killed bacteria induces protective immunity against gastrointestinal pathogens. *Infection and immunity* **77**, 2962-2970.

Damge, C., Aprahamian, M., Marchais, H., Benoit, J., and Pinget, M. (1996). Intestinal absorption of PLAGA microspheres in the rat. *Journal of anatomy* **189**, 491.

Delie, F. (1998). Evaluation of nano-and microparticle uptake by the gastrointestinal tract. *Advanced Drug Delivery Reviews* **34**, 221-233.

Desai, M.P., Labhasetwar, V., Amidon, G.L., and Levy, R.J. (1996). Gastrointestinal uptake of biodegradable microparticles: effect of particle size. *Pharmaceutical research* **13**, 1838-1845.

Eldridge, J.H., Hammond, C.J., Meulbroek, J.A., Staas, J.K., Gilley, R.M., and Tice, T.R. (1990). Controlled vaccine release in the gut-associated lymphoid tissues. I. Orally administered biodegradable microspheres target the Peyer's patches. *Journal of Controlled Release* **11**, 205-214.

Ermak, T.H., Dougherty, E.P., Bhagat, H.R., Kabok, Z., and Pappo, J. (1995). Uptake and transport of copolymer biodegradable microspheres by rabbit Peyer's patch M-cells. *Cell and tissue research* **279**, 433-436.

Ermak, T.H., and Giannasca, P.J. (1998). Microparticle targeting to M-cells. *Advanced drug delivery reviews* **34**, 261-283.

Eyles, J., Alpar, H., Field, W., Lewis, D., and Keswick, M. (1995). The transfer of polystyrene microspheres from the gastrointestinal tract to the circulation after oral administration in the rat. *Journal of pharmacy and pharmacology* **47**, 561-565.

Fasano, A. (1998). Innovative strategies for the oral delivery of drugs and peptides. *Trends in biotechnology* **16**, 152-157.

Florence, A.T. (1997). The oral absorption of micro-and nanoparticulates: neither exceptional nor unusual. *Pharmaceutical Research* **14**, 259-266.

Foster, N., Clark, M.A., Jepson, M.A., and Hirst, B.H. (1998). Ulex europaeus 1 lectin targets microspheres to mouse Peyer's patch M-cells *in vivo*. *Vaccine* **16**, 536-541.

Gilley, R., Eldridge, J., Opitz, J., Hanna, L., Staas, J., and Tice, T. (1988). Development of secretory and systemic immunity following oral administration of microencapsulated antigens. Paper presented at: Proc Int Symp Rel Bioact Mater.

Griebel, P.J., and Hein, W.R. (1996). Expanding the role of Peyer's patches in B-cell ontogeny. *Immunology today* **17**, 30-39.

Gruber, P., Longer, M.A., and Robinson, J.R. (1987). Some biological issues in oral, controlled drug delivery. *Advanced Drug Delivery Reviews* **1**, 1-18.

Gupta, P.N., Khatri, K., Goyal, A.K., Mishra, N., and Vyas, S.P. (2007). M-cell targeted biodegradable PLGA nanoparticles for oral immunization against hepatitis B. *Journal of drug targeting* **15,** 701-713.

Herbst, E.F. (1844). Das lymphgefäßsystem und seine verrichtung.

Hultgren, S.J., Abraham, S., Caparon, M., Falk, P., Geme, J.W.S., and Normark, S. (1993). Pilus and nonpilus bacterial adhesins: assembly and function in cell recognition. *Cell* **73,** 887-901.

Hunter, A.C., Elsom, J., Wibroe, P.P., and Moghimi, S.M. (2012). Polymeric particulate technologies for oral drug delivery and targeting: a pathophysiological perspective. *Nanomedicine: Nanotechnology, Biology and Medicine* **8,** S5-S20.

Hussain, N., and Florence, A.T. (1998). Utilizing bacterial mechanisms of epithelial cell entry: invasin-induced oral uptake of latex nanoparticles. *Pharmaceutical research* **15,** 153-156.

Jang, M.H., Kweon, M.-N., Iwatani, K., Yamamoto, M., Terahara, K., Sasakawa, C., Suzuki, T., Nochi, T., Yokota, Y., and Rennert, P.D. (2004). Intestinal villous M-cells: an antigen entry site in the mucosal epithelium. *Proceedings of the National Academy of Sciences of the United States of America* **101,** 6110-6115.

Jani, P., Halbert, G., Langridge, J., and Florence, A. (1989). The uptake and translocation of latex nanospheres and microspheres after oral administration to rats. *Journal of Pharmacy and Pharmacology* **41,** 809-812.

Jenkins, P., Howard, K., Blackhall, N., Thomas, N., Davis, S., and O'Hagan, D. (1994). The quantitation of the absorption of microparticles into the intestinal lymph of Wistar rats. *International journal of pharmaceutics* **102,** 261-266.

Jepson, M., Simmons, N., O'hagan, D., and Hirst, B. (1993). Comparison of poly (DL-lactide-co-glycolide) and polystyrene microsphere targeting to intestinal M-cells. *Journal of drug targeting* **1,** 245-249.

Jones, B.D., Ghori, N., and Falkow, S. (1994). Salmonella typhimurium initiates murine infection by penetrating and destroying the specialized epithelial M-cells of the Peyer's patches. *The Journal of experimental medicine* **180,** 15-23.

Kabok, Z., Ermak, T.H., and Pappo, J. (1995). Microdissected domes from gut-associated lymphoid tissues: a model of M-cell transepithelial transport *in vitro*. In Advances in Mucosal Immunology (Springer), pp. 235-238.

Kernéis, S., Bogdanova, A., Kraehenbuhl, J.-P., and Pringault, E. (1997). Conversion by Peyer's patch lymphocytes of human enterocytes into M-cells that transport bacteria. *Science* **277,** 949-952.

Kozlowski, P.A., Williams, S.B., Lynch, R.M., Flanigan, T.P., Patterson, R.R., Cu-Uvin, S., and Neutra, M.R. (2002). Differential induction of mucosal and systemic antibody responses in women after nasal, rectal, or vaginal immunization: influence of the menstrual cycle. *The Journal of Immunology* **169**, 566-574.

Kraehenbuhl, J.-P., and Neutra, M.R. (2000). Epithelial M-cells: differentiation and function. *Annual review of cell and developmental biology* **16**, 301-332.

Kreuter, J. (1991). Peroral administration of nanoparticles. *Advanced Drug Delivery Reviews* **7**, 71-86.

Landsverk, T. (1988). Phagocytosis and transcytosis by the follicle-associated epithelium of the ileal Peyer's patch in calves. *Immunol Cell Biol* **66**, 261-268.

Lavelle, E., Grant, G., Pusztai, A., Pfüller, U., and O'Hagan, D. (2000). Mucosal immunogenicity of plant lectins in mice. *Immunology* **99**, 30-37.

Leong, J.M., Fournier, R.S., and Isberg, R. (1990). Identification of the integrin binding domain of the Yersinia pseudotuberculosis invasin protein. The *EMBO journal* **9**, 1979.

Levine, M.M. (2000). Immunization against bacterial diseases of the intestine. *Journal of pediatric gastroenterology and nutrition* **31**, 336-355.

Marcial, M.A., and Madara, J.L. (1986). Cryptosporidium: cellular localization, structural analysis of absorptive cell-parasite membrane-membrane interactions in guinea pigs, and suggestion of protozoan transport by M-cells. *Gastroenterology* **90**, 583-594.

McNeela, E.A., O'Connor, D., Jabbal-Gill, I., Illum, L., Davis, S.S., Pizza, M., Peppoloni, S., Rappuoli, R., and Mills, K.H. (2000). A mucosal vaccine against diphtheria: formulation of cross reacting material (CRM(197)) of diphtheria toxin with chitosan enhances local and systemic antibody and Th2 responses following nasal delivery. *Vaccine* **19**, 1188-1198.

Modlin, J.F. (2004). Poliomyelitis in the United States: the final chapter. *Jama* **292**, 1749-1751.

Neutra, M.R., and Kozlowski, P.A. (2006). Mucosal vaccines: the promise and the challenge. *Nature Reviews Immunology* **6**, 148-158.

O'Hagan, D.T., ed. (1994). Microparticles as oral vaccines.

Owen, R.L., Pierce, N.F., Apple, R., and Cray, W.C. (1986). M-cell Transport of Vibrio cholerae from the Intestinal. Lumen into Peyer's Patches: A Mechanism for Antigen Sampling and for Microbial Transepithelial Migration. *Journal of Infectious Diseases* **153**, 1108-1118.

Pappo, J., and Ermak, T. (1989). Uptake and translocation of fluorescent latex particles by rabbit Peyer's patch follicle epithelium: a quantitative model for M-cell uptake. *Clinical and experimental immunology* **76**, 144.

Pappo, J., Ermak, T., and Steger, H. (1991). Monoclonal antibody-directed targeting of fluorescent polystyrene microspheres to Peyer's patch M-cells. *Immunology* **73**, 277.

Pascopella, L., Raupach, B., Ghori, N., Monack, D., Falkow, S., and Small, P. (1995). Host restriction phenotypes of Salmonella typhi and Salmonella gallinarum. *Infection and immunity* **63,** 4329-4335.

Perdomo, O., Cavaillon, J., Huerre, M., Ohayon, H., Gounon, P., and Sansonetti, P. (1994). Acute inflammation causes epithelial invasion and mucosal destruction in experimental shigellosis. *The Journal of experimental medicine* **180,** 1307-1319.

Pinto-Alphandary, H., Balland, O., Laurent, M., Andremont, A., Puisieux, F., and Couvreur, P. (1994). Intracellular visualization of ampicillin-loaded nanoparticles in peritoneal macrophages infected *in vitro* with Salmonella typhimurium. *Pharmaceutical research* **11,** 38-46.

Porta, C., James, P., Phillips, A., Savidge, T., Smith, M., and Cremaschi, D. (1992). Confocal analysis of fluorescent bead uptake by mouse Peyer's patch follicle-associated M-cells. *Experimental physiology* **77,** 929-932.

Prego, C., Torres, D., and Alonso, M.J. (2005). The potential of chitosan for the oral administration of peptides.

Salman, H.H., Gamazo, C., Campanero, M.A., and Irache, J.M. (2005). Salmonella-like bioadhesive nanoparticles. *Journal of controlled release*: official journal of the Controlled Release Society **106,** 1-13.

Scherer, D., Mooren, F.C., Kinne, R., and Kreuter, J. (1993). *In vitro* permeability of PBCA nanoparticles through porcine small intestine. *Journal of drug targeting* **1,** 21-27.

Siciński, P., Rowiński, J., Warchoł, J., Jarzabek, Z., Gut, W., Szczygieł, B., Bielecki, K., and Koch, G. (1990). Poliovirus type 1 enters the human host through intestinal M-cells. *Gastroenterology* **98,** 56.

Tawde, S.A., Chablani, L., Akalkotkar, A., D'Souza, C., Chiriva-Internati, M., Selvaraj, P., and D'Souza, M.J. (2012). Formulation and evaluation of oral microparticulate ovarian cancer vaccines. *Vaccine* **30,** 5675-5681.

Trantolo D.J, Gresser J.D, Yang L, Wise D.L, Smith J.F, and P.J, G. (1996). Delivery of vaccines by biodegradable polymeric microparticles with bioadhesion properties. Paper presented at: Proceedings of the Fifth World Congress of Chemical Engineering, American Institute of Chemical Engineers (New York).

Volkheimer, G. (1964). Durchlaessigkeit der Darmschleimhaut fuer grosskorpuskulaere Elemente. *Gastroenterol* **2,** 57-64.

Volkheimer, G. (1977). Persorption of particles: physiology and pharmacology. *Adv Pharmacol Chemother* **14,** 163-187.

Wang, X., Kochetkova, I., Haddad, A., Hoyt, T., Hone, D.M., and Pascual, D.W. (2005). Transgene vaccination using Ulex europaeus agglutinin I (UEA-1) for targeted mucosal immunization against HIV-1 envelope. *Vaccine* **23,** 3836-3842.

Wells, C., Maddaus, M., Erlandsen, S., and Simmons, R. (1988). Evidence for the phagocytic transport of intestinal particles in dogs and rats. *Infection and immunity* **56,** 278-282.

Weltzin, R., Lucia-Jandris, P., Michetti, P., Fields, B., Kraehenbuhl, J., and Neutra, M. (1989). Binding and transepithelial transport of immunoglobulins by intestinal M-cells: demonstration using monoclonal IgA antibodies against enteric viral proteins. *The Journal of cell biology* **108,** 1673-1685.

Wolf, J.L., and Bye, W.A. (1984). The membranous epithelial (M) cell and the mucosal immune system. *Annual review of medicine* **35,** 95-112.

Yoo, M.-K., Kang, S.-K., Choi, J.-H., Park, I.-K., Na, H.-S., Lee, H.-C., Kim, E.-B., Lee, N.-K., Nah, J.-W., and Choi, Y.-J. (2010). Targeted delivery of chitosan nanoparticles to Peyer's patch using M-cell-homing peptide selected by phage display technique. *Biomaterials* **31,** 7738-7747.

Zhou, F., Kraehenbuhl, J.-P., and Neutra, M.R. (1995). Mucosal IgA response to rectally administered antigen formulated in IgA-coated liposomes. *Vaccine* **13,** 637-644.

Zychlinsky, A., Prevost, M.C., and Sansonetti, P.J. (1992). Shigella flexneri induces apoptosis in infected macrophages. *Nature* **358,** 167-169.

5 Drug Delivery Systems based on Multiple Emulsions

Vinod K. Dhote[1], Kanika Dhote[1], Piush Khare[2] and Sharad P. Pandey[1]

[1]Truba Institute of Pharmacy, Karond - Gandhi Nagar Bypass Road, Bhopal-462 038, India.

[2]Eiman Pharma Pvt Limited, 1/1 Palm Road, Shipra Sun City (Gaziabad), National Capital Region, 201 014, India.

5.1   Introduction

Emulsion science and technology has been used for many years to create a diverse range of commercial products, including pharmaceuticals, foods, agrochemicals, lubricants, personal care products, and cosmetics (Cunha et al., 1997). The majority of these products are conventional emulsions consisting of droplets of one liquid dispersed in another immiscible liquid, e.g., oil-in-water emulsions. Recently, there has been growing interest in extending the functional performance of emulsion-based products using structural design principles. Emulsions are utilized in industrial and medical applications for a variety of reasons: encapsulation and delivery of active components; modification of rheological properties; alteration of optical properties; lubrication; modification of organoleptic attributes (Geiger et al., 1998).

An **emulsion** is a two-phase system consisting of at least two immiscible liquids (or two liquids that are saturated with each other), one of which is dispersed as globules (internal or dispersed phase) within the other liquid phase (external or continuous phase), generally stabilized by an emulsifying agent. Emulsions have been widely used in many areas, including the petroleum industry, agriculture, food technologies, pharmaceutics and cosmetics. Pharmaceutical emulsions are also used internally for the administration of drugs and diagnostic agents.

Emulsions discussed in this chapter include macroemulsions, multiple emulsions, microemulsions, and a special emulsion type (Baroli et al., 2000).

Traditionally, conventional emulsions consisting of small spherical droplets of one liquid dispersed in another immiscible liquid are used in industrial applications. The two immiscible liquids are typically an oil phase and an aqueous phase, although other immiscible liquids can sometimes be used (Eccleston, 2002). The droplets in conventional emulsions usually have diameters in the range of 100 nm to 100 μm, and are coated by a single layer of surface active components ("emulsifiers") that stabilize them against aggregation (Peltola et al., 2003). These systems are thermo-dynamically unstable and tend to breakdown over time due to physicochemical mechanisms such as gravitational separation, flocculation, coalescence, Ostwald ripening, and phase inversion. Conventional emulsions are usually classified according to the arrangement of the two immiscible liquids as either oil-in-water (O/W) or water-in-oil (W/O) systems.

5.1.1 Multiple Emulsions

Multiple emulsions are the emulsion system in which the dispersed phases in the form of smaller droplet have the same composition as external phase. This is made possible by double emulsification, so these systems are also called double emulsion.

Multiple emulsions are also called as liquid membrane system. In which liquid membrane which separated the liquid phase act as a thin semipermeable film through which solute must diffuse from one phase to another. As phase distribution W/O/W or O/W/O emulsions are possible. Multiple emulsions were observed as a laboratory curiosity in former times but these systems have now been evaluated systematically and could prove to be suitable as an interesting delivery system with potential for biopharmaceutical application and as vehicles for various drugs. The droplets of the dispersed phase contain even smaller dispersed droplets themselves, therefore also called as **"emulsions of emulsions"**. Each dispersed globule in the double emulsion forms a vesicular structure with single or multiple aqueous compartments separated from the aqueous phase by a layer of oil phase compartments. In multiple emulsions system, solute has to transverse from inner miscible phase to outer miscible phase through the middle immiscible organic phase, so it also called as liquid membrane system.

The two major types of multiple emulsions are the water-oil-water (W/O/W) and oil-water-oil (O/W/O) double emulsions. The most common multiple emulsions are of W/O/W type, although some specific applications O/W/O emulsions can also be prepared.

Multiple emulsions may find many potential applications in various fields such as chemistry, pharmaceutics, cosmetics and food (Patel and Sawant, 2007). These emulsions have been investigated as controlled-release drug delivery systems (DDS), as 'emulsion liquid membranes' for simultaneous liquid extraction and stripping of metals, organic acids and antibiotics, as microcapsules for the protection and controlled release of functional food ingredients, for the formulation of reduced-calorie food emulsions, etc (Shah et al., 1994). Other applications include the use of multiple emulsions as intermediate products to the preparation of lipid nanoparticles, gel microbeads, polymeric microspheres, biodegradable microspheres, inorganic particles, and vesicles such as polymerosomes

Although multiple emulsions have not been commercially exploited because of their inherent thermodynamic instability, a number of attempts have been made in last two decades for improving stability by several investigators. These attempts are: polymerization gelling, additives in different phases, surfactant concentration modulation, interfacial complexation, pro-multiple emulsion approach and steric stabilization (Kang et al., 2004).

5.2 Formulation Considerations

The choice of oil, emulsifier, and emulsion type (O/W, W/O, or multiple) is limited by its ultimate use and route of administration. Potential toxicity and chemical incompatibilities in the final formulation must be taken into account as most processing details for these also affect the variables that control emulsion stability and therapeutic response such as droplet size distributions and rheology (Florence and Whitehill, 1982; Kommuru et al., 2001).

5.2.1 Pharmaceutical Oils

Oils used in the preparation of pharmaceutical emulsions are of various chemical types, including simple esters, fixed and volatile oils, hydrocarbons, and turpenoid derivatives. The oil itself may be the medicament, it may function as a carrier for drug, or even form part of a mixed emulsifier system as in the case of some fixed oils that contain sufficient free fatty acids (Joshi and Patravale, 2006).

Many oils, particularly those of vegetable origin, are liable to auto oxidation with subsequent rancidity, and it is frequently necessary to add an antioxidant and/or preservative to inhibit this degradation process. For externally applied emulsions, mineral oils, either alone or combined with soft or hard paraffin, are widely used both as the vehicle for the drug and for their occlusive and sensory characteristics. The most widely used oils in oral preparations are non-biodegradable mineral and castor oils that provide a local laxative effect, and fish liver oils or various fixed oils of vegetable origin (e.g., arachis, cottonseed, and maize oils) as nutritional supplements (Lawrence and Rees, 2000).

5.2.2 Pharmaceutical Emulsifiers

Emulsifying agents are used both to promote emulsification at the time of manufacture and to control stability during a shelf life that can vary from days for extemporaneously prepared emulsions to months or years for commercial preparations. In practice, combinations of emulsifiers rather than single agents are used. The emulsifier also influences the *in vivo* fate of lipid parenteral emulsions by its influence on the surface properties of the droplets and on the droplet size distributions. For convenience, most pharmacy texts classify emulsifiers into three groups:

(i)   surface active agents;

(ii)   natural (macromolecular) polymers; and

(iii)   finely divided solids (Lee et al., 2005).

5.2.3 Surface Active Agents

Surfactants are manufactured from a variety of natural and synthetic sources and consequently they show considerable batch-to-batch variations in their homologue compositions and in trace impurities from the starting material. For example, batch variations in the number of neutral phospholipids occur in lecithin surfactants and non-ionic polyethylene surfactants show variations in the number of moles of ethylene oxide (Korhonen et al., 2000; Lin and Lui, 1992).

In general, cationic surfactants are the most toxic and irritant and non-ionic surfactants the least. Surfactants are therefore used mainly at relatively low concentrations in topical preparations. The quaternary ammonium compounds constitute an important group of cationic emulsifiers in dermatological preparations because they have antimicrobial properties in addition to their O/W emulsifying action.

5.2.4 Preservatives

It is essential that emulsions are formulated to resist microbial attack, as this not only can affect the physicochemical properties of the formulation, causing color, odor, or pH changes and even phase separation, but may also constitute a health hazard. The potential sources of contamination can be from raw materials (especially if these are natural products), water, manufacturing and packaging equipment, or patients themselves. W/O emulsions are less susceptible to attack than o/w emulsions because the aqueous continuous external phase can produce ideal conditions for the growth of bacteria, moulds, and fungi. Preservatives are not used in parenteral emulsions, which are sterilized, generally by autoclaving, but sometimes by using sterile components and aseptically assembling the final emulsion.

There is no simple way of predicting the ideal preservative for a particular emulsion. In addition to requiring a wide spectrum of activity against bacteria, yeasts, and molds, the preservative should be free from toxic, irritant, or sensitizing activity. Some commonly used preservatives in oral and topical preparations include phenoxyethanol, benzoic acid, parabenzoates, and chlorcresol. Emulsions are heterogeneous products, and the preservative partitions between the oil and aqueous phases. As a sufficient aqueous concentration of the active (usually unionized) form must be present to ensure proper preservation, pH is an additional factor to be considered. Problems often arise because many of the materials used in emulsion formulation, for example hydrocolloids or polyoxyethylene surfactants, can interact with the preservatives, thus depleting their activity.

5.2.5 Antioxidants and Humectants

Antioxidants are added to many pharmaceutical preparations to prevent oxidative deterioration on storage of the oil, emulsifier, or the drug itself. Such deterioration, as well as destabilizing the formulation, imparts an unpleasant odor or taste. Butylated hydroxyanisole (BHA) and butylated hydroxytoluene (BHT) at concentrations up to 0.2%, and the alkyl gallates are commonly used antioxidants. Humectants such as propylene glycol, glycerol, and sorbitol (5%) are often added to dermatological preparations to reduce the evaporation of water from the emulsion during storage and use.

5.3   Formulation of Multiple Emulsions

There are essentially two major considerations in emulsification: first, the formation of emulsions of the correct type, oil-in-water, water-in-oil, or multiple emulsion with the required droplet size distribution and second, the stabilization of the dispersed droplets so formed. When given amounts of two immiscible liquids are mixed or mechanically agitated in the absence of other additives, both phases tend to form droplets of various sizes. The size distributions are related to the forces involved during the agitation process, and the number of droplets of each liquid depends on its relative volume. Fig. 5.1 shows various method for formulation of multiple emulsion.

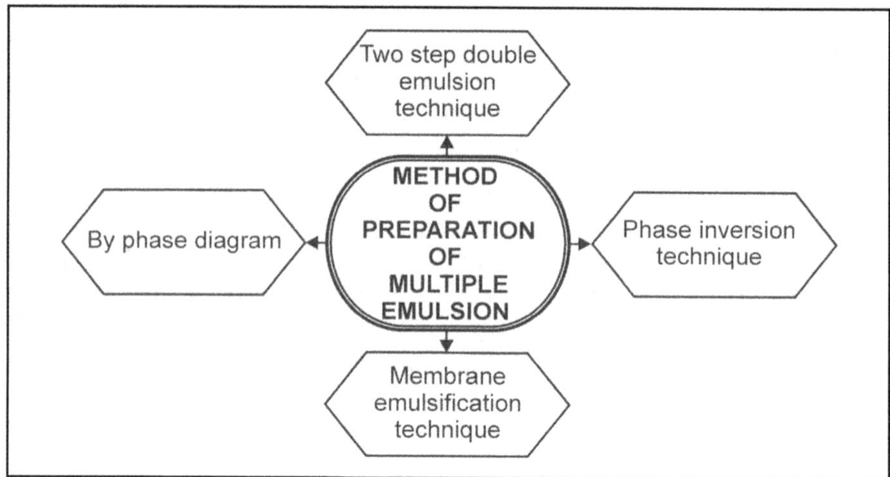

FIGURE 5.1 Various methods of formulation of multiple emulsion.

The type of emulsion that forms, either O/W or W/O, depends on the relative rates of coalescence of each type of droplet, with the more rapidly coalescing droplets forming the continuous phase. Generally, this is the liquid present in the larger amount because higher number of droplets increases the probability of collision and coalescence. With phase volumes of oil and water close to 50%, other factors such as the order and rate of addition of each liquid are important. If agitation ceases, coalescence will continue until complete phase separation the state of minimum free energy is reached. Thus, emulsification can be considered as the result of two competing processes, namely the disruption of bulk liquids to produce fine droplets and the recombination of the droplets to give back the original bulk liquids.

5.3.1 Double Emulsification Technique (Two Step Technique)

In the first step, an aqueous phase is added to an oily phase containing a lipophilic surfactant. Upon mixing, a W/O type emulsion is formed. In the second step, this W/O emulsion is poured into a second aqueous phase containing a hydrophilic surfactant which upon mixing results in formation of multiple W/O/W emulsion. Multiple emulsions can be end products or serve as intermediate products, as during the preparation of drug-loaded microparticles. The use of multiple emulsions, such as W/O/W, O/W/O and W/O/O can for example, help to reduce drug loss into an outer aqueous phase and thus, increase the resulting drug encapsulation efficiency. The same has been depicted in Fig. 5.2.

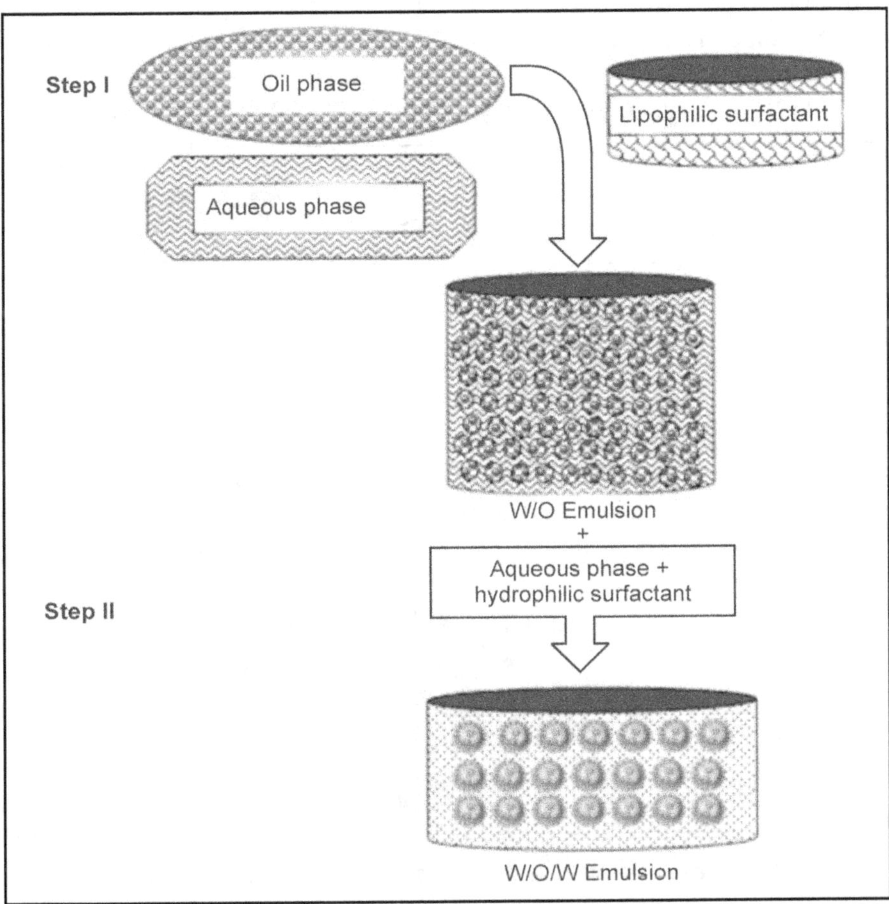

FIGURE 5.2 Double emulsification technique displays preparation of water-in-oil-in-water (W/O/W) emulsion.

5.3.2 Phase Inversion Technique

An increase in volume concentration of dispersed phase may cause an increase in the phase volume ratio, which subsequently leads to formation of multiple emulsions. The method typically involves the addition of an aqueous phase containing a hydrophilic emulsifier (Tween 80/sodium dodecyl sulphate or cetyl trimethyl ammonium salt) to an oil phase consisting of liquid paraffin along with lipophilic emulsifier (Span 80). A well-defined volume of oil phase is placed in a vessel of pin mixer. An aqueous solution of emulsifier is then successively introduced to the oil phase in the vessel at a fixed rate, while the pin mixer rotates steadily at room temperature. When volume fraction of the aqueous solution of hydrophilic emulsifier exceeds 0.7, the continuous oil phase is substituted by the aqueous phase containing a number of the vesicular globules among the simple oil droplets, leading to phase inversion and formation of W/O/W multiple emulsion (Fig. 5.3).

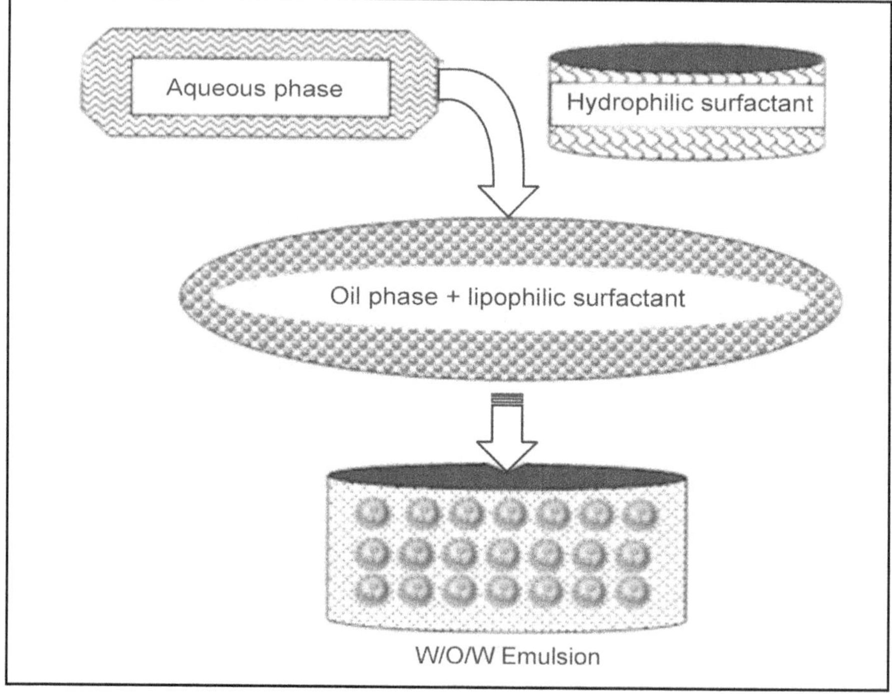

FIGURE 5.3 Phase inversion technique showing preparation of water-in-oil-in-water (W/O/W) emulsion.

5.3.3 Membrane Emulsification Technique

In this process, the dispersed phase is forced through the pores of a microporous membrane directly into the continuous phase. Emulsified droplets are formed and detached at the end of the pores with a drop-by-drop mechanism as shown in Fig 5.4. The advantages of membrane emulsification over conventional emulsification processes is that it enables to obtain very fine emulsions of controlled droplet sizes and narrow droplet size distributions. Successful emulsification can be carried out with much less consumption of emulsifier and energy, and because of the lowered shear stress effect, membrane emulsification allows the use of shear-sensitive ingredients, such as starch and proteins. The membrane emulsification process is generally carried out in cross-flow (continuous or batch) mode or in a stirred cell (batch).

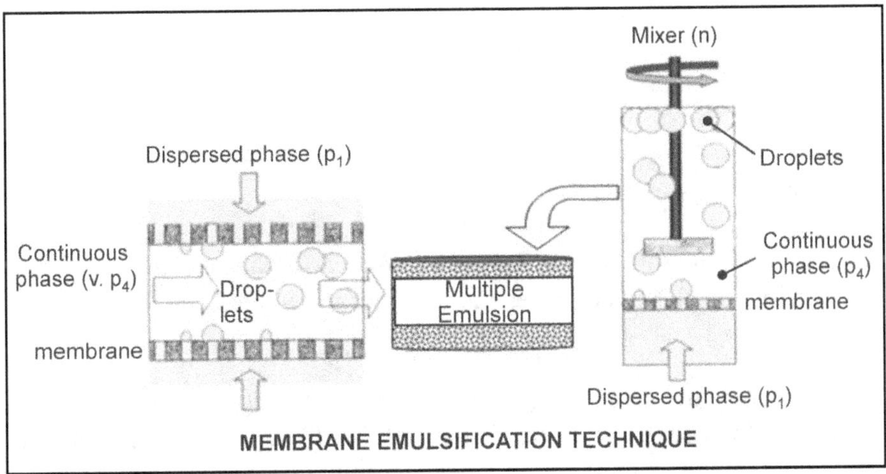

FIGURE 5.4 Membrane emulsification technique.

5.4 Instability in Multiple Emulsions

The process by which an emulsion completely breaks (coalescence), i.e., the system separates into bulk oil and water phases, is generally considered to be governed by four different droplet loss mechanisms, i.e., Brownian flocculation, creaming, sedimentation flocculation and disproportionation, shown schematically in Fig. 5.5. The first three are the primary methods by which emulsions are destabilized but all four processes may occur simultaneously and in any order. The processes of creaming, flocculation and coalescence are well demonstrated by taking an emulsion of limited stability and centrifuging it at low speeds or various lengths of time (Laugel et al., 1996).

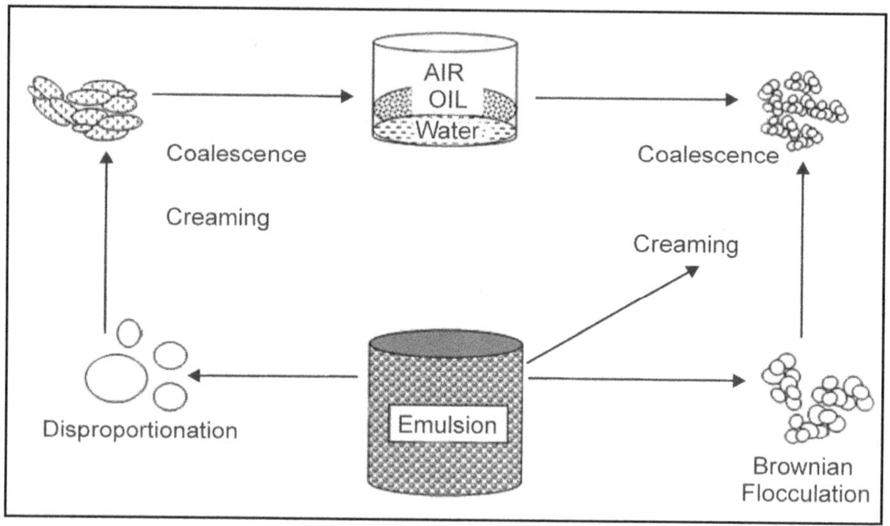

FIGURE 5.5 Instability in multiple emulsions.

The creaming rate (or settling rate for disperse phases more dense than the continuous phase) can be estimated from the Stokes' equation:

$$\upsilon = 2\,r^2\,(\rho - \rho_o)\,g\,/\,9\eta$$

where, υ is the creaming (settling) rate, r is the droplet radius, ρ is the density of the droplet, ρ_o is the density of the dispersion medium, η is the viscosity of the dispersion medium (continuous phase) and g is the acceleration due to gravity (Magdassi and Garti, 1986).

The density difference, $(\rho - \rho_o)$, is negative for creaming (an O/W emulsion) but positive for settling (a W/O emulsion). The Stokes' equation shows that creaming is inhibited by a small droplet radius, a highly viscous continuous phase and a low density difference between the oil and water phases. Substituting "typical" values into the equation, i.e., $r \sim 1$ μm, $\Delta\rho \sim 0.2$ g·cm^{-3} and $\eta \sim 1$ mPa·s gives a creaming rate of ~ 5 cm per day which is substantial. Role of ingredients plays a vital role in formulation and storage of multiple emulsion and various strategies are available to overcome instability (Itoh et al., 2002) (Table 5.1).

TABLE 5.1

Role of ingredients and strategies to overcome instability of multiple emulsion

Component	Role	Strategies
Emulsifying equipment	The primary emulsion can be prepared using a laboratory mixer or homogenizer to provide a good dispersion of droplets within the appropriate continuous phase. Excessive mixing, especially at high shear, can cause the primary emulsion droplets to rupture.	Ultrasonic homogenizers must be used with care for the secondary emulsi-fication step.
Nature of the oil Phase	The oil phase to be employed in a pharmaceutical emulsion must be nontoxic. The various oils of vegetable origin (soybean, sesame, peanut, safflower, etc.) are acceptable if purified correctly. Refined hydrocarbons such as light liquid paraffin, squalane, as well as esters of fatty acids (ethyl oleate and isopropyl myristate) have also been used in double emulsions.	Mineral oils produced more stable multiple emulsions (w/o/w) than those produced from vegetable oils. **light liquid paraffin > squalane > sesame oil > maize or peanut oil.**
Volumes of the dispersed phases	The quantity of water dispersed in the initial w/o emulsion [expressed as a phase volume ratio, (w/o/w)] can have an influence on both the yield and stability of the final emulsion system.	It should be optimized.
Nature and quantity of emulsifying agents	It adversely affect the stability of the emulsion system, too little emulsifier may result in unstable systems, whereas too much emulsifier may lead to toxic effects and can even cause destabilization.	Two different emulsifiers (lipohilic and hydrophilic) are required to form a stable emulsion. In general, for a w/o/w emulsion the optimal HLB value will be in the range 2-7 for the primary surfactant and in the range 6-16 for the secondary surfactant. The concentration of the emulsifiers can also be varied.
Effect of lipophilic emulsifier	Increase in concentration of lipophilic surfactant causes swelling capacity of oil globule to increase leading to more delay in release	In an increase of the rigidity of the second interface by the progressive migration of the lipophilic surfactant.
Nature of entrapped materials	Electrolytes and nature of the drug (hydrophilic or hydrophobic etc.) affect the stability of the formulation.	When formulating a w/o/w system the presence of the drug and other components (especially electrolytes) needs to be considered.

TABLE 5.1 *Contd...*

Component	Role	Strategies
Stabilizers	The stabilizers are added to improve the stability of multiple emulsions. These include gelling or viscosity-increasing agents added to internal and/or external aqueous phases.	The nature of drug (hydrophilic or hydrophobic) is also given due consi-deration Viscosity-enhancing agents (e.g., 10-20% gelatin, methylcellulose), and similar thickening agents, as well as complexing agents that will lead it to liquid crystalline phase at the o/w interface.

5.5　Multiple Emulsion Stability Testing

Stability testing is an integral part of emulsion development work. The emulsion formulator is generally concerned with understanding the effects of storage and shipping conditions on shelf-life which may include extremes of temperatures and exposure to sunlight, vibration and humidity (Kita et al., 1977). Hence, formulations are stored under standardized test conditions and carefully examined at periodic intervals. Table 5.2. lists general conditions commonly and historically used to evaluate emulsion stability though regulated emulsion products must be tested in compliance with applicable ICH guidelines (Nakhare and Vyas, 1995, 1996). Further, although freeze-thaw has been widely used as an accelerated path to judge emulsion stability, it is not truly appropriate to rely solely on it to make those judgements. The cycling of temperature in freeze-thaw experiments affects parameters other than those that directly relate to creaming which is the actual mechanism of emulsion instability (Florence and Whitehill, 1982).

TABLE 5.2

Storage conditions for multiple emulsion

Test conditions for multiple emulsion stability testing	
Storage conditions	Storage period
Ambient temperature	25 °C for 3 years (or) projected shelf-life of the product
Elevated temperature	37 °C for 6 months and 45 °C for 6 months
Refrigerator	Approximately 4 °C for 3 months
Freeze/thaw cycles (5)	Approximately −10 °C to ambient
Cycling chamber	4 °C to 45 °C in 48 hours for 1 month
Light exposure	1 month exposure to north-facing daylight or light cabinet

Laboratory batches are generally stored in glass jars to evaluate the inherent stability of the emulsion. The use of glass jars permits easy observation and physical measurements at regular intervals (Laugel et al., 1996). However, ultimately the emulsion must also be evaluated in the intended final packaging, as this may impact the stability due to interfacial wetting behaviour, permeation, or leaching of components into or out of the packaging material. Table 5.3. lists properties that are important to fully understand, including the characteristics and stability of an emulsion formulation (Rayner et al., 2004). The number of parameters is quite extensive, and all the instrumentation required may not be available to many formulators. Ideally, all these tests should be conducted on final formulations but it is not practical, nor necessary, to conduct all the tests on all preliminary formulations. Typically, initial formulations are screened for changes in pH, viscosity, flow behaviour, odour and physical separation at elevated temperatures (Table 5.2, Table 5.3).

TABLE 5.3

Stability testing parameter for multiple emulsion

Stability testing parameter	
Property	Test method
pH	pH meter
Viscosity	Rotational viscometer
Flow behaviour	Oscillatory shear viscosity with a cone/plate rheometer
Tack/Texture	Extensional and compressional deformation
Color	Visual or colorimeter
Odor	Organoleptic
Specific gravity	Pycnometer
Separation	Creaming value - visual or instrumental
Conductivity	Conductivity meter
Droplet size distribution	Microscopic examination (image analysis) and instrumental
Preservation	Microbial challenge and/or assay
Vibration	Shipping test or shaker table
Active ingredient(s)	Chemical or bio-assay

5.6 Drug Release Mechanism from Multiple Emulsions (Vaziri and Warburton, 1994)

In multiple emulsions, the drug is released from internal to external phase through the oily layer by different mechanisms. The release rates are affected by the various factors such as droplet size, pH, phase volume and viscosity etc (Ma et al., 1993).

5.6.1 Diffusion Mechanism

This is most common transport mechanism where unionized hydrophobic drug diffuses through the oil layer in the stable multiple emulsions. Drug transport has been found to follow first order kinetics and obeyed Fick's law of diffusion.

5.6.2 Facilitated Diffusion (Carrier-Mediated Transport)

This mechanism involves a special molecule (carrier) which combines with the drug and makes it compatible to permeate through the oil membrane. These carriers can be incorporated in internal aqueous phase or oil membrane.

5.6.3 Thinning of the Oil Membrane

Due to osmotic pressure difference, the oil membrane becomes thin leading to easy diffusion of water and drug. This pressure difference also provides force for the transverse of molecule therefore it should be taken into consideration.

5.6.4 Photo-Osmotic Transport

The mechanism of this transport process is not very clear. Transport of the drug through the oil membrane takes place with the help of the light.

5.6.5 Rupture of Oil Phase

According to this mechanism rupturing of oil membrane can unite both aqueous phases and thus, drug could be released easily.

5.6.6 Solubilization of Internal Phase in the Oil Membrane

It is a conspicuous transport mechanism. In this solubilization of minute amounts of the internal phase in the membrane phase results in the transport of very small quantities of materials.

5.6.7 Micellar Transport

Inverse micelles consisting of non-polar part of surfactant lying outside and polar part inside encapsulate hydrophilic drug in core and permeate through the oil membrane because of the outer lipophilic nature. Inverse micelles can encapsulate both ionized and unionized drugs.

5.7 Application of Multiple Emulsions

Emulsions have a long history of use and are widely used in many products encountered in everyday life. Understanding the theoretical considerations in emulsion formulation and having the ability and proper instrumentation to fully characterize and monitor stability of an emulsion system is highly beneficial to provide a superior product in a more time efficient manner. Some of the applications are listed the Table 5.4.

TABLE 5.4

Application of multiple emulsions in various fields

S. No.	Contributors	Contribution
		Multiple emulsions in cancer therapy
1	Higashi and co-workers (Higashi et al., 1995)	Developed such a new drug delivery system for treating hepatocellular carcinoma (HCC) using W/O/W emulsions prepared with iodinated poppy-seed oil and water soluble epirubicin. The emulsion accumulated in the small vessels in the tumor when injected to the liver via the hepatic artery.
2.	(Nakajima M et al., 2003)	Prepared ethanol-in-oil-in water (E/O/W) emulsions which are capable to encapsulate functional components that have a low solubility with respect to water and oil but are soluble in ethanol. An example is taxol which is an anticancerous terpenoid can be used in cancer treatment by incorporating it in E/O/W emulsion.
3.	(Khopade and Jain, 1999)	prepared multiple emulsion of 6-mercaptopurine by incorporation of sphingomyelins (SM) and monosialogangliosides (GM1) in the oily phase and by coating with lipidgrafted polyethylene glycol (PEG-PC) and concluded that PEG-PC-coated multiple emulsions are superior as prolonged release and extended blood circulating carriers compared to multiple emulsions having GM1 or SM.
4.	(Khopade and Jain, 1999)	Prepared PEG-PC coated multiple emulsion bearing 6-mercaptopurine and studied antitumor activity on the murine leukemia cell line L-1210 *in vitro* and showed that decreased uptake and cytotoxicity were observed and mean survival time was increased due to sustained release and effective delivery of drug from the formulation.
5.	(Takahashi et al., 1973)	Prepared multiple emulsion of bleomycin, studied and found that the concentration of bleomycin in tumour tissues of rats was 2 to 7 times higher after intratumoral injection of w/o or w/o/w emulsions than those produced by local administration of an aqueous solution of the drug.

TABLE 5.4 *Contd...*

S. No.	Contributors	Contribution
6.	(Takahashi et al., 1973)	They utilized the lipid absorbing ability of the lymphatic system to facilitate delivery of the drug especially to the regional lymph nodes. A comparison of the radioactivity in the regional lymph nodes after intratesticular injection of various types of preparation containing the labeled anticancer agent 5-FU showed that the highest value was observed in w/o/w emulsion followed by w/o, o/w emulsions, and aqueous solution
7.	(Yanagie et al., 2011)	Treated the hepatocellular carcinoma by neutron capture therapy using intra-arterial administration of boron-entrapped w/o/w emulsion. In this therapy tumour cell destruction takes place when there is a nuclear reaction between 10 boron atoms and thermal neutrons, and concluded that it is necessary to accumulate efficient 10 boron atoms to tumour cells for effective results.

Multiple emulsions in herbal drugs

S. No.	Contributors	Contribution
10.	(Jiang and Zhou, 2003)	Studied the influence of the elemenum emulsion on the human lung adenocarcinoma cell line A549 and protein expression. Results showed that the elemenum emulsion has a significant inhibition on the growth and proliferation of the A549 *in vitro* and it showed a time and dose dependent relationship. Elemenum emulsion is a type of new anti-cancer drug with great application prospects. Furthermore, it has no marrow inhibition and no harm to the heart and liver.

Vaccine/vaccine adjuvant

S. No.	Contributors	Contribution
11.	(Herbert, 1965)	The use of w/o/w multiple emulsion as a new form of adjuvant for antigen was first reported by him. These emulsions elicited better immune response than antigen alone.
12.	(Verma and Jaiswal, 1997)	Developed a multiple emulsion vaccine against Pasteurella multocida infection in cattle. This vaccine contributed both humoral as well as cell-mediated immune responses in protection against the infection. It was concluded that this multiple emulsion based vaccine can be successfully used in the effective control of haemorrhagic septicaemia.

Oxygen substitute

S. No.	Contributors	Contribution
13.	(Zheng et al., 1993)	Studied multiple emulsion of aqueous oxygen carrying material in oil in outer aqueous phase and found suitable for provision of oxygen for oxygen transfer processes. A hemoglobin multiple emulsion in physiologically compatible oil in an outer aqueous saline solution is provided in sufficiently small droplet size to provide oxygen flow through blood vessels to desired body tissues or organs thereby providing a blood substitute.

Inverse targeting

S. No.	Contributors	Contribution
14.	(Talegaonkar and Vyas, 2005)	Prepared poloxamer 403 containing sphere in- oil-in-water (s/o/w) multiple emulsion of diclofenac sodium by gelatinization of inner aqueous phase and they examined the effect of poloxmer 403 on surface modification for inverse

TABLE 5.4 Contd...

S. No.	Contributors	Contribution

Inverse targeting

targeting to reticuloendothelial system-rich organs. They concluded that the multiple emulsion system containing poloxamer has capability to retards the RES uptake of drugs mainly to liver, brain and targeting to non-RES tissues such as lungs, inflammatory tissue.

Multiple emulsions in diabetes

15.	(Toorisaka et al., 2003)	Developed a S/O/W emulsion for oral administration of insulin. Surfactant-coated insulin was dispersed in the oil by ultrasonication, this dispersion was mixed with the outer water phase with a homogenizer and finally, the S/O/W emulsion thus obtained was adjusted to a constant particle size by passage through a SPG membrane. The S/O/W emulsion showed hypoglycemic activity for a long period after oral administration to rats.

Multiple emulsions in food

16.	(Rayner et al., 2004)	Showed another possible application of double emulsions is in the food industry. Preliminary studies have been performed in the field of entrapment of a flavour component in a release system. Sensitive food materials and flavours can be encapsulated in W/O/W emulsions. Sensory tests have indicated that there is a significant taste difference between W/O/W emulsions and O/W emulsions containing the same ingredients, and that there is a delayed release of incorporated drug.

Drug over dosage treatment

17.	(Chiang et al., 1978)	Showed utilization of multiple emulsion for the over dosage treatment by utilizing the difference in the pH e.g. barbiturates. In these emulsions, the inner aqueous phase of emulsion has the basic buffer and when emulsion is taken orally, acidic pH of the stomach acts as an external aqueous phase. In the acidic phase barbiturate remains mainly in unionized form which transfers through oil membrane into inner aqueous phase and gets ionized. Ionized drug has less affinity to cross the oil membrane thereby getting entrapped. Thus, entrapping excess drug in multiple emulsion cures over dosage condition.

Taste masking

18.	(Vaziri and Warburton, 1994)	Multiple emulsions of chloroquine, an antimalarial agent has been successfully prepared and demonstrated to mask the bitter taste efficiently. Also taste masking of chlorpromazine, an antipsychotic drug has also been reported by multiple emulsions.

References

Baroli, B., López-Quintela, M.A., Delgado-Charro, M.B., Fadda, A.M., and Blanco-Méndez, J. (2000). Microemulsions for topical delivery of 8-methoxsalen. *Journal of Controlled Release* **69,** 209-218.

Chiang, C.W., Fuller, G.C., Frankenfeld, J.W., and Rhodes, C. (1978). Potential of liquid membranes for drug overdose treatment: *in vitro* studies. *Journal of pharmaceutical sciences* **67,** 63-66.

Cunha, A.S., Grossior, J., Puisieux, F., and Seiller, M. (1997). Insulin in W/O/W multiple emulsions: preparation, characterization and determination of stability towards proteases *in vitro*. *Journal of microencapsulation* **14,** 311-319.

Eccleston, G. (2002). Emulsion and Microemulsions In Encyclopedia of Pharmaceutical Technology,; Ed: Swarbrick, J., Boylan, JC (Marcel Dekker, Inc., New York).

Florence, A., and Whitehill, D. (1982). The formulation and stability of multiple emulsions. *International journal of pharmaceutics* **11,** 277-308.

Geiger, S., Tokgoz, S., Fructus, A., Jager-Lezer, N., Seiller, M., Lacombe, C., and Grossiord, J.-L. (1998). Kinetics of swelling–breakdown of a W/O/W multiple emulsion: possible mechanisms for the lipophilic surfactant effect. *Journal of controlled release* **52,** 99-107.

Herbert, W. (1965). Multiple emulsions: a new form of mineral-oil antigen adjuvant. *The Lancet* **286,** 771.

Higashi, S., Shimizu, M., Nakashima, T., Iwata, K., Uchiyama, F., Tateno, S., Tamura, S., and Setoguchi, T. (1995). Arterial-injection chemotherapy for hepatocellular carcinoma using monodispersed poppy-seed oil microdroplets containing fine aqueous vesicles of epirubicin. Initial medical application of a membrane-emulsification technique. *Cancer* **75,** 1245-1254.

Itoh, K., Matsui, S., Tozuka, Y., Oguchi, T., and Yamamoto, K. (2002). Improvement of physicochemical properties of N-4472: Part II: characterization of N-4472 microemulsion and the enhanced oral absorption. *International journal of pharmaceutics* **246,** 75-83.

Jiang, S.J., and Zhou, X.J. (2003). Examination of the mechanism of oleic acid-induced percutaneous penetration enhancement: an ultrastructural study. *Biological and Pharmaceutical Bulletin* **26,** 66-68.

Joshi, M., and Patravale, V. (2006). Formulation and evaluation of nanostructured lipid carrier (NLC)-based gel of valdecoxib. *Drug development and industrial pharmacy* **32,** 911-918.

Kang, B.K., Lee, J.S., Chon, S.K., Jeong, S.Y., Yuk, S.H., Khang, G., Lee, H.B., and Cho, S.H. (2004). Development of self-microemulsifying drug delivery systems (SMEDDS) for oral bioavailability enhancement of simvastatin in beagle dogs. *International journal of pharmaceutics* **274,** 65-73.

Khopade, A., and Jain, N. (1999). Fine Multiple Emulsions Bearing 6-Mercaptopurine: *In vitro* and *In vivo* Antitumor Studies. *Drug Delivery* **6**, 181-185.

Kita, Y., Matsumoto, S., and Yonezawa, D. (1977). Viscometric method for estimating the stability of W/O/W-type multiple-phase emulsions. *Journal of Colloid and Interface Science* **62**, 87-94.

Kommuru, T., Gurley, B., Khan, M., and Reddy, I. (2001). Self-emulsifying drug delivery systems (SEDDS) of coenzyme Q 10: formulation development and bioavailability assessment. *International journal of pharmaceutics* **212**, 233-246.

Korhonen, M., Niskanen, H., Kiesvaara, J., and Yliruusi, J. (2000). Determination of optimal combination of surfactants in creams using rheology measurements. *International journal of pharmaceutics* **197**, 143-151.

Laugel, C., Chaminade, P., Baillet, A., Seiller, M., and Ferrier, D. (1996). Moisturizing substances entrapped in W/O/W emulsions: analytical methodology for formulation, stability and release studies. *Journal of controlled release* **38**, 59-67.

Lawrence, M.J., and Rees, G.D. (2000). Microemulsion-based media as novel drug delivery systems. *Advanced drug delivery reviews* **45**, 89-121.

Lee, J., Lee, Y., Kim, J., Yoon, M., and Choi, Y.W. (2005). Formulation of microemulsion systems for transdermal delivery of aceclofenac. *Archives of pharmacal research* **28**, 1097-1102.

Lin, S.Y., and Lui, W.Y. (1992). Zero-order of first-order release kinetics of water-in-oil-in-water (W/O/W) multiple emulsions of lipiodol dependent on the types of surfactants. *Chemical and pharmaceutical bulletin* **40**, 2860-2863.

Ma, J.-L., Xiong, Q.-M., and Tao, T. (1993). Physico-chemical Properties and its Release *in vitro* of Multiple Emulsion Containing Etoposide. *Chinese Journal of Pharmaceuticals* **24**, 357-357.

Magdassi, S., and Garti, N. (1986). A kinetic model for release of electrolytes from W/O/W multiple emulsions. *Journal of controlled release* **3**, 273-277.

Nakajima M, Nabetani H, Ichikawa S, and QY, X. (2003). Functional emulsions, U.S. Patent, ed. (US).

Nakhare, S., and Vyas, S. (1995). Prolonged release of rifampicin from multiple W/O/W emulsion systems. *Journal of microencapsulation* **12**, 409-415.

Nakhare, S., and Vyas, S. (1996). Preparation and characterization of multiple emulsion based systems for controlled diclofenac sodium release. *Journal of microencapsulation* **13**, 281-292.

Patel, D., and Sawant, K.K. (2007). Oral bioavailability enhancement of acyclovir by self-microemulsifying drug delivery systems (SMEDDS). *Drug development and industrial pharmacy* **33**, 1318-1326.

Peltola, S., Saarinen-Savolainen, P., Kiesvaara, J., Suhonen, T., and Urtti, A. (2003). Microemulsions for topical delivery of estradiol. *International journal of pharmaceutics* **254,** 99-107.

Rayner, M., Bergenstahl, B., Massarelli, L., Tragaradh, G., and Dickinson, E. (2004). Double emulsion prepared by membrane emulsification: Stability entrapment degree in a flavour release system. Paper presented at: Abstract Food Colloids Conference, Harrogate.

Shah, N., Carvajal, M., Patel, C., Infeld, M., and Malick, A. (1994). Self-emulsifying drug delivery systems (SEDDS) with polyglycolyzed glycerides for improving *in vitro* dissolution and oral absorption of lipophilic drugs. *International journal of pharmaceutics* **106,** 15-23.

Takahashi, T., Mizuno, M., Fujita, Y., Ueda, S., and Nishioka, B. (1973). Increased concentration of anticancer agents in regional lymph nodes by fat emulsions, with special reference to chemotherapy of metastasis. *Gann Gan* **64,** 345.

Talegaonkar, S., and Vyas, S. (2005). Inverse targeting of diclofenac sodium to reticuloendothelial system-rich organs by sphere-in-oil-in-water (S/O/W) multiple emulsion containing poloxamer 403. *Journal of drug targeting* **13,** 173-178.

Toorisaka, E., Ono, H., Arimori, K., Kamiya, N., and Goto, M. (2003). Hypoglycemic effect of surfactant-coated insulin solubilized in a novel solid-in-oil-in-water (S/O/W) emulsion. *International journal of pharmaceutics* **252,** 271-274.

Vaziri, A., and Warburton, B. (1994). Slow release of chloroquine phosphate from multiple taste-masked W/O/W multiple emulsions. *Journal of microencapsulation* **11,** 641-648.

Verma, R., and Jaiswal, T. (1997). Protection, humoral and cell-mediated immune responses in calves immunized with multiple emulsion haemorrhagic septicaemia vaccine. *Vaccine* **15,** 1254-1260.

Yanagie, H., Kumada, H., Nakamura, T., Higashi, S., Ikushima, I., Morishita, Y., Shinohara, A., Fijihara, M., Suzuki, M., and Sakurai, Y. (2011). Feasibility evaluation of neutron capture therapy for hepatocellular carcinoma using selective enhancement of boron accumulation in tumour with intra-arterial administration of boron-entrapped water-in-oil-in-water emulsion. *Applied Radiation and Isotopes* **69,** 1854-1857.

Zheng, S., Zheng, Y., Beissinger, R.L., Wasan, D.T., and McCormick, D.L. (1993). Hemoglobin multiple emulsion as an oxygen delivery system. *Biochimica et Biophysica Acta (BBA)-General Subjects* **1158,** 65-74.

6   Site Specific Oral Drug Delivery Systems

Pankaj K. Singh[1] and Priya Singh Kushwaha[2]

[1]Pharmaceutics Division, CSIR-Central Drug Research Institute,
Lucknow-226 031, India.

[2]Babasaheb Bhimrao Ambedkar University, Lucknow-226 025, India.

6.1   Introduction

Despite tremendous advancements in drug delivery, oral route remains the most considered one for administration of drugs in various therapeutic areas, and many patients prefer standard oral dosage forms as well as advanced oral drug delivery systems over other dosage forms. Several reasons can be pointed out to support this fact, namely ease of administration and full control of administration by the patient, together with a high degree of flexibility on dosing.

Drug efficacy generally depends upon the ability of the drug to reach its target in sufficient quantity to maintain therapeutic levels for the desired time period. Oral delivery of large molecular weight drug as well as macromolecules through GIT still remains one of the major hurdles to be surmounted before they can produce systemic effect after oral administration. This group of drugs is usually administered parenterally with some obvious disadvantages such as poor patient acceptance, invasiveness, expensive and unwieldy treatment. Though, several drugs have to be administered parenterally over a long period of time when necessary.

The very intricate absorption process of drugs from oral administration to its site of action is schematically represented in Fig. 6.1. In general, absorption of drugs through GI tract varies on account of many factors like the nature and surface area of the GI mucosal membrane varying from the stomach to the rectum, as well as the physicochemical properties of the pharmaceutical dosage form along with the luminal content. Hence, a balance among these factors would have a notable effect on how much of the administered drug reaches to the bloodstream that is summed up by the term bioavailability.

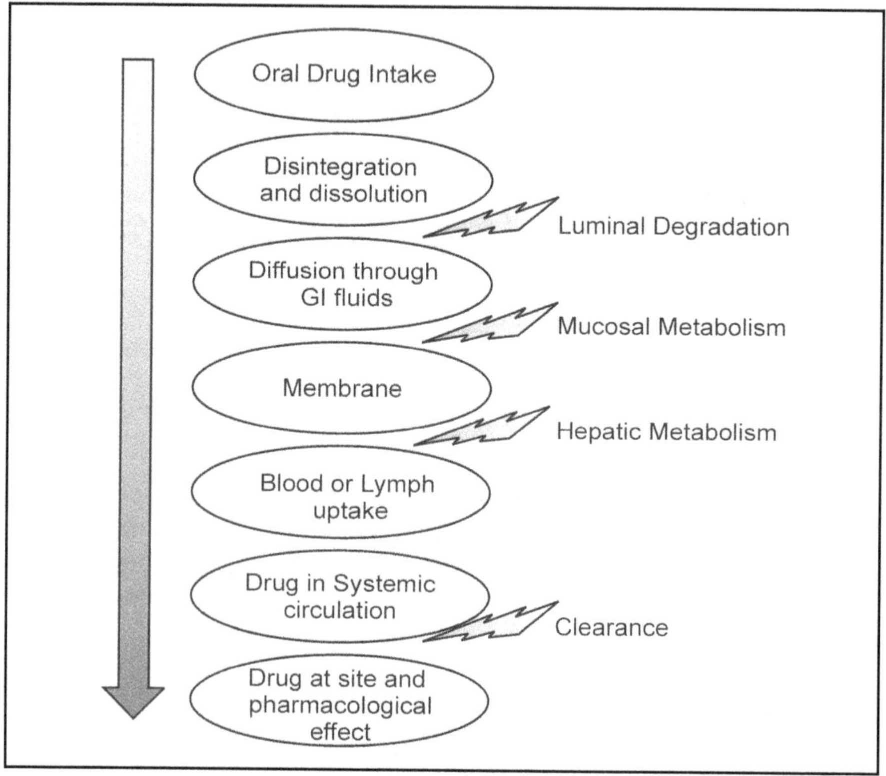

FIGURE 6.1 Schematic representation of fate of an oral dosage form.

However, there is a huge difference in physiology, preferential site of drug absorption, as the same time many systems in the human body such as cardiovascular, pulmonary, hepatic and renal systems show variation in their function throughout a typical day, dosage forms must be tailored to a site specific organ or even a part of the organ. Site specific delivery is usually driven by environmental factors, like the pH or enzymes present in the lumen, whereas the drug delivery from time controlled systems is controlled primarily by the delivery system and ideally not by the environment. Sometimes controlled delivery system based on the transit time to specific location in the gastro intestinal tract also assist in designing of site specific drug delivery systems such as colon targeting.

Although there have been several advantages of oral drug delivery, some major obstacles come along a way in to systemic circulation, such as underprivileged absorption profiles, incomplete drug release, shorter residence time of dosage forms in absorption window and etc. For example, targeted delivery to the colon represents an advantageous approach for the treatment of widespread inflammatory bowel disease (IBD) including ulcerative colitis and crohn's disease and tumoral, infective or neurovegetative colonic pathologies. Other commercial benefits can be the ever-greening of already existing patents and the ability to promote new claims. Scientists and research groups have been pushing the margins of traditional oral drug delivery for many decades, and in addition to all the premature advances in this area, progress in several domains of oral drug delivery has come to fruition over the ancient times. With objective of minimizing higher peaks and valleys of drug concentration in body fluid, constant/sustained drug output, reduced dosing frequency and improved patient compliance and ultimate goal of reduction in side effect, oral delivery system has moved towards site specific, pulsatile, constant/sustained and chronotherapeutic oriented formulation development. The shift from conventional oral delivery approach to modern site specific delivery of drugs can be credited to the following facts:

(a) *First pass metabolism*: Drugs, such as beta blockers and salicylamide, undergo extensive first pass metabolism and require fast drug input to saturate metabolizing enzymes in order to minimize pre-systemic metabolism.

(b) *Local activity*: Sometimes local delivery of drug is required for treatment at specific site in GIT such as inflammatory bowel disease, the site specific delivery toward inflammatory tissue is required to achieve the therapeutic effect and to minimize side effects.

(c) *Absorption site*: Absorption of drug is slow in stomach as compare to small intestine and slower in large intestine. Absorption variability characteristic is beneficial for some drug. For example, it is required for some site specific delivery system to pump out the drug much faster when the system reaches the distal segment of the intestine, to avoid the interment of the drug in the feces.

(d) *Chronopharmacological factor*: It has been well notorious commencement of many disease such as angina pectoris, asthma were occur during specific time periods of the 24 hour day, most frequently in the morning hours.

(e) ***Gastric pH:*** GI tract showing variation in pH from stomach to colon and groups of drug showing instability and degradation at acidic pH of the stomach, in such case site specific delivery system requires delivering drug in unchanged form.

6.2 Designing of Oral Mucosal Drug Delivery System

Designing of oral mucosal drug delivery system depends on lot of limitation and factor to be considered simultaneously for effective and site specific delivery of drug. Even drugs have favorable physiochemical properties, a tiny amount can cross mucosal barrier so to deliver high amount of drug, a suitable designing of drug delivery system is needed. Some physiochemical properties of candidate drug should be unique to traverse transmucosally. For example, drug should have a balance of solubility and lipophilicity. HLB value of drug candidate is one of the essential key for its selection during designing of oral delivery. Release of the drug from the delivery system is one of the considerable factors for effective delivery of drug candidate orally. The release kinetics of a given drug from a system could be governed predominantly by the polymer characteristics and excipients present in the system. Selection of drug, excipient and solvents should be done on the basis of biocompatibility with mucosa. An ideally designed site specific drug delivery should rapidly attach to the target site and maintain a strong interaction to prevent displacement and should not be affected by surrounding environmental pH. In this unit designing, components, principle, function and application of following site specific drug delivery system elaborated.

- Buccal tablets
- Buccal patches
- Osmotic tablets
- Pulsincaps
- Lozenges
- Medicated chewing gum
- Egalet® technology
- Enterion technology
- Hydrophillice sandwich

6.3   Buccal Tablets

Buccal drug delivery can be defined as the administration of drug via the buccal mucosa to the systemic circulation. Absorption of drugs was noted as early as 1847 by Sobrero via the mucous membranes of the oral cavity. The presence of nitroglycerine and systemic studies of oral cavity absorption were first reported by Walton in 1935 & 1944. The buccal region of the oral cavity is an attractive target for administration of the drug due to advantages associated with the bypass of first-pass metabolism and the avoidance of pre-systemic elimination within the gastrointestinal tract (Smart, 1993). Moreover, rapid onset of action can be achieved relative to the oral route and the formulation can be removed if therapy is required to be discontinued. It is also possible to administer drugs to patients who are unconscious and less cooperative. To avoid swallowing, various adhesive delivery systems are used including buccal tablets, buccal patches, lozenges and many other dosage forms with different combinations of polymers and absorption enhancers. Buccal route offers a passive system of drug absorption and does not require any activation. The presence of saliva ensures relatively large amount of water for drug dissolution unlike in case of rectal or transdermal routes. Systemic absorption is rapid as buccal mucosa is thin and highly perfused with blood and it provides an alternative route for the administration of various hormones, narcotics, analgesics, steroids, enzymes, cardiovascular agents etc. It allows the local modification of tissue permeability, inhibition of protease activity and reduction in immunogenic response. Thus, delivery of therapeutic agents like peptides, proteins and ionized species can also be done easily.

The oral mucosa is made up of an outermost layer of stratified squamous epithelium, which is covered with mucus and consists of stratum distendum, stratum filamentosum, stratum suprabasale, and a stratum basale (Fig. 6.2). Below this layer lies a basal lamina, the lamina propria followed by the submucosa as the innermost layer. The epithelium serves as a mechanical barrier protecting the underlying tissues whereas the lamina propria acts as a mechanical support and carries blood vessels and nerves. The stratified squamous epithelium has a mitotically active basal layer and produces different cell layers, where cells are shed from the surface of the epithelium. The epithelium is about 40-50 cell layers thick, while sublingual epithelium contains somewhat fewer layers. The epithelial cells increase in size and become flatter as they differentiate from the basal layers to the superficial layers. The turnover time for the oral mucosal epithelium has been estimated at 5-6 days. The oral mucosal thickness varies depending on the site: the buccal mucosa measures at 500-800 μm, while the mucosal thickness of the hard and soft palates, the floor of the mouth, the ventral tongue, and the gingival measure at about 100-200 μm. The non-keratinized regions of oral mucosa are soft sublingual palate, sublingual and buccal mucosa. These are more permeable than keratinized regions such as that of hard palate due to the composition of intercellular lipids comprising those particular regions. The keratinized epithelium contains predominantly the neutral lipids like ceramides and acylceramides which have been associated with the barrier function. These epithelia are relatively impermeable to water. The non-keratinized epithelia are composed of small amounts of neutral but polar lipids, mainly cholesterol sulfate and glucosyl ceramides. These epithelia have been found to be considerably more permeable to water than keratinized epithelia. Structure of oral mucosa consists of numerous racemose, mucous or serons glands present in the sub mucous tissue of the cheeks (Salamat-Miller et al., 2005).

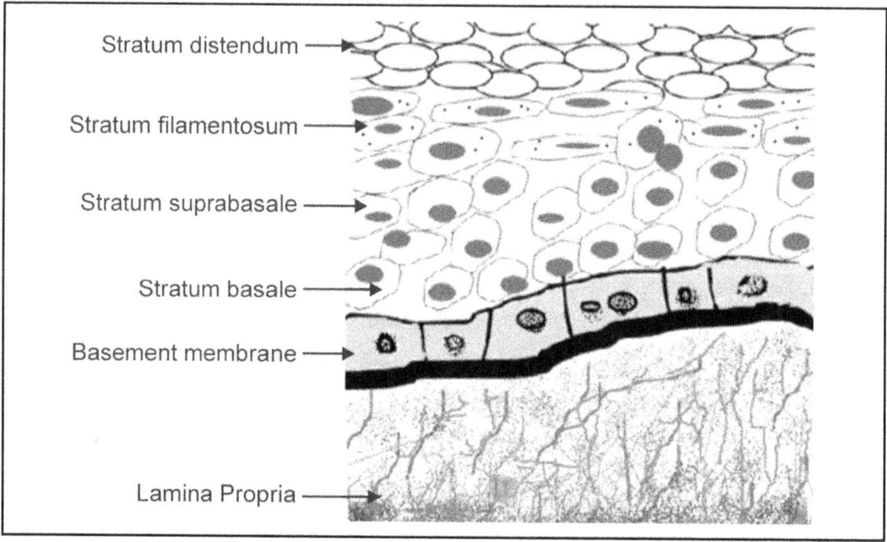

FIGURE 6.2 Structure of oral mucosa.

6.3.1 Mucoadhesion

Mucoadhesion may be defined as the state in which two materials, at least one of which is biological in nature, are held together for long period of time by interfacial forces. In the pharmaceutical sciences, when the adhesive attachment is to mucous or a mucous membrane, the phenomenon is referred to as mucoadhesion. Several theories have been developed in the formation of bioadhesive bonds and are based on the formation of mechanical bonds, while others focus on chemical interactions (Salamat-Miller et al., 2005; Woolfson et al., 2011).

6.3.1.1 The Electronic Theory

This assumes that bioadhesive material and the glycol-protein mucin network have different electronic structures. A charged double layer is formed at the interface of the mucus and the polymer due to the electron transfer. It results in attraction in the interface region and contributes to the inter diffusion of the two surfaces.

6.3.1.2 The Adsorption Theory

This is the most widely accepted theory of bioadhesion. According to the adsorption theory, these two surfaces adhere to each other due to a surface force between chemical structures of two surfaces after the initial contact. When polar molecules or groups are present, they change their orientation at the interface. Chemisorption can occur when adhesion is particularly strong. The theory maintains that adherence to tissue is due to the net force of one or more secondary factors i.e., Van der Waal's forces, hydrogen bonding, or hydrophobic bonding.

6.3.1.3 The Wetting Theory

It describes the ability of bioadhesive polymer to spread over a biological surface to develop intimate contact with the corresponding substrate for bond formation. This theory is used predominantly in liquid adhesives.

6.3.1.4 The Diffusion Theory

This theory is based on the formation of semi-permanent adhesive bonds due to interpenetration and entanglement of bioadhesive polymer chains and mucus polymer chain. The depth of penetration of polymer chains increase with the bond strength. The bioadhesive polymers and mucus should have similar chemical structures for the formation of strongest bioadhesive bond. For the diffusion to occur, it is important to have good solubility of one component in the other.

6.3.1.5 The Fracture Theory

This theory explains the force required for the detachment of polymers from the mucus which depends on the strength of the adhesive bond. This is the most useful theory for studying bioadhesion strength through tensile experiments. The maximum tensile stress produced during detachment is the ratio of maximum force of detachment and the total surface area involved in the adhesive interaction.

6.3.2 Basic Components of Mucoadhesive Buccal Tablets and Patches

The basic components of buccal drug delivery system are drug substance, bioadhesive polymers, permeation enhancers and backing membrane.

6.3.2.1 Drug Substance

While formulating buccal mucoadhesive tablets, one has to decide whether the intended action is for rapid release, prolonged release or for local or systemic effect. The selection of suitable drug for the design of buccal mucoadhesive tablets should be based on the pharmacokinetic properties. The drug should have following properties in order to be formulated as buccal tablets and patches:

(a) Drug should have molecular weight 1000 dalton or less.
(b) It should possess lipophilic and hydrophilic properties.
(c) Drug should be potent in nature.
(d) Half-life of the drug should be shorter.
(e) Drug should be non-irritant to oral mucosa.

6.3.2.2 Mucoadhesive Polymers

The first step in the development of mucoadhesive tablet is the selection and characterization of appropriate mucoadhesive polymers in the formulation. Mucoadhesive polymers play a major role in formulation of adhesive drug delivery systems. Polymers are also used in matrix devices in which the drug is embedded in the polymer matrix that controls the duration of release of drugs. These polymers are often water soluble and in a dry form attract water from the biological surface and this water transfer leads to a strong interaction. It also forms viscous liquids when hydrated with water that increases their retention time over mucosal surfaces and may lead to adhesive interactions. Mucoadhesive polymer should possess certain physicochemical properties like hydrophilicity, numerous hydrogen bond-forming groups, flexibility for interpenetration with mucus and epithelial tissue, and visco-elastic properties. The drug is released into the mucous membrane by means of rate controlling layer or core layer. Mucoadhesive polymers which adhere to the epithelial surface are effective and lead to significant improvement in the oral drug delivery. Table 6.1 depicts various mucoadhesive polymers used for the formulation of buccal tablets and patches (Morales and McConville, 2011; Sudhakar et al., 2006).

The mucoadhesive polymers used for the formulation of buccal tablets should have following characteristic:

(a) Mucoadhesive polymer should be compatible with the drug and other excipients.

(b) Polymer and its degradation products should be non-toxic and non-irritant.

(c) It should have good spreadability, wetting, swelling, solubility and bio-degradability.

(d) Mucoadhesive polymer should adhere quickly to buccal mucosa and should possess sufficient mechanical strength.

(e) It should possess peel, tensile and shear strengths at the mucoadhesive range.

(f) It should show mucoadhesive properties in both dry and liquid state and should possess adhesively active groups.

(g) Mucoadhesive polymer should be sufficiently cross-linked but not to the degree of suppression of bond forming groups.

(h) Polymer must be easily available and non-expensive.

(i) It should demonstrate local enzyme inhibition and penetration enhancement properties.

(j) It should have optimum molecular weight, required spatial conformation and acceptable shelf life.

TABLE 6.1

Mucoadhesive polymers used in formulation of mucoadhesive tablets and patches

Criteria	Category	Examples
Source	Natural	Agarose, chitosan, gelatin, hyaluronic acid and various gums (guar gum, hakea, xanthan gum, gellan gum, carragenan, pectin and sodium alginate)
	Synthetic	**Cellulose derivatives** Carboxymethyl cellulose (CMC), thiolated CMC, sodium CMC, hydroxy ethyl cellulose (HEC), hydroxy propyl cellulose (HPC), hydroxy propyl methyl cellulose (HPMC), methyl cellulose, methyl hydroxyl ethyl cellulose.

TABLE 6.1 *Contd...*

Criteria	Category	Example
		Poly(acrylic acid)-based polymers Carbopol (CP), propyl cellulose, *Poly(acrylic acid)*, polyacrylates, poly (methylvinylether-co-methacrylic acid), poly (2-hydroxyethyl methacrylate), poly (acrylic acid-co-ethylhexylacrylate), poly (methacrylate), poly (alkylcyanoacrylate), poly (isohexylcyanoacrylate), poly (isobutylcyanoacrylate), copolymer of acrylic acid and PEG, polyoxyethylene, Poly vinyl alcohol (PVA), Poly vinyl pyrrolidone (PVP), thiolated polymer.
Aqueous solubility	Water soluble	CP, HEC, HPC, HPMC (in cold water), *Poly (acrylic acid)*, sodium CMC, sodium alginate.
	Water insoluble	Chitosan (soluble in dilute aqueous acids), ethyl cellulose, propyl cellulose.
Charge	Cationic	Aminodextran, chitosan, (DEAE)-dextran, trimethylene carbonate (TMC)
	Anionic	Chitosan-EDTA, CP, CMC, pectin, sodium alginate, sodium CMC, xanthan gum
	Non-ionic	Hydroxyethyl starch, HPC, poly (ethylene oxide), PVA, PVP, Scleroglucan.
Potential mucoadhesive forces	Covalent	Cyanoacrylate
	Hydrogen bond	Acrylates [hydroxylated methacrylate, poly(methacrylic acid)], CP, propyl cellulose, PVA
	Electrostatic interaction	Chitosan

6.3.2.3 Permeation Enhancers

These are the substances which facilitate or increase the permeation of drugs through mucosa. Table 6.2 summarizes various permeation enhancers which are used to increase permeation (Morales and McConville, 2011; Sudhakar et al., 2006). Membrane permeation is the limiting factor for many drugs in the development of mucoadhesive delivery system. The epithelium that lines the mucosa is an effective barrier to the absorption of drugs especially buccal mucosa. The efficacy of enhancer at one site is not same to the other site because of the differences in cellular morphology, membrane thickness, enzymatic activity, lipid composition and potential protein interactions as well as structural and functional properties. The mechanism of permeation enhancer should be one of the following:

(a) Some permeation enhancers act by reducing the viscosity of the mucus and saliva which ultimately increase the dissolution and absorption.

(b) By increasing the fluidity of lipid bilayer membrane due to change in the intracellular lipid packing by interaction with either lipid or protein components.

(c) Acting on the components at tight junction of the lipid layer by inhibiting the various peptidases and proteases present within buccal mucosa, thereby overcoming the enzymatic barrier.

(d) Some enhancers increase the solubility of drug and thereby alter the partition coefficient.

TABLE 6.2

List of various permeation enhancers

Category	Examples
Chelators	EDTA, citric acid, sodium salicylates, methoxy salicylates
Surfactants	Sodium lauryl sulphate, polyoxyethylene, polyoxyethylene-9-laurylether, polyoxythylene-20-cetylether, benzalkonium chloride, 23-lauryl ether, cetylpyridinium chloride, cetyltrimethyl ammonium bromide.
Bile Salts	Sodium glycocholate, sodium deoxycholate, sodium taurocholate, sodium glycodeoxycholate, sodium taurodeoxycholate.
Fatty Acids	Oleic acid, capric acid, lauric acid, lauric acid with propylene glycol, methyloleate, lysophosphatidylcholine, phosphatidylcholine.
Thiolated Polymers	Chitosan-4-thiobutylamide, chitosan-cysteine, poly (acrylic acid)-homocysteine, polycarbophil-cysteine, polycarbophil-cysteine with glutathione, chitosan-4-thioethylamide with glutathione, chitosan- 4-thioglycholic acid.
Others	Aprotinin, azone, cyclodextrin, dextran sulfate, menthol, polysorbate 80, sulfoxides and various alkyl glycosides.

6.3.2.4 Backing Membrane

Backing membrane plays a major role in the attachment of mucoadhesive devices to the mucus membrane. The materials used as backing membrane should be inert and impermeable to the drug and penetration enhancer. Such impermeable membrane on buccal mucoadhesive patches prevents the drug loss and offers better patient compliance. The commonly used materials in backing membrane include CB, magnesium stearate, HPMC, HPC, CMC and polycarbophil.

6.3.3 Advantages of Buccal Tablets and Buccal Patches

(a) Drugs, which show poor bioavailability via the oral route, can be administered conveniently, e.g., drugs which are unstable in the acidic environment of the stomach or are destroyed by the enzymatic or alkaline environment of the intestine.

(b) Bypass of the gastrointestinal tract and hepatic portal system, increasing the bioavailability of orally administered drugs that otherwise undergo hepatic first-pass metabolism.

(c) Patient compliance due to the elimination of associated pain with injections.

(d) A relatively rapid onset of action can be achieved compared to the oral route.

(e) Can be used in case of unconscious and less co-operative patients.

(f) A sustained drug delivery system be formulated using various combinations of biodegradable polymers.

(g) Formulation can be removed if therapy is required to be discontinued.

(h) Increased ease of drug administration.

(i) The large contact surface of the oral cavity contributes to rapid and extensive drug absorption.

6.3.4 Formulation of Mucoadhesive Buccal Tablet

Buccal tablets are small, flat, oval shaped and are retained in position until dissolution and release is complete. Tablets can be applied to different regions of oral cavity, such as cheeks, lips, gums, and palate. Unlike conventional tablets, buccal tablets allow drinking, eating, and speaking without any major discomfort. Mucoadhesive polymer is used for the tablet to adhere the tablet to oral cavity.

The formulation of mucoadhesive buccal tablet can be done by three processes same as conventional tablet formulation i.e., wet granulation, dry granulation, and direct compression. Mucoadhesive tablets are usually prepared by direct compression, but wet granulation techniques can also be used. Tablets intended for buccal administration by insertion into the buccal pouch may dissolve or erode slowly; therefore, they are formulated and compressed with sufficient pressure only to give a hard tablet. In order to achieve unidirectional release, every face of the tablet, except the one that is in contact with the buccal mucosa, can be coated with water impermeable materials backing membrane, such as ethyl cellulose or hydrogenated castor oil, using either compression or spray coating. Multilayered tablets may be prepared by sequentially adding and compressing the ingredients layer by layer. If necessary, the drug may be formulated in certain physical states, such as microspheres, prior to direct compression in order to achieve some desirable properties, e.g., enhanced activity and prolonged drug release. Some newer approaches use tablets that melt at body temperatures. The matrix of the tablet is solidified while the drug is in solution. After melting, the drug automatically appears in solution form and is available for absorption, thus eliminating dissolution as a rate-limiting step in the absorption of poorly soluble compounds. Table 6.3 comprised the various marketed products based on buccal tablets technology along with name of their manufactures (Madhav et al., 2009; Robinson, 2005; Sudhakar et al., 2006).

TABLE 6.3

Various products based on buccal tablets available in market

Marketed brand	Drug	Manufacturer	Uses
Striant®	Testosterone	Columbia Labs	Hormone replacement in hypogonadal men.
Buccastem	Prochlorperazine	Alliance Pharmaceuticals	Treatment and prevention of nausea and vomiting due to any cause, including migraine.
Asftach®	Triamcinolone acetonide		Treatment of aphthous ulcers
Effentora	Fentanyl	Cephalon Inc, France	Opioid analgesic
Suscard	Glyceryl trinitrate	Forest Laboratories Limited, UK	Prevent chest pain caused by angina pectoris
Oravig	Miconazole	Par Pharmaceuticals	Treatment of Oropharyngeal Candidiasis
Striant SR	Testosterone	Columbia Labs	Hormone replacement in hypogonadal men
Fentora®	Fentanyl citrate	Cephalon Inc, France	Potent opioid analgesic

6.3.5 Evaluation of Buccal Tablets

The buccal tablets are to be evaluated for the following studies after preparation.

6.3.5.1 Weight Variation

The weight of the prepared tablets is routinely measured to help ensure that a tablet contains the proper amount of drug. Composite samples of the tablets are to be taken and weighed throughout the compression process. The tablets should pass the weight variation limits provided by Indian Pharmacopoeia or other regulatory guidelines.

6.3.5.2 Thickness

The thickness of three randomly selected buccal tablets from every batch needs to be determined in mm using vernier callipers. The average thickness is calculated.

6.3.5.3 Hardness

The hardness test of tablets is performed by placing the tablet in between the two anvils, force is then applied and the crushing strength that just causes the tablet to break is recorded. Several devices operating in this manner to test the tablet hardness are the Monsanto tester, the Strong-Cobb tester, the Pfizer tester and the Erweka tester. Newer machines have been introduced in the markets which are completely automatic in nature. The tablet sample is to be kept in the machine and the result of hardness test is retrieved from the computer attached with the machine.

6.3.5.4 Friability

The laboratory friability tester known as the Roche friabilator can be used to test the friability of tablets where the tablets are subjected to abrasion and shock by utilizing a revolving plastic chamber.

6.3.5.5 Drug Content

The drug content is determined by dissolving the tablets in appropriate solvent. The amount of drug present in the solvent is estimated after filtration using a UV spectrophotometer or HPLC.

6.3.5.6 Stability Studies

Stability studies are performed as per ICH guidelines by placing the tablets in an amber colored bottle by wrapping them in an aluminium foil. The tablets are to be stored at 40 °C, 75 ± 5% RH for 6 months. Every month the sample tablets should be taken out and tested for physical characteristics, bioadhesion strength, drug content and *in vitro* drug release. Stability study data obtained is to be compared with that obtained at zero time at ambient temperature. The results are analyzed with statistical correlation.

6.4 Buccal Patches

Buccal-adhesive patches may be up to 10-15 cm^2 in size, but are more usually 1-3 cm^2 so as to be convenient and comfortable for the patient (Fig. 6.3). An ideal buccal film should be flexible, elastic, soft yet adequately strong to withstand breakage due to stress from mouth activities. Moreover, it must possess good bioadhesive strength so that it can be retained in the mouth for a desired duration. Buccal patches consist of two laminates, with an aqueous solution of the adhesive polymer being cast onto an impermeable backing sheet. The backing sheet is used to control the direction of drug release, prevent drug loss, and minimize deformation and disintegration of the device during the application period (Robinson, 2005). A novel mucosal adhesive film called "Zilactin" consisting of an alcoholic solution of HPC and three organic acids, if applied to the oral mucosal, can be retained in place for at least 12 hours even when it is challenged with fluids.

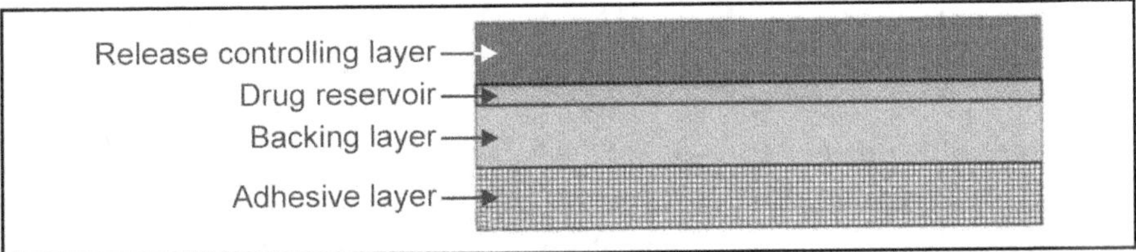

FIGURE 6.3 Various layers of buccal patches.

6.4.1 Method of Preparation

There are two methods to prepare adhesive patches.

6.4.1.1 Solvent Casting

In this method, all patch excipients including the drug is co-dispersed in an organic solvent and coated onto a sheet of release liner. After solvent evaporation a thin layer of the protective backing material is laminated onto the sheet of coated release liner to form a laminate that is die-cut to form patches of the desired size and geometry.

6.4.1.2 Direct Milling

In this, patches are manufactured without the use of solvents. Drug and excipients are mechanically mixed by direct milling or by kneading, usually without the presence of any liquid(s). After mixing process, the resultant material is rolled on a release liner until the desired thickness is achieved. The backing material is then laminated as previously described.

While there are only minor or even no differences in patch performance between patches fabricated by the two processes, the solvent-free process is preferred because there is no possibility of residual solvents and consequent health issues.

Laminated patches to deliver drugs (specifically peptides) through the oral mucosa have been described by Anders and Merkle. They developed patches consisting of two-ply laminates, with an aqueous solution of the adhesive polymer being cast onto an impermeable backing sheet which was then cut to the required oval shape. The adhesive polymers used were HPMC, HEC, PVA and PVP and contained in addition a plasticiser and the active drug. These patches adhered to the buccal mucosa in vivo for up to an hour, although this may be considered too short period with regard to the optimal delivery of peptides.

Adhesive plaster have been described in literature consisting of a mucosal adhesive drug reservoir formulation attached to an inert backing, which achieved a sustained delivery of a prostaglandin to the gingival mucosa of an animal model for over 8 hours without any sign of irritation. A three-layered tape dosage form has been described that consists of a backing layer of EC and castor oil, a middle layer of butyl rubber, and an adhesive layer containing karaya gum. This was prepared by casting a solution containing EC and castor oil dissolved in butanone onto a glass plate, allowing the solvent to evaporate and then casting the components of the second two layers dissolved in the appropriate solvents on top of this. The active drug (e.g., an antibiotic) is either included in the adhesive layer or deposited onto the tape prior to application. Such tape has been successfully used to treat stomatitis and other oral conditions (Nagai and Konishi, 1987). A bioadhesive multilayered extruded film [containing HPC, poly(ethylene oxide), EC (or another water-insoluble polymer), a plasticizer and a drug] has also been investigated with a view to achieve local therapy in the oral cavity.

6.4.2 Evaluation of Buccal Patches

6.4.2.1 Surface pH

Patches are left to swell for 2 hr on the surface of an agar plate. The surface pH is measured by means of a pH paper placed on the surface of the swollen patch.

6.4.2.2 Thickness

The thickness of each film is measured at five different locations (center and four corners) using an electronic digital micrometer.

6.4.2.3 Swelling Index

Buccal patches are weighed individually, and placed separately in 2% agar gel plates, incubated at 37 ± 1°C, and examined for any physical changes. At regular 1 hour time intervals until 3 hours, patches are removed from the gel plates and excess surface water is removed carefully using the filter paper. The swollen patches are then reweighed and the swelling index (SI) is calculated using the following formula.

$$SI = \frac{Wf - Wi}{Wi} \times 100$$

Where SI: swelling index, Wf: final weight, Wi: initial weight

6.4.2.4 Common Parameters for Evaluation of Buccal Tablets and Buccal Patches

There are some parameters which are used to evaluate both buccal tablet and buccal patches such as disintegration test, dissolution, residence time and permeation study.

6.4.2.4.1 Disintegration Test

Disintegration tests are usually performed for rapid dissolving tablets and patches to determine the disintegration rate when they come in contact with the mucus and saliva. There are two approaches which are used to check disintegration time. First approach disintegration test using a texture analyzer (TA), consisting of a 35 mm tall flat-ended acrylic cylindrical probe with 2 kg load cell (Fig. 6.4). The tablet is attached to a cylindrical probe and placed under a constant force to promote disintegration. The tablet is immersed into a defined volume of medium (200 µl) and the time for complete tablet disintegration versus distance traveled is determined. The main drawback of this method is one side of the tablet or patches is attached to the probe and cannot come in contact with the disintegrating medium, but in the oral cavity it is moistened on all sides.

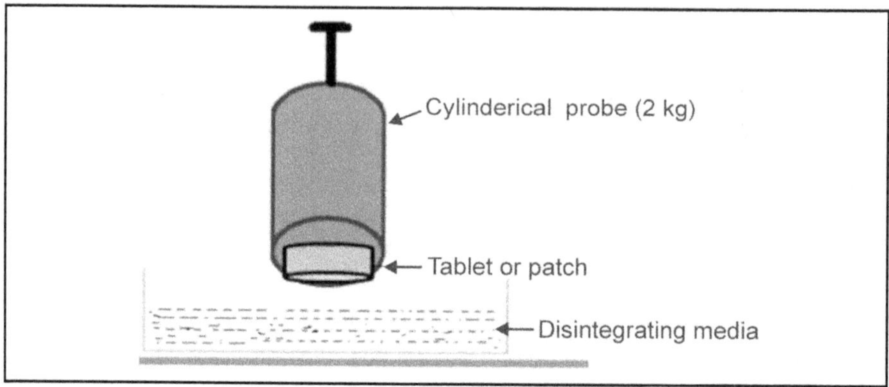

FIGURE 6.4 Disintegration test apparatus based on texture analyser.

To overcome the limitations, researcher modified the operation of the TA to mimic the *in vivo* movement of tablets in the mouth (Abdelbary et al., 2005). In this method tablet or patch is placed on a perforated grid where the tablet is completely dry and is not in contact with the disintegration medium. The flat ended cylindrical probe descends and comes in contact with water and pushes the whole system downwards into the liquid medium and tablet disintegration starts. At this point, the TA apparatus is set to maintain a predetermined nominal force (50 g) for a given period of time (60 s). Typical time-distance profiles generated by the texture analysis software are obtained, thus enabling the calculation of the starting and ending disintegration times. In this method as the tablet disintegrates, the particles that are detached during the process pass through the holes of the grid. This simulates an *in vivo* oral disintegration pattern where these particles are progressively swallowed or diffused through the oral mucosa.

6.4.2.4.2   Dissolution Test

Several studies have been performed to investigate drug dissolution in smaller volumes or using different apparatus. Franz diffusion cell were used to study the release of nicotine from buccal tablets (Fig. 6.5) (İkinci et al., 2004). The dissolution medium is 22 ml phosphate buffer saline (PBS) pH 7.4 at 37 °C. Uniform mixing of the medium is provided by magnetic stirring at 300 rpm. To provide unidirectional release, each bioadhesive tablet is embedded into paraffin wax which is placed on top of a bovine buccal mucosa as membrane.

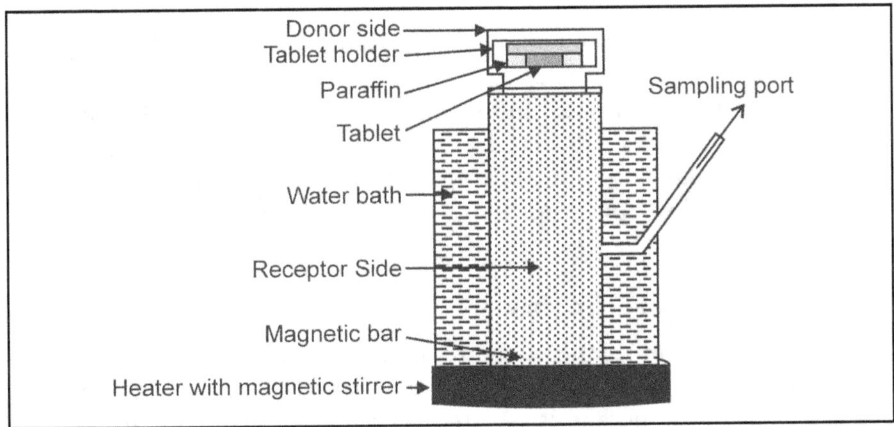

FIGURE 6.5 Dissolution test apparatus.

One another approach based on the circulation of pre-warmed dissolution medium through a cell. Here the buccal tablet is attached on the tissue collected from chicken. Samples are removed at different time intervals for drug content analysis (Patel et al., 2012).

6.4.2.4.3 Residence Time

A modified USP dissolution apparatus is used for the determination of residence time in which 800 ml isotonic phosphate buffer (pH 6.75) dissolution medium is maintained at 37°C. A segment of rabbit intestinal mucosa (3 cm long), is glued to the surface of a glass slab, vertically attached to the apparatus (Fig. 6.6). Hydrated surface from buccal tablet is brought in contact with the membrane and the time necessary for complete erosion or detachment of the tablet from the mucosal surface is recorded (Nair et al., 2013).

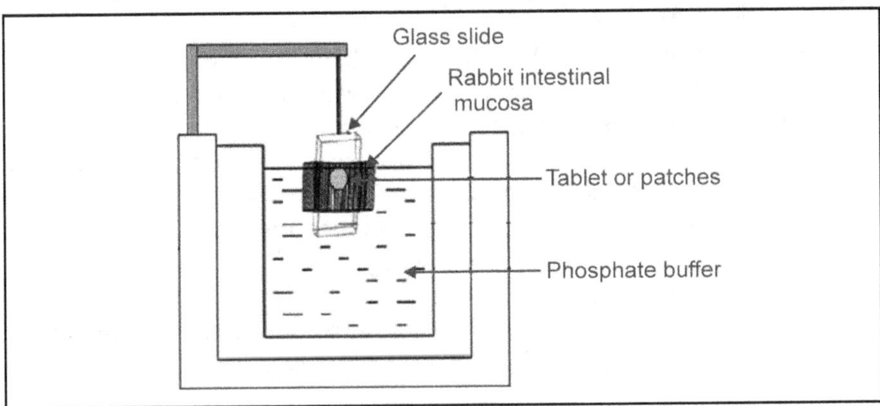

FIGURE 6.6 Apparatus for determination of residence time.

In vivo residence test is performed by placing the formulation on the buccal mucosa between the cheek and gingiva in the region of the upper canine and gently pressed onto the mucosa for about 30 seconds. Afterwards volunteers are asked to note any tendency for detachment. The time necessary for complete erosion of the tablet is monitored by carefully observing for residual polymer on the mucosa (Patel et al., 2012).

6.4.2.4.4   Permeation Studies

Buccal mucosa of experimental animal species with underlying connective tissue is surgically removed from the oral cavity and the buccal mucosal membrane is isolated. The membrane is mounted in the diffusion cells for *in-vitro* permeation experiments.

6.5   Osmotic Tablet

Osmotic drug delivery systems and devices are an advanced drug delivery technology that uses osmotic pressure as the driving force to deliver pharmacotherapy in several therapeutic areas. Osmosis can be defined as the net movement of water across a selectively permeable membrane driven by a difference in osmotic pressure across the membrane. The pressure applied to the higher-concentration side to inhibit solvent flow is called the osmotic pressure. It is driven by a difference in solute concentrations across the membrane that allows passage of water, but rejects most solute molecules or ions (Malaterre et al., 2009; Verma et al., 2004).

6.5.1 Osmosis and its Principal

Osmotic tablets are designed on the principle of osmotic pressure for drug delivery. The first osmotic effect was reported by Abbe Nollet in 1748. Later in 1877, Pfeffer performed an experiment using semi-permeable membrane to separate sugar solution from pure water. He showed that the osmotic pressure of the sugar solution is directly proportional to the solution concentration and the absolute temperature. In 1886, Vant Hoff identified an underlying proportionality between osmotic pressure, concentration and temperature. According to that osmotic pressure is proportional to concentration and temperature and the relationship can be described by following equation (Sastry Srikonda, 2006).

$$\Pi = pc\,RT \qquad\qquad .....(1)$$

Where,

p = Osmotic pressure Π = osmotic coefficient

c = molar concentration R = gas constant

T = Absolute temperature

Osmotic pressure is a colligative property, which depends on concentration of solute that contributes to osmotic pressure. Solutions of different concentrations having the same solute and solvent system exhibit an osmotic pressure proportional to their concentrations. Thus a constant osmotic pressure and thereby a constant influx of water can be achieved by an osmotic delivery system that results in a constant zero order release rate of drug.

6.5.2 Historical Aspects of Osmotic Pumps

About 75 years after discovery of the osmosis principle, it was first used in the design of drug delivery systems. Rose and Nelson, the Australian scientists, were initiators of osmotic drug delivery. In 1955, they developed an implantable pump as shown below Fig. 6.7, which consisted of three chambers: a drug chamber, a salt chamber contains excess solid salt and a water chamber. The drug and water chambers are separated by rigid semipermeable membrane. The difference in osmotic pressure across the membrane moves water from the water chamber into the salt chamber. The volume of the salt chamber increases because of this water flow, which distends the latex diaphragm separating the salt and drug chambers, thereby pumping drug out of the device. The design and mechanism of this pump is comparable to modern push-pull osmotic pump. The major disadvantage of this pump was the water chamber, which must be charged before use of the pump. The pumping rate of this push-pull pump is given by the equation (Eckenhoff, 1987; Gupta et al., 2010; Sastry Srikonda, 2006).

$$\frac{dM}{dt} = \frac{dV}{dt} \times C$$

.....(2)

Where,

dM/dt = Mass release

dV/dt = Volumetric pumping rate

c = Concentration of drug

But,

$$\frac{dV}{dt} = \left(\frac{A}{h}\right) L_p \ (\sigma\Delta\Pi - \Delta p) \qquad\qquad .....(3)$$

Where,

A = membrane area,

h = thickness of membrane

L_p = mechanical permeability

σ = reflection coefficient

$\Delta\Pi$ = osmotic pressure difference

Δp = hydrostatic pressure difference

As the size of orifice delivery increases, Δp decreases, so $\Delta\Pi \gg \Delta p$ and equation becomes

$$\frac{dV}{dt} = \left(\frac{A}{h}\right) L_p \ (\sigma\Delta\Pi) \qquad\qquad .....(4)$$

When the osmotic pressure of the formulation is large compared to the osmotic pressure of the environment, p can be substituted for Δp.

$$\frac{dV}{dt} = \left(\frac{A}{h}\right) L_p \ (\sigma\Pi) = \left(\frac{A}{h}\right) k\Pi \qquad\qquad .....(5)$$

($k = L_p\sigma$ = membrane permeability)

Now, equation (5) can be given as

$$\frac{dV}{dt} = \left(\frac{A}{h}\right) k\Pi c = \left(\frac{A}{h}\right) k\Pi S \qquad\qquad .....(6)$$

(S = solubility of drug, c taken as S)

In general, this equation, with or without some modifications, applies to all other type of osmotic systems.

Several simplifications in Rose-Nelson pump were made by Alza Corporation in early 1970s. The Higuchi-Leeper pump is modified version of Rose-Nelson pump. It has no water chamber, and the device is activated by water imbibed from the surrounding environment. The pump is activated when it is swallowed or implanted in the body. This pump consists of a rigid housing, and the semipermeable membrane is supported on a perforated frame. It has a salt chamber containing a fluid solution with excess solid salt. Recent modification in Higuchi-Leeper pump accommodated pulsatile drug delivery. The pulsatile release is achieved by the production of a critical pressure at which the delivery orifice opens and releases the drug.

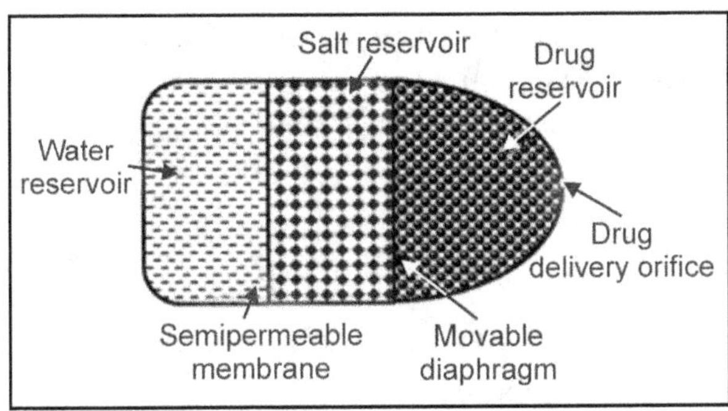

FIGURE 6.7 Rose-Nelson pump.

Further simplified variant of Rose-Nelson pump was developed by Higuchi and Theeuwes. This pump comprises a rigid, rate controlling outer semipermeable membrane surrounding a solid layer of salt coated on the inside by an elastic diaphragm and on the outside by the membrane. In use, water is osmotically drawn by the salt chamber, forcing drug from the drug chamber.

In 1975, the major leap in osmotic delivery occurred with the introduction of the elementary osmotic pump (EOP) for oral delivery of drugs was introduced.

Apart from oral osmotic pumps, the development of miniature implantable osmotic pumps in the mid-1970s was a major breakthrough to deliver wide range of drugs and hormones, including peptides at constant and programmed rate in mice, rat and larger animals. These implants provide a convective stream of drug solution that can be directed through suitable catheter connections to sites in the animal, remote from itself. Most recently the implantable pumps for human use are developed to deliver the drug for targeting or systemic application.

6.5.3 Advantages of Osmotic Tablets

(a) The delivery rate of zero-order is achievable with osmotic systems.

(b) Delivery may be delayed or pulsed, if desired.

(c) Drug release independent from physicochemical property of drug.

(d) Higher release rates are possible with osmotic systems compared to conventional diffusion-controlled drug delivery systems.

(e) The release rate of osmotic systems is highly predictable and can be programmed by controlling the release control parameters.

(f) For oral osmotic systems, drug release is independent of gastric pH and hydrodynamic conditions.

(g) The release from osmotic systems is minimally affected by the presence of food in gastrointestinal tract.

(h) A high degree of *in vivo-in vitro* correlation is obtained in osmotic systems.

6.5.4 Disadvantages

(a) Osmotic systems are expensive.

(b) Drug toxicity can occur due to dose dumping.

(c) Rapid development of tolerance.

(d) Reduce potential for dose adjustments

6.5.5 Components of Osmotic Tablets

The basic components for formulation of an osmotic tablet are drug, osmotic agent, semipermeable membrane, plasticizer, hydrophilic and hydrophobic polymer, wicking agent and flux regulators (Patra et al., 2012).

6.5.5.1 Drug

Drugs which are having short biological half-life (2-6 hr) and which are used for prolonged cure of diseases are suitable for osmotic tablet formulation. Moreover drug should be potent in nature. Various drugs such as nifedipine, glipizide, carbamazepine, metoprolol, oxprenolol, verapamil and chlorpromazine hydrochloride have been formulated as osmotic tablet.

6.5.5.2 Osmotic Agent

Osmotic agents or osmogen are essential ingredients of osmotic pump. Osmotic components usually are ionic compounds consisting of either inorganic salts or hydrophilic polymers. Osmotic pressures for concentrated solution of soluble solutes commonly used in controlled release formulations are extremely high, ranging from 30 atm for sodium phosphate up to 500 atm for a lactose-fructose mixture. Osmotic agents can be any salt such as sodium chloride, potassium chloride, or sulfates of sodium or potassium and lithium. Additionally, sugars such as glucose, sorbitol, or sucrose or inorganic salts of carbohydrates as well as hydrophilic polymers encompass osmopolymers, osmogels, or hydro-gels can act as osmotic agents. These materials maintain a concentration gradient across the membrane. They also generate a driving force for the uptake of water and assist in maintaining drug uniformity in the hydrated formulation. The polymers may be formulated along with poly (cellulose), osmotic solutes, or colorants such as ferric oxide. Further, hydrogels such as carbopol, cyanamer, and Aqua-Keeps may also be used. Finally, tableting aids such as binders, lubricants, and antioxidants may be added to aid in the manufacture of the osmotic systems. Different osmotic agents are classified in two categories with their osmotic pressure of saturated solution (Table 6.4) (Sastry Srikonda, 2006).

TABLE 6.4

Osmotic agents with osmotic pressure in their saturated solution.

Inorganic water soluble osmogen	Osmotic pressure (atm)	Organic water soluble osmogen	Osmotic pressure (atm)
Sodium chloride	356	Fructose	355
Potassium Chloride	245	Sucrose	150
Potassium phosphate	105	Dextrose	82
Potassium Sulphate	39	Mannitol	138
Sodium phosphate tribasic	36	Lactose-fructose	500
Sodium phosphate dibasic	31	Dextrose-fructose	450
Sodium phosphate dibasic anhydride	29	Sucrose- fructose	430
Sodium phosphate monobasic	28	Mannitol-fructose	415
		Mannitol- lactose	130
		Dextrose-sucrose	190
		Latose-sucrose	250

6.5.5.3 Semipermeable Membrane

Release of drug from the osmotic tablets is totally independent to the pH and movement of GIT, because of semipermeable membrane which only allows water to move across the membrane, and on the basis of osmotic pressure of water the drug is released. Selection of polymer is based on the solubility of drug as well as amount and rate of drug to be released from the pump. The permeability is the most important criteria for the selection of semi permeable membrane (Theeuwes; Felix 1974). The membrane must have certain performance criteria mentioned below:

(a) It should be adequately thick to withstand the pressure generated within the device.

(b) It should have enough wet strength and water permeability.

(c) It should be biocompatible.

(d) It should be rigid and non-swelling.

Cellulose polymers are mostly used as a semipermiable membrane because its nature is permeable to water but impermeable to solute (drug, organic and inorganic ions). The cellulosic polymers have a degree of substitution (DS) of 0 to 3 on the anhydroglucose unit. The DS is the number of hydroxyl groups present on the anhydroglucose unit being replaced by a substituting group. Examples of this group include cellulose acylate, cellulose diacylate, cellulose triacylate, cellulose acetate, cellulose diacetate, and mono-, di-, and tricellulose alkanylates. Different grades of cellulose acetate with different acetyl content usually 32 and 38% are mostly used as cellulosic polymers such as cellulose ethers, cellulose esters, and cellulose ester ethers. Cellulose acetate is available in different grades, such as cellulose acetate having a DS of 1 to 2 and an acetyl content of 21 to 35% or 32 to 39.8% (Eckenhoff, 1987).

6.5.5.4 Plasticizers

Plasticizers have a crucial role to play in the formation of a film coating and its final structure. Permeability and flexibility of membranes can be increased by adding plasticizer, which increases the water diffusion coefficient. Plasticizer is used from 0.001 to 50 parts or a mixture of plasticizers is incorporated into 100 parts of semipermeable film forming materials. They can change viscous-elastic behavior of polymers and these changes may affect the permeability of the polymeric films. Plasticizers can have a marked effect on the release of active materials from modified release dosage forms where they are incorporated into the rate controlling membrane. Some of the plasticizers used are polyethylene glycols, glycolate, glycerolate, myristates, ethylene glycol monoacetate, and diacetate for low permeability and tri ethyl citrate, diethyl tartarate or diacetin for more permeable film.

6.5.5.5 Hydrophilic and Hydrophobic Polymers

Osmotic pumps are suitable for delivery of drugs having intermediate water solubility. This is because the kinetics of osmotic drug release is directly related to solubility of drug within the core. Drugs for osmotic delivery should have water solubility in the desired range to get optimum drug release. However, by modulating the solubility of these drugs within the core, effective release patterns may be obtained, which might otherwise appear to be poor for osmotic delivery. Both hydrophilic and hydrophobic polymers are used to modulate the solubility of these drugs within the core. The selection of polymer is done on the basis of solubility of drug as well as the amount and rate of drug to be released from the pump. The highly water soluble API can be co-entrapped in hydrophobic matrices and moderately water soluble compounds can be co-entrapped in hydrophilic matrices to obtain optimum controlled release. Hydrophilic polymers such as hydroxyl ethyl cellulose, carboxy methyl cellulose, hydroxyl propyl methyl cellulose, polysaccharides and hydroxyl propy methyl cellulose are commonly used.

Hydrophobic polymers which are commonly used include ethyl cellulose, wax materials, Kollicoat, SR latex, Eudragit, styrene, butadiene, calcium phosphate, polysilicone, nylon, Teflon, polytetrafluoroethylene and halogenated polymers.

6.5.5.6 Wicking Agents

The wicking agent is one, which helps to increase the contact surface area of the drug with the incoming aqueous fluid. It is defined as a material with the ability to draw water into the porous network of a delivery device. The function of the wicking agent is to draw water to surfaces inside the core of the tablet, thereby creating channels or a network of increased surface area. Examples are colloidal silicon dioxide, kaolin, titanium dioxide, alumina, niacinamide, sodium lauryl sulphate, low molecular weight polyvinyl pyrrolidone, bentonite, magnesium aluminium silicate, polyester and polyethylene.

6.5.5.7 Flux Regulators

Flux regulating agents are added to the wall forming materials which assist in regulating the fluid permeability through membrane. Delivery systems can be designed to regulate the permeability of the fluid by incorporating flux-regulating agents in the layer. Hydrophilic substances such as polyethethylene glycols (300-6000 Da), polyhydric alcohols and polyalkylene glycols are generally used to improve the flux, whereas hydrophobic materials such as phthalates substituted with an alkyl or alkoxy (e.g., diethyl phthalate or dimethoxy ethylphthalate) tend to decrease the flux. Insoluble salts or insoluble oxides, which are substantially water-impermeable materials also, can be used for this purpose.

6.5.6 Classification of Osmotic Tablets

Osmotic tablets can be broadly classified into two categories:

A. Single chamber osmotic pump
- (a) Elementary osmotic pump
- (b) Controlled porosity osmotic pump
- (c) Osmotic bursting osmotic pump

B. Multi-chamber osmotic pump
- (a) Push pull osmotic pump
- (b) Sandwich osmotic tablets

6.5.6.1 Elementary Osmotic Pump

It was developed in the year 1975 by Theeuwes (Santus et al,1995). The Elementary Osmotic Pump (EOP) consists of single layered tablet core containing a water soluble drug with or without other osmotic agent (Fig 6.8). EOP is the most basic device made up of a compressed tablet. The EOP consists of an osmotic core with the drug, surrounded by a semipermeable membrane. The semipermeable membrane is provided with a hole for the controlled delivery of the saturated solution of the drug formed as a result of imbibition of water. The delivery rate is determined by the fluid permeability of the membrane and the osmotic pressure of the compressed tablet when the dosage form is placed in the aqueous environment. Normally, the EOP delivers 60-80% of its content at a constant rate with gradual hydration. EOP showed small lag time (30-60 min) before zero order drug release. The main limitation of the EOP is that semipermeable membrane should be 200-300 μm thick to withstand pressure & thick coatings lowers the water permeation rate. EOP is mostly applicable for water soluble drugs (Theeuwes, 1975).

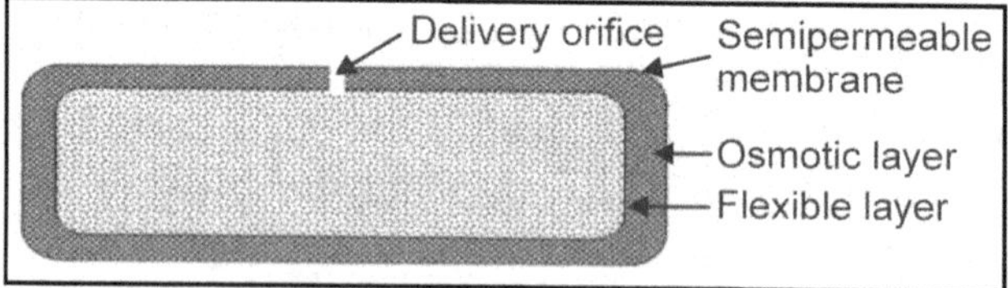

FIGURE 6.8 Diagram of elementary osmotic pump.

6.5.6.2 Controlled Porosity Osmotic Pump

The controlled porosity osmotic pump does not have any orifice initially but contains a semipermeable membrane with water soluble additives (Fig. 6.9). When placed in aqueous environment the water soluble component of coating dissolves and forms micropores in the membrane.

Water diffuses inside the core through microporous membrane, setting up an osmotic gradient and thereby controlling the release of drug. Generally, materials producing from 5 to 95% pores with a pore size ranging from 10Å-100 μm can be used. The resulting membrane is substantially permeable to both water and dissolved solute. Water-soluble additives used for this purpose are dimethyl sulfone, saccharides, amino acids and sorbitol (Qiu, 2009).

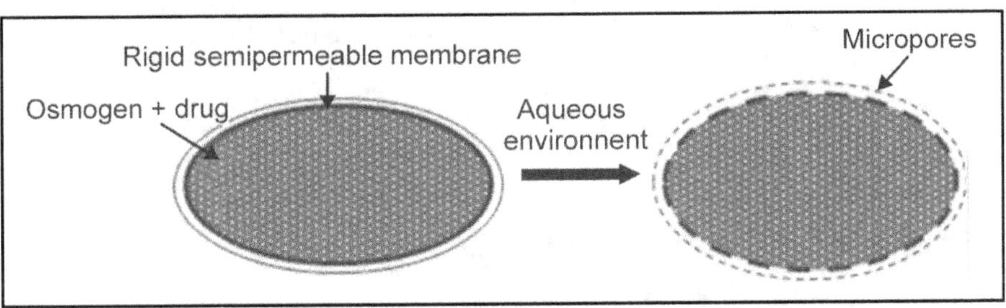

FIGURE 6.9 Controlled porosity osmotic pump.

6.5.6.3 Osmotic Bursting Osmotic Pump

This system is similar to an EOP except delivery orifice is absent and size may be smaller. When it is placed in an aqueous environment, water is imbibed and hydraulic pressure is built up inside until the wall rupture and the contents are released to the environment. Varying the thickness as well as the area the semi permeable membrane can control release of drug. This system is useful to provide pulsated release.

6.5.6.4 Push Pull Osmotic Pump

Push pull osmotic pump (PPOP) is a modified EOP (Fig. 6.10). EOP is limited to the delivery of relatively soluble drugs with solubility greater than about 2-10%, depending on dose. Through PPOP it becomes possible to deliver both poorly water soluble and highly water soluble drugs at a constant rate. This system has two layers like bilayer tablet. Upper layer contains drug in a matrix of polymer, osmotic agent and other tablet excipients and lower layer matrix contains all ingredients except drug. These layers are bonded together by tablet compression to form a single bilayer core. The tablet core is then coated with a semipermeable membrane. After the coating has been applied, a small hole is drilled through the membrane by a laser or mechanical drill on the drug layer side of the tablet. When the system is placed in aqueous environment water is attracted into the tablet by an osmotic agent in both the layers. The osmotic attraction in the drug layer pulls water into the compartment to form *in situ* a suspension of drug. The osmotic agent in the non-drug layer simultaneously attract water into that compartment, causing it to expand volumetrically and the expansion of non-drug layer pushes the drug suspension out of delivery orifice (Qiu, 2009).

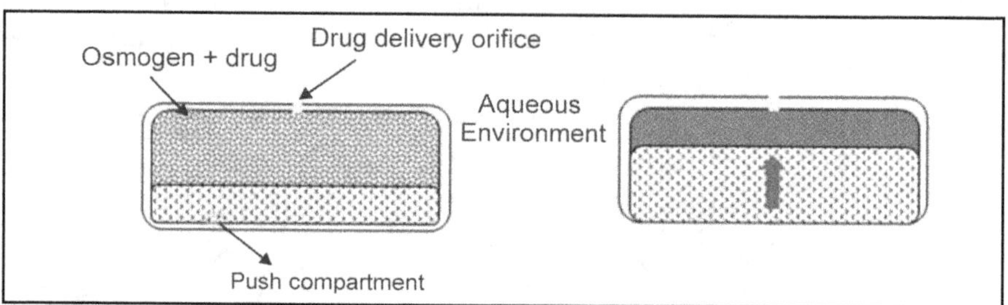

FIGURE 6.10 Push pull osmotic pump.

6.5.6.5 Sandwich Osmotic Tablets

Sandwich Osmotic Tablets (SOTS) composed of polymeric push layer sandwiched between two drug layers with two delivery orifices (Fig. 6.11). When placed in the aqueous environment the middle push layer containing the swelling agent swells and the drug is released from the two orifices situated on opposite sides of the tablet. SOTS can be suitable for drugs prone to cause local irritation of the gastric mucosa (Liu et al., 1999; Liu et al., 2000; Verma et al., 2002).

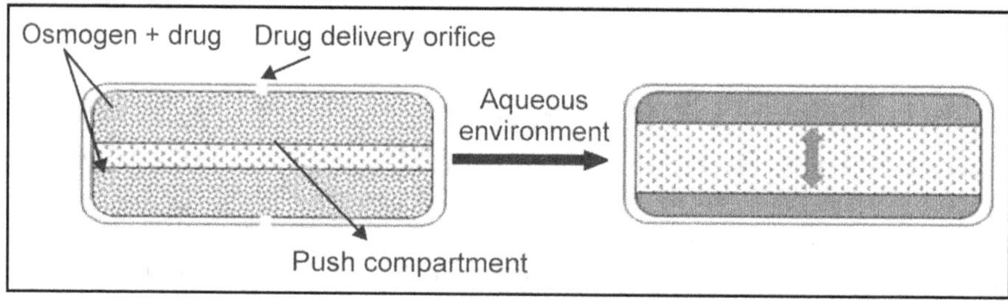

FIGURE 6.11 Sandwich osmotic pump.

6.5.7 Marketed Osmotically Controlled Tablets

ALZA Corporation (Mountain View, CA) pioneered the solid tablet osmotic dosage form in the 1970s. Currently, more than 10 products using EOS technology are marketed for the treatment of various conditions. Table 6.5 illustrates various formulations which are commercially available in market and are based on osmotic principle of delivery (Wong et al., 2003).

TABLE 6.5

List of commercially available osmotically controlled formulations (Gupta et al., 2010)

Brand name	Drug	Manufacturer	Uses
Alpress[R] LP	Prazosin	Novartis Pharmaceuticals	Treatment of hypertension
Cardura XL[R]	Doxazosin mesylate	Pfizer	Attention deficit hyperactivity disorder
Covera-HS[R]	Verapamil	GD Searle & Co.	Management of hypertension and angina
CalanSR	Verapamil	Pfizer	Management of essential hyper-tension
Ditropan XL[R]	Oxybutynin chloride	ALZA Pharmaceuticals	Treatment of overactive bladder with symptoms of urge urinary incontinence, urgency, and frequency
DynaCirc CR[R]	Isradipine	Novartis Pharmaceuticals	Treatment of hypertension
Efidac 24	Pseudoephiderine	Novartis Pharmaceuticals	Treatment of common cold, sinusitis, and hay fever and other respiratory allergies.
Glucotrol XL[R]	Glipizide	Pfizer	Treatment of hyperglycemia in patients with non-insulin-dependent diabetes.
Procardia XL[R]	Nifedipine	Pfizer	Treatment of angina and hypertension
Sudafed[R]	Pseudoephedrine HCL	Warner-Lambert Consumer Healthcare	Common cold, hay fever, and other respiratory allergies, and nasal congestion associated with sinusitis
Volmax[R]	Albuterol sulfate	Muro Pharmaceutical	Treatment of broncho-spasm in patients with reversible obstructive airway disease
Tegretol[R] XL	Carbamazepine	Novartis Pharmaceuticals	Anticonvulsant
Acutrim	Phenylpropanolamine	ALZA Pharmaceuticals	Treatment of congestion associ-ated with allergies, hay fever, sinus irritation, and the common cold.

6.6 Pulsincap

Pulsincap systems are based on the concept of pulsatile drug delivery system (PDDS). PDDS is defined as the rapid and transient release of certain amount of molecules within a short period of time, immediately after predetermined off-release periods i.e., lag time. Significant advantages of the PDDS are reduced dosing frequency, reduced side effects and drug targeting to specific sites like colon. PDDS deliver the drug at the required site of action at the right time and in the desired amount, thus providing spatial and temporal delivery, consequently enhance patient compliance. PDDS shows potential benefits for the diseases which are associated with circadian rhythms viz. rheumatoid arthritis, cardiovascular diseases, asthma, peptic ulcer and allergic rhinitis (Ahuja et al., 2006; Sharma et al., 2011; Stevens, 1998).

6.6.1 Types of Pulsincaps

A. Predetermined PDDS
  (a) Osmosis dependent
  (b) Erodible or rupturable layer dependent
  (c) Capsule shell dependent

B. Induced PDDS
  (a) pH induced
  (b) Temperature induced
  (c) Chemically induced
  (d) Externally induced

Pulsincap device comes under erodible or rupturable layer dependent PDDS. Pulsincap system consists of a water insoluble capsule body and water soluble cap having an acid insoluble coating. This capsule encloses a drug reservoir and the capsule body is closed at one end by a hydrogel plug (Fig. 6.12). Hydrogel plug is swellable and degradable in nature. Plug is made-up of substances such as hydrophilic polymer or lipid. It begins to swell when the capsule comes in contact with the dissolution fluid, after a specific time period of time, known as lag time. After this lag time the plug pushes itself outside the capsule and the drug is rapidly released. The lag time of the plug basically depends on the dimension, insert thickness and position of the plug. The plug material consists of insoluble but permeable and swellable polymers (e.g., poly-methacrylates), erodible compressed polymers (eg. hydroxypropylmethyl cellulose, polyvinyl alcohol, polyvinyl acetate, polyethylene oxide) and congealed melted polymers (e.g., saturated polyglycolated glycerides, glyceryl monooleate) (Stevens, 2003).

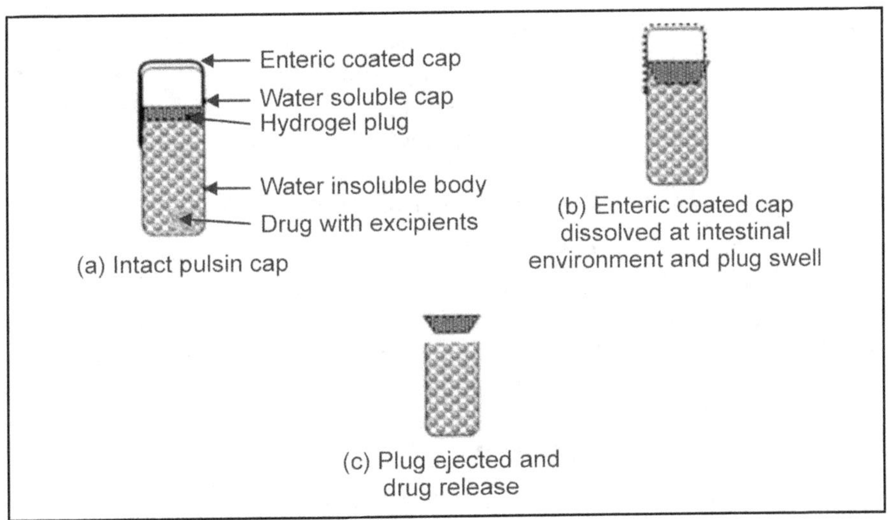

FIGURE 6.12 Release of drug from Pulsincap.

These formulations are well tolerated in animals and healthy volunteers, and there have been no reports of gastro-intestinal irritation or any other side effects. However, there is a potential problem of variable gastric residence time, which is solved by enteric coating layer at the outer coat. The system allows its dissolution in the basic pH region of intestine. Physicochemical characterization parameters of hydrogel plug include hardness, lag time, swelling Index and water uptake study. Release of the drug from the system is mainly determined by the swelling index of the plug (Bussemer et al., 2003).

6.6.1.1 Osmosis Dependent Pulsincap

It consists of a gelatin capsule coated with a semi permeable membrane (e.g.: cellulose acetate) housing an insoluble plug and an osmotically active agent along with the drug and excipients. When it comes in contact with the aqueous medium, water diffuses across the semi permeable membrane, resulting in increased inner pressure that ejects the plug after a time lag. The time lag is controlled by the thickness of semipermeable membrane.

6.6.1.2 Erodible or Rupturable Layer Dependent Pulsincap

This is a multiparticulate system in which drug is coated on non-pareil sugar seeds followed by a swellable layer and a rupturable insoluble top layer. The swelling agents used include sodium carboxymethyl cellulose, sodium starch glycollate and L-hydroxypropyl cellulose. Upon ingress of water, the swellable layer expands, resulting in rupture of film with subsequent rapid drug release. The release is independent of environmental factors like pH and drug solubility. The lag time can be varied by changing coating thickness or adding high amounts of lipophilic plasticizer in the outermost layer (Ueda et al., 1994).

6.6.1.3 Capsule Shell Dependent Pulsincap

Capsule based pulsincap system consists of an insoluble capsule body and swellable and degradable plug which is made of approved substances such as hydrophilic polymers or lipids. The lag time is controlled by plug, which is pushed away by swelling or erosion and drug is released as a pulse from the insoluble capsule (Krogel and Bodmeier, 1999)

6.6.1.4 pH Induced Pulsincap

Such type of pulsatile drug delivery system contains two components one is of immediate release type and other one is pulsed release type which releases the drug in response to change in pH. In the case of pH dependent system advantage has been taken of the fact that there exists a different pH environment at different parts of the GI tract. Thus, by selecting the pH dependent polymers, drug release at specific locations can be obtained. Examples of pH-dependent polymers include cellulose acetate phthalate, Eudragit L100, Eudragit S100, HPMC phthalate, HPMC trimellitate, HPMC acetate maleate and polyvinyl acetate phthalate. These polymers are used as enteric coating materials so as to provide release of drug in the small intestine (Sharma et al., 2011).

6.6.1.5 Temperature Induced Pulsincap

Thermo responsive hydrogel systems have been developed for pulsatile release. In these systems the polymer undergoes swelling or deswelling phase in response to the temperature which modulate drug release in swollen state.

6.6.1.6 Chemically Induced Pulsincap

Chemical stress is one of the most widely utilized triggering signals for a variety of triggered or PDDS. A biochemical change in the physiology of human beings is utilized as a stimulus for triggering drug release from the pulsatile system. They are further classified into glucose-responsive insulin release devices, inflammation-induced pulsatile release and drug release from intelligent gels responding to antibody concentration (Gandhi et al., 2011).

6.6.1.7 Externally Induced Pulsincap

For releasing the drug in a pulsatile manner, another way can be the externally regulated systems in which drug release is programmed by external stimuli like magnetism, ultrasound, electrical effect and irradiation.

6.6.2 Evaluation of Pulsincap

6.6.2.1 Swelling Index

In order to determine the swelling index of the plug, it is kept in different pH conditions and then plug is taken out after different time intervals and is weighed carefully[5]. The following formula is used for the calculation of swelling index.

$$\% \ SI = \frac{W_w - W_d}{W_w} \times 100$$

Where,   SI: Swelling Index, W_w: Wet weight, W_d: Dry weight

6.6.2.2 Lag Time and Drug Release

Lag time and drug release of pulsatile capsule is determined by USP Dissolution Apparatus 2 (Paddle Method) at 37°C with rotation speed of 100 rpm. Capsules are tied to the paddle with a cotton thread in each dissolution vessel to prevent floating. To simulate the pH changes along the gastrointestinal tract, three dissolution media with pH 1.2 simulated to gastric fluid (SGF) used for 2 hr, pH 7.4 simulated intestinal fluid (SIF) used for 3 hr and 6.8 simulated colonic fluid (SCF) for subsequent hours. Nine hundred milliliters of the dissolution medium is used each time. Ten milliliters of the sample is withdrawn from the dissolution media at suitable time intervals and the same amount is replaced with fresh dissolution media and drug content is measured using appropriate technique.

6.6.2.3 Water Uptake Study

Pulsatile capsules are exposed to phosphate buffer pH 7.4 (37°C, 50 ml-flask, shaker-incubator at 50 rpm) for predetermined period of time. The capsules are carefully blotted with tissue paper to remove the excess surface water and then weighed. The water uptake is calculated using following formula

$$\% \ Water \ uptake = \frac{W_{wet} - W_{dry}}{W_{wet}} \times 100$$

Where W_{wet}: weight of wet sample, W_{dry}: weight of dry sample

6.6.2.4 Hardness

Capsules, optionally after incubation in phosphate buffer USP, pH 7.4 at 37°C, is fixed on a metal plate. A metal probe connected to *tensile tester* equipment (Instron 4466) is positioned on the surface of the capsules. The metal probe is then moved downward at a constant speed of 5 mm/min. The maximum force when the coating of the capsule is cracked is recorded as hardness of the capsules (Bussemer et al., 2003).

6.6.2.5 Thickness of Enteric Coated Layer

Thickness of the enteric coated layer is measured using a vernier caliper and is expressed in mm.

Some researchers were eliminated reliance on hydrogel polymers and developed a Pulsincap formulation using a simple erodible compressed tablet instead of using the swelling hydrogel plug (Ross et al., 2000; Stevens et al., 1994). Precise dimensional tolerances between plug and capsule required by the sliding mechanism of the plug in the earlier pulsincap formulations was improved by the later technique, since the tablet remains at fixed position until complete erosion.

The Port® system consists of a gelatin capsule coated with a semipermeable membrane (eg. cellulose acetate) housing an insoluble plug (e.g., lipidic) and an osmotically active agent along with the drug formulation. When in contact with the aqueous medium, water diffuses across the semipermeable membrane, resulting in increased inner pressure that allows ejecting the plug after a lag time. Coating thickness controls the lag time. The system shows good correlation in lag times of *in vitro* and *in vivo* experiments in humans. The system was proposed to deliver methylphenidate for the treatment of attention deficit hyperactivity disorder in school-age children.

6.7 Lozenges

Lozenges are flavored medicated dosage forms that dissolve slowly in the mouth and so release the drug dissolved in the saliva. Lozenges are used to relieve oropharyngeal problems caused by local infection. They can thus be described as slow-release tablets for local drug delivery. Lozenges may contain antibiotics, antiseptics, local anesthetics, antihistamines, decongestants, corticosteroids or combinations of these ingredients. Lozenges have the advantage of easy administration to pediatric and geriatric patients. Moreover, the drug remains in contact with oral cavity for an extended period of time (Aulton and Taylor, 2013; Jambhekar, 1990).

6.7.1 Classification of Lozenges

Lozenges can be categorized or classified as represented in Fig. 6.13.

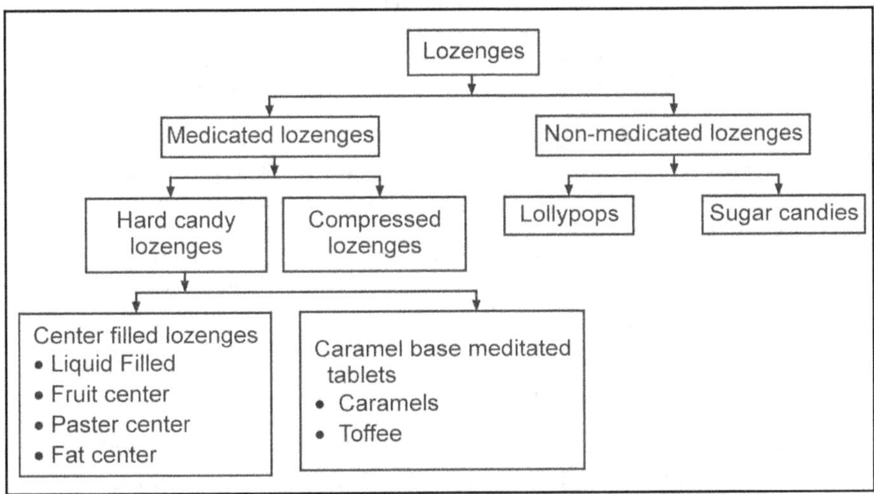

FIGURE 6.13 Classification of lozenges.

6.7.1.1 Medicated Lozenges

Medicated lozenges are confections consisted medicament or combination of medicament designed for local chemotherapy. Most of the preparations are available as OTC products and are very economic dosage forms. Medicated lozenges are classified into following sub categories:

6.7.1.1.1 Hard Candy Lozenges

Hard candy lozenges are mixtures of sugar and other carbohydrates in an amorphous (noncrystalline) or glassy state. They can also be regarded as solid syrups of sugars. The moisture content and weight of hard candy lozenge should be between, 0.5 to 1.5% and 1.5-4.5 g, respectively. These should undergo a slow and uniform dissolution or erosion over 5-10 min, and should not disintegrate. The temperature requirements for their preparation is usually high hence heat labile materials cannot be incorporated. The essential ingredient of hard candy lozenges are summarized in Table 6.6.

TABLE 6.6

Essential component of hard candy lozenges

S. No.	Ingredient	Function	Example
1.	Candy base	To control crystallization To supply solids at a reduced cost To adjust sweetness level	Corn syrup, invert sugar, reducing sugars
2.	Acidulents	Fortifiers to strengthen the flavor characteristics	Citric, tartaric, fumaric, and malic acid.
3.	Colors	To provide color To improve organoleptic sophistication	FD & C colors
4.	Flavors	Suppression of unwanted taste To improve organoleptic elegance	Menthol, eucalyptus oil, spearmint, cherry flavor, etc.
5.	Medicaments	To treat local complication	Local anesthetics, antihistamines, antitussives, analgesics, and decongestants etc.

6.7.1.1.1.1   Manufacturing of hard candy lozenges

Manufacturing of hard candy lozenges starts in candy base cooker. The essential steps of manufacturing are summarized in Fig. 6.14 (Jambhekar, 1990; Remington and Osol, 1980).

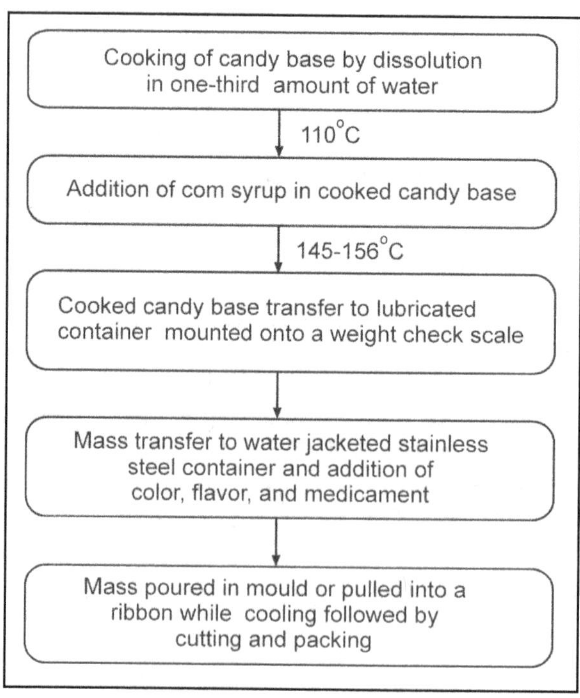

FIGURE 6.14 Flow chart of essential steps of commercial production of hard candy lozenges.

6.7.1.1.1.2 Center filled lozenges

Center filled lozenges are developed with intention to solve incompatibilities issue as well as to improve and get subtle flavorings in lozenges. Main difficulty arises during development of liquid center hard candy is content uniformity of the medicament. Center filled lozenges are formulated with different flavors in outer shell and in center filled area. The sophistication of the product can be enhanced by having excipients like high-impact flavors in the center in contrast with subtle flavorings included in the shell. Aromatics can give a burst of flavor or perceived efficacy to the user, thus increasing the over-all organoleptic presentation of the product. However, medicament must be uniformly distributed between the shell and the center to eliminate the problem of non-uniformity of center fill. Center filled lozenges can be divided in following four categories:

6.7.1.1.1.2.1 Liquid fill

Fruit juice, sugar syrup, hydro alcoholic solutions and sorbitol solution etc., type of materials are filled in center of these types of lozenges. The liquid is filled in these lozenges in varying concentrations from 10 to 20%. Only a noticeable sensation of liquid goes to patient throat after burst. There are some disadvantages associated with liquid fill lozenges such as the tendency for the product to leak if the shell cracks or the ends of the tablet are not properly sealed, higher chance of degradation due to the liquid center. Moreover, the processing of liquid fill lozenges is difficult as compared to other center filled lozenges.

6.7.1.1.1.2.2 Fruit center

These types of lozenges are used for encapsulating confectionary type products. Center of these lozenges is rich with sugar, jellies and flavor and viscosity is maintained with sucrose solution or corn syrup. Internal graining and melting characteristics are retard with higher viscosity and low moisture content. Average fill weight of fruit center is high (20-25%) as compare to liquid fill.

6.7.1.1.1.2.3 Paste center

Materials of high specific gravity are filled in these types of lozenges. It allows filling of up to 40% w/w and the high viscosity of material also reduces the tendency for the center material to leak out of the lozenge, if cracking occurs. Paste center lozenges are more difficult to fill as compared to other types of lozenges. The lower moisture content in paste center helps retard graining and internal candy base melting, so typical shelf life of paste center can be as long as 24 months.

6.7.1.1.1.2.4 Fat center

Fat center lozenges are mostly used to fill medicament in center of hard shell. Medicament and flavor were dissolved in hydrogenated vegetable oil and incorporated in the lozenge center. Vegetable oil also serves as lubricant for equipment and rollers in case of leak out of center material. Fats can be incorporated in lozenges at 25-32% w/w fill. Shelf life of fat filled lozenges are more than 3 year since the candy base is insoluble in the oil and will not grain or melt from the inside. Disadvantage associated with fat center lozenges vegetable oil retard the flavor impact so the reduced flavor impact in center can differentiate the outer shell and center.

6.7.1.1.1.3   Caramel base medicated tablets

Unlike hard candy lozenges, caramel based lozenges are chewed instant of sucking. Medicament is incorporated into a caramel base which is chewed instead dissolved in mouth. Carmel based lozenges are suitable for drugs intended for systemic action. It reduces the chances of degradation of drug in oral cavity because of low time of contact of drug with enzymes present in oral mucosa in comparison to other types of lozenges. The essential ingredients (Table 6.7) of caramel lozenges are somewhat similar to hard candy lozenges (Rachana Maheshwari, 2013).

TABLE 6.7

Essential components of caramel base medicated tablets

S. No.	Ingredient	Function	Example
1.	Candy base	To control crystallization To supply solids at a reduced cost To adjust sweetness level	Sugar to corn syrup ratio of 50:50 to 75:25
2.	Whipping agent	To incorporate air to achieve soft chew	Milk protein, egg albumin, gelatin, xanthan gum, starch, pectin, algin and carageenen
3.	Humectants	To improve chew and mouth feel properties	Glycerin, propylene glycol and sorbitol
4.	Lubricants	Avoid sticking	Vegetable oils and fats
5.	Seeding crystals	Reduce time of crystallization	Powdered sugar (3-10%)
6.	Flavors	Suppression of unwanted taste Improvement of organoleptic elegance	Menthol, eucalyptus oil, spearmint, and cherry flavor, etc.
7.	Medicaments	To treat local complications	Local anesthetics, antihistamines, antitussives, analgesics, and decongestants etc.

6.7.1.1.1.4 Manufacturing of caramel base medicated tablets

Essential steps involved in the manufacturing of caramel candy lozenges are summarized in Fig. 6.15 (Jambhekar, 1990).

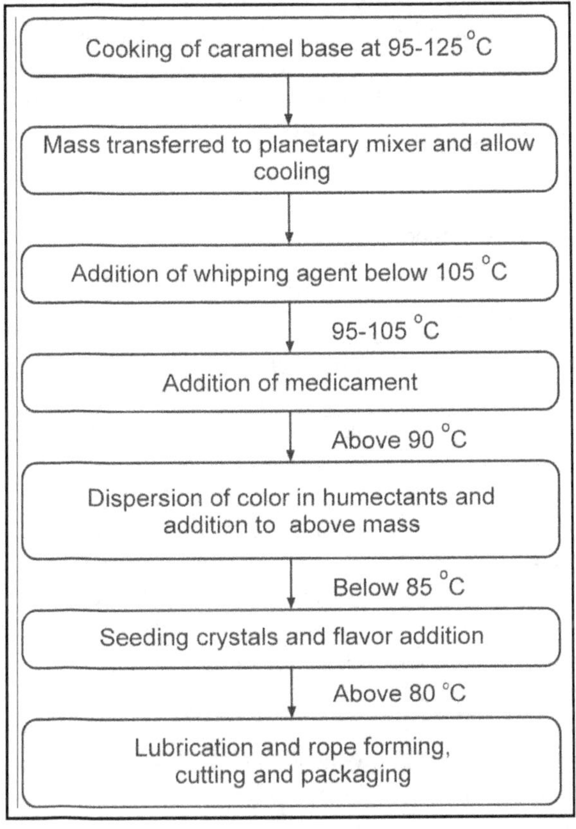

FIGURE 6.15 Flow chart of essential steps involved in commercial production of caramel based lozenges.

6.7.1.1.2 Compressed Lozenge

The rationale of manufacturing compressed lozenges is to eliminate the limitations associated with preparation of hard candy lozenge. These limitations may be one or many of the following:

(a) Requirement of high temperature which is not suitable for thermo labile medicament.

(b) Compatibility of candy base with other ingredients (flavor, colorant, acidulents)

(c) Higher therapeutic dose of medicament or combination of medicaments.

The compressed lozenges can be prepared either by wet granulation or direct compression technique. The lozenge is made using heavy compression equipment to give a tablet that is harder than normal compressed tablet, as it is desirable for the troche to dissolve slowly in the mouth. They are usually flat faced with sizes, weight, hardness, and erosion time ranging between, 5/8-3/4 inch, 1.5-4 g, 30-50 Kg/inch^2 and 5-10 min, respectively (Ghosh and Pfister, 2005). The essential components of compressed lozenges are summarized in Table 6.8.

TABLE 6.8

Essential components of compressed lozenges

S. No.	Ingredient	Function	Example
1.	Compression base or diluents	Provide bulk and base	Sugar- dextrose, sucrose Sugar-free vehicles: mannitol, sorbitol, PEG 6000 and 8000 Other fillers – di calcium phosphate, calcium sulfate, calcium carbonate, lactose, microcrystalline cellulose
2.	Binder	To formulate granules	Acacia, corn syrup, sugar syrup, gelatin, polyvinyl pyrrolidone, tragacanth, and methylcellulose
3.	Flavor	Suppression of unwanted taste and improvement of organoleptic elegance	Liquid flavors, and spray dried flavors.
4.	Colors	To provide color To improve organoleptic elegance	Water-soluble colours and lakolene dyes
5.	Lubricants	Improved powder flow properties	Magnesium stearate, calcium stearate, and stearic acid
6.	Medicaments	To treat local complications	Anesthetics, antihistamines, antitussives, analgesics etc.

6.7.1.1.2.1   Manufacturing of compressed lozenges

Methods that are used to manufacture conventional tablets i.e., wet and dry granulation method are used to formulate compressed lozenges.

6.7.2 Commercially Available Lozenges

Lot of medicated lozenges is commercially available in market. Some of the common marketed lozenges are summarized in Table 6.9.

TABLE 6.9

Common lozenges available in market

Brand	Active pharmaceutical ingredient	Type of lozenges
Suplical+D	Calcium carbonate and Vit. D3	Caramel based lozenges
Mediquell	Dextromethorphan Hydrobromide	Caramel based lozenges
Equate	Nicotine	Caramel based lozenges
Vapodrops	Menthol	Hard candy lozenges
TheraZinc®	Zinc and Vitamin A	Caramel based lozenges
Chloraseptic	Benzocaine	Caramel based lozenges
Difflam	Benzydamine hydrochloride and cetylpyridinium chloride	Caramel based lozenges

6.8 Medicated Chewing Gum

Medicated chewing gum (MCG) represents innovative drug delivery system that can provide new competitive benefits for a drug and thus increases revenue. Oral route is the most preferred route amongst the patients and clinicians due to various advantages and most important is its way of administration. Intraoral dosage forms that deliver the drug to the target sites for local or systemic drug delivery include the following:

- buccal,
- sublingual,
- periodontal,
- periodontal pocket,
- peribuccal,
- perlingual,
- tongue (i.e., lingual) and
- Gum (i.e., gingival).

The intraoral dosage forms include liquid (solution, sprays, syrups, injection, etc) semisolids (i.e., ointment pastes, etc.) and solid dosage forms (i.e., quick-dissolve and slow-dissolve tablets, sublingual tablet, lozenges, films, filament, gums, patches, micro particles, drug delivery devices, etc.) based on their advantages & disadvantages.

A medicated chewing gum is solid, single-dose preparation that is chewed (remaining mass after chewing is discarded) for a certain period of time to deliver the drug. It may contain one or more than one active pharmaceutical ingredient with various compositions. During chewing the drug contained in the gum is released into the saliva. The released drug has got two fates; either it could be absorbed through the oral mucosa or may reach the stomach for GI absorption (Imfeld, 1999; Rassing and Jacobsen, 2002).

6.8.1 Advantages of MCG over Conventional Drug Delivery System

It offers various benefits over other solid oral dosage form which may be summarized as below (Pagare et al., 2012; Surana, 2010; William and Millind, 2012):

(a) Medicated chewing gum can be used without solvent, at any time, and everywhere.

(b) Finished product is stable as the intended therapeutic agents are protected from oxygen, light, and water.

(c) Medicated chewing gum shows its action, both locally and systemically with good bioavailability, since it avoids metabolism of the drug in the gastrointestinal tract and the so called liver-first-pass effect.

(d) Fast/rapid onset of action in comparison to other oral dosage form.

(e) High acceptance by children and patients because of its easy administration (without swallowing)

(f) Excellent dosage form for acute medication

(g) Reducing the risk of intolerance of gastric mucosa (avoid direct gastricintestinal tract contact).

6.8.2 Disadvantages of MCG

(a) MCGs sometimes consist of sorbitol which may cause flatulence and diarrhea.

(b) In medicated chewing gum flavoring agents like cinnamon can cause ulcers in oral cavity and liquorice causes hypertension.

(c) Due to unpleasant taste and staining properties to teeth and tongue, oromucosal chlorhexidine cannot be administered for longer period of time.

(d) Chewing gum has been shown to adhere to different degrees to enamel dentures and fillers.

(e) Prolonged chewing may result in pain in facial muscles and ear ache in children.

6.8.3 Composition

The most important material is the gum base which is an inert and insoluble component. The other materials may be grouped as water soluble bulk portion. Table 6.10 illustrates various components required for preparation of MCGs (D.J. et al., 2003; Pagare et al., 2012).

TABLE 6.10

Components required for medicated chewing gum formulation

Component	Function	Example
Water insoluble gum base		
Elastomers	Provides elasticity and controls gummy texture	Natural (chicle gum, nispero, rosadinha, jelutong, periollo, sorva) and synthetic rubbers (butadiene, styrene copolymers, polyiso-butylene, polyethylene mixtures, polyvinyl alcohol)
Elastomer solvents	Softening the elastomer base component	Terpinene resins (polymers of alpha-pinene or beta-pinene), modified resins or gums (hydro-genated, dimerized or polymerized resins)
Plastisizers	To obtain a variety of desirable textures and consistency properties	Lanolin, palmitic acid, oleic acid, stearic acid, glyceryl triacetate, propylene glycol monostearate, sorbital monostearate, glycerine, propylene glycol, natural and synthetic waxes, hydrogenated vegetable oils, paraffin waxes
Fillers or texturizers or mineral adjuvant	Provide texture, improve chewability and reasonable size of the gum lump with low dose drug	Calcium carbonate, magnesium carbonate, aluminum hydroxide, talc, aluminum silicate
Water soluble portions		
Softners and emulsifiers	These are added to the chewing gum in order to optimize the chewability and mouth feel of the gum	Glycerin, lecithin, tallow, hydro-genated tallow and mono/di/tri glycerides
Water soluble portions		
Colorants and whiteners	Gives the formulation soothing color and improves acceptability of the formulation	Titanium dioxide, natural food colors and dyes suitable for food, drug and cosmetic applications
Sweeteners	To provide the desired sweetness of the product	Water soluble sweetening agents (xylose, ribulose, glucose, mannose, galactose, sucrose, fructose, maltose, sugar alcohols like sorbitol

TABLE 6.10 Contd...

Component	Function	Example
		and mannitol), water soluble artificial sweeteners (sodium or calcium saccharin salts and cyclamate salts), di-peptide based sweeteners (aspartame and alitame), naturally occurring water soluble sweeteners, chlorinated derivatives of ordinary sugar (sucralose), protein based sweeteners (thaumatin I and II)
Antioxidants	Prevents any possible microbial growth	Butylated hydroxytoluene, butylated hydroxyanisole, propyl gallate
Flavoring agents	To enhance consumer acceptability	Essential oils (citrus oil, fruit essences, peppermint oil, spearmint oil and clove oil) and synthetic or artificial flavors
Bulking agents	Used if low calorie gum is desired	Polydextrose, oligofructose, inulin, fructo-oligosaccharides, guar gum hydrolysate, indigestible dextrin
Compression adjuvant	To ease the compression process	Silicon dioxide, magnesium stearate, calcium stearate, talc

6.8.4 Manufacturing and Evaluation

MCGs are manufactured by following three methods (Keizo and Fumio, 1976; Morjaria et al., 2004; N.K. and A, 2001; Pagare et al., 2012):

6.8.4.1 Conventional/Traditional Method (Melting)

Components of gum base are melted together and placed in a kettle mixer to which sweeteners, syrups, active ingredients and other excipient are added at proper time. The melted gum is sent through a series of rollers to form a thin, wide ribbon. During this process, to reduce gum sticking and to enhance the flavor, a light coating of finely powdered sugar substitutes is added. The gum is allowed to set proper in a carefully controlled room and is cooled up to 48 hours. Finally the gum is cut to the desired size and stored in controlled temperature and humidity conditions. A brief process of conventional method of manufacturing is given in flow diagram (Fig. 6.16):

6.8.4.1.1 Limitations

(a) Elevated temperature used in this method is not suitable for thermolabile drugs.

(b) Melting and mixing of highly viscous gum mass makes difficulty in accuracy and uniformity of drug dose.

(c) Stringent manufacturing conditions not so easily adaptable for production of pharmaceutical products.

(d) Because of their moisture content (2-8%), the risk of jamming of machine is high.

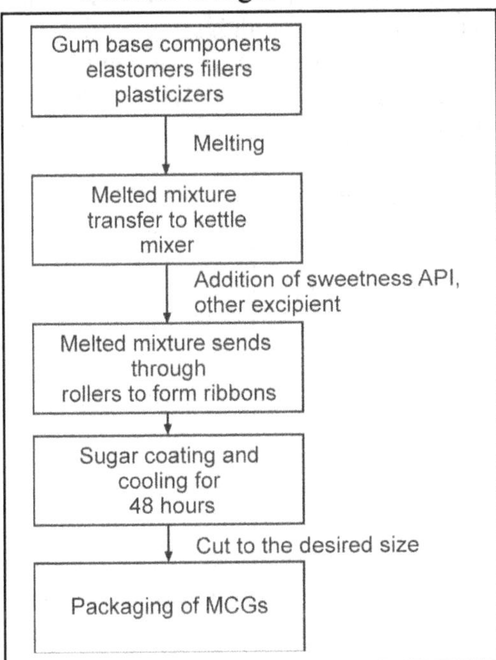

FIGURE 6.16 Flow diagram of conventional method for manufacturing MCGs.

6.8.4.2 Cooling, Grinding and Tableting Method

6.8.4.2.1 Cooling and Grinding

The MCGs composition is cooled to a temperature at which the composition is sufficiently brittle without adhesion to the grinding apparatus. Amongst the various coolants solid carbon dioxide is preferred as it can give temperatures as low as -78.5°C, sublimes readily and is not absorbed by the chewing gum composition. It does not interact adversely with the processing apparatus and does not leave behind any residue which may be undesirable or potentially hazardous. An anti-caking agent such as precipitated silicon dioxide can be mixed prior to grinding to prevent agglomeration of the ground chewing gum particles. A grinding agent such as alkaline metal phosphate, alkaline earth metal phosphate or maltodextrin, is added to prevent the gum from sticking to the grinding apparatus. However, these substances are limited because of their highly alkaline nature which would be incompatible with acidic ionisable therapeutic agents.

6.8.4.2.2 Tableting

After the coolant has been removed from the powder, it is mixed with other excipients such as binders, lubricants, coating agents and sweeteners, which are mixed with the components of the chewing gum base using suitable blender such as sigma mill or a high shear mixer. The powder mixture is then converted to granules using fluidized bed reactor. The granules are blended with an antiadherent like talc in blender and screened by desired mesh size followed by compression using simple rotary machine. A brief process of cooling, grinding and tabletting method of manufacturing given in flow diagram below (Fig. 6.17).

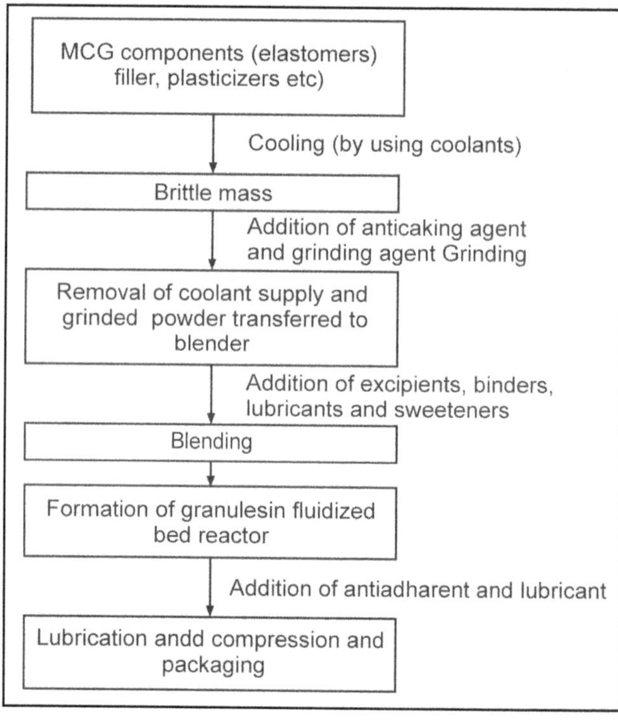

FIGURE 6.17 Flow diagram of cooling, grinding and tabletting method.

6.8.4.2.3 Limitations

(a) It requires equipment other than conventional tabletting equipment.

(b) Careful monitoring of humidity during the tabletting process.

6.8.4.3 Use of Directly Compressible Chewing Gum Excipients

The limitations of melting and freezing can be overcome by the use of this method and also we can accelerate the rate of manufacturing of chewing gum. This particular method uses directly compressible excipients available in the market such as "Pharmagum". Pharmagum is available in the form of directly compressible powder which is a mixture of chewing gum base and sugars. The directly compressible powder and active constituent are transferred into mass mixer for mixing. Mixed powder is transferred into the blender and blended with antiadherent followed by transfer of the blended mass for compression. Pharmagum is available in three forms namely S, M and C which are differentiated in terms of amount of gum and other excipients. Chewing gums formed using direct compressible method are 10 times harder and crumble when pressure is applied resulting in faster release and are more cost effective in comparison to those manufactured by traditional methods. Fig. 6.18 demonstrates the step by step manufacturing of MCGs using directly compressible excipients.

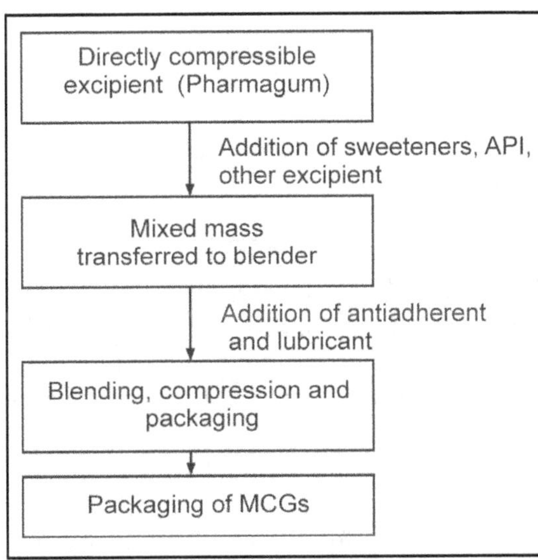

FIGURE 6.18 Flow diagram of directly compressible excipients method.

6.8.5 Factors affecting Release of Active Ingredient

6.8.5.1 Contact Time

The local or systemic effect is dependent on time of contact of MCGs in oral cavity and it is close to 30 minutes on ordinary use.

6.8.5.2 Physicochemical Properties of Active Ingredient

Physicochemical properties especially solubility has impact on the release of active ingredient from chewing gum formulation. The saliva soluble ingredients are released immediately within few minutes whereas lipid soluble drugs are released first into the gum base followed by slow release into oral cavity.

6.8.5.3 Inter Individual Variability

The chewing frequency and intensity may vary from person to person thus affect the drug release and onset of action.

6.8.5.4 Composition of Gum Base

Composition and amount of gum base affect rate of release of lipid soluble active ingredient to a greater extent. Use of solubilizers is more effective to change the release properties in comparison to gum base. However use of solubilizers requires specially designed gum bases as the solubilizer affects the texture and become soft to an unacceptable degree after a very short period of chewing.

6.8.6 Evaluation of MCG

Medicated chewing gum needs to be evaluated in terms of compliance requirements of the European pharmacopoeia.

6.8.6.1 Uniformity of Mass (Weight Variation Test)

This test is specifically used for uncoated compressed dosage forms. Twenty MCGs are randomly taken and weigh individually followed by calculation of the arithmetic mean weight. The formulation complies with the test; if not more than two of the individual masses deviate from the average mass by more than 5%.

6.8.6.2 Uniformity of Content

Ten MCGs are selected randomly for assay for content. The preparation complies with the test if each individual content is between 85 percent and 115 percent of the average content. The preparation fails to comply with the test if more than one individual content is outside these limits or if one individual content is outside the limits of 75 percent to 125 percent of the average content. If one individual content is outside the limits of 85 percent to 115 percent but within the limits of 75 percent to 125 percent, determine the individual contents of another 20 dosage units taken at random. The preparation complies with the test if not more than one of the individual contents of the 30 units is outside 85 percent to 115 percent of the average content and none is outside the limits of 75 percent to 125 per cent of the average content (European Pharmacopoeia, 2007).

6.8.6.3 *In-Vitro* Drug Release Study

The modified dissolution apparatus as per European Pharmacopoeia for assessing drug release from MCGs is represented in Fig. 6.19. The amount of drug released from MCGs is estimated by applying a mechanical kneading procedure to a piece of gum placed in a small chewing chamber containing a known volume of buffer solution.

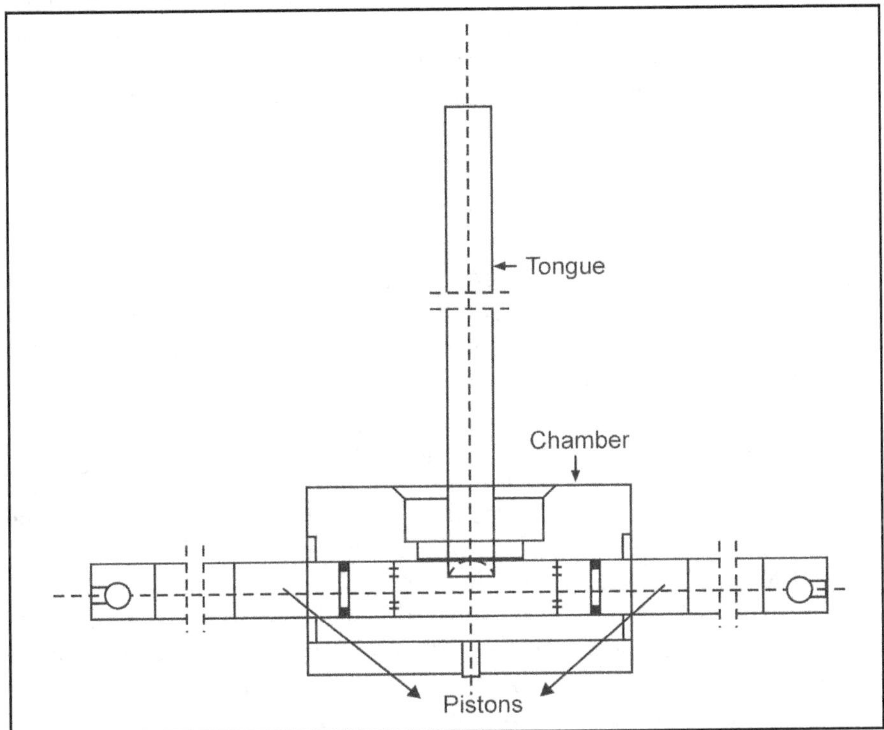

FIGURE 6.19 Apparatus for the determination of drug release from medicated chewing gum.

The chewing apparatus consists of a chewing chamber in which the gum is artificially chewed with the help of two horizontal pistons. The volume of the chewing chamber is approximately 40 ml and both the pistons are operated together at constant speed. The gum is subjected to maximum chewing which is ensured by the fact that at the end of each chewing the pistons are rotated around their own axis in opposite direction to each other. Another vertical piston is also provided operating alternately with the two horizontal pistons and the purpose is to make sure that gum resides in the right place between chews. Stainless steel is used to fabricate all the materials and pistons are operated by compressed air and their mutual movements are controlled. 20 ml of buffer (generally close to pH 6) is added into the chewing chamber and the machine is run for 2 min without placing chewing gum. The buffer is completely removed using pipette and fresh 20 ml buffer is added into the chamber. The buffer which has been taken out is analyzed and serves as control for cleaning procedure. After placing a precisely weighed piece of chewing gum in the chamber, the machine is run. At various time intervals a definite volume of buffer is removed and is analyzed using appropriate analytical method i.e., UV spectorphotometry or HPLC. The temperature of the chewing chamber is maintained at $37 \pm 0.5°C$ and the chewing frequency is usually fixed at 60 cycles/min (Azarmi et al., 2007; European Pharmacopoeia, 2007; Kvist et al., 1999; Rømer Rassing, 1994).

6.8.7 Applications

Sugar free chewing gum is probably the most successful innovation in confectionery in recent years. Combining a tooth-friendly image with a softer, chewy texture and a cleaner refreshing taste, it appeals to the desire of today's consumer for healthier and tastier sweets. Target of MCGs is prevention and cure of oral diseases. MCGs can control the release of the drug and can provide a prolonged release for local effect. It re-elevates plaque pH which lowers intensity and frequency of dental caries. Gums that contain fluoride have been useful in preventing dental caries with xerostomia. Chewing gum formulated with chlorhexidine can be used to treat gingivitis, periodontitis, oral and pharyngeal infections. Chlorhexidine offers numerous flexibility in its formulation as it gives less staining of the teeth and is distributed evenly in the oral cavity (Pagare et al., 2012; Surana, 2010). The bitter taste of drugs can be masked quite well in a chewing gum formulation. Table 6.11 comprises various marketed products based on buccal tablets technology along with name of manufactures (Dodds et al., 1991; Gadhavi et al., 2011; Gavaskar et al., 2011; William and Millind, 2012).

6.8.8 Systemic Therapy

MCGs have applications in the management of pain, smoking cessation, treatment of obesity and some other indications. These are used to control minor pains, headache and muscular aches. Formulations containing nicotine and lobeline have been clinically tested as aids to smoking cessation. Active substances contained in the chewing gum like chromium (reduces craving for food due to an improved blood-glucose balance), guaran and caffeine (stimulate lipolysis) are proved to be efficient in treating obesity. Xerostomia, allergy, motion sickness, acidity, anxiety, cold and cough are all indications for which chewing gum as drug delivery system could be beneficial (Gavaskar et al., 2011; Stefan et al., 1974).

TABLE 6.11

List of various products (MCGs) available in the market

Brand name	Drug	Uses	Manufacturer
Nicorette	Nicotine	Smoking cessation	GlaxoSmithkline
Aapergum	Asprin	Pain relief	Insight pharmaceuticals
Trawell	Dimenhydrinate	Travel illness	Meda Pharma
Nicotinell	Nicotine	Smoking cessation	Novartis
Chooz	Calcium carbonate	Antacid	Insight pharmaceuticals
NiQuitin CQ	Nicotine	Smoking cessation	GlaxoSmithkline
Fluorette	Fluoride	Prevation of dental caries	Fertin pharma A/S
Vitaflow CHX	Chlorhexidine	Treatment of gingivitis and plaeue	Fertin pharma A/S
Stay Alert	Caffeine	Anti bacterial	Stay Alert Safety Services.
Travvell	Dimenhydrinate	Motion Sickness	Asta Medica

6.9 Egalet® Technology

Injection Molding (IM) is a rapid and versatile manufacturing technique used in the plastics industry to produce objects with different size, shape and, if needed, many details. The great potential of IM for producing drug delivery systems is demonstrated by the multiplicity of patents filled over the last ten years, although the number of products at an advanced development stage or already on the market is still limited (e.g., Capill®, Chronocap™, Egalet®, Septacin™); hence, there is still room for improvement and indepth investigation (Zema et al., 2012). Egalet Ltd. has developed one of the world's first erosion based pill that allows for the controlled release of drugs. The unconventionally shaped pill is made up of an inner matrix which contains the active ingredient and an outer coating shell made up of specific polymers. Egalet® technology is used for a series of controlled release products developed by Egalet Ltd. UK.

6.9.1 Mechanism of Action

The Egalet® technology enables the controlled release of drugs through gradual erosion of a tablet. The matrix is designed to erode when it comes into contact with water but not until the desired point of release in order to avoid hydrolysis and the reduction of enzymatic activity. The active substance is then released with a zero order release which ensures that a steady amount of the drug is released over time. This minimizes fluctuations while maximizing the amount of time the drug remains within the therapeutic window. The uniquely shaped, user-friendly tablet consists of an impermeable shell with two lag plugs, enclosing a plug of active drug in the middle of the unit. Time of release can then be modulated by the length and composition of the plugs. The shells are made of cetostearyl alcohol and ethyl cellulose while the matrices of the plugs are composed of a mixture of polyethylene glycol monostearates and polyethylene oxides. The shell also contains a second cellulose derivative which is soluble in an aqueous solution, a plasticizer which promotes plasticity and reduces brittleness, and filler which increases volume. The outer shell protects the inner matrix making it an ideal system for chemically unstable substances, those with low melting and boiling points, and water insoluble compounds. Also, this protective shell significantly increases the shelf life of the substance. The drug is distributed throughout the matrix, which is eroded by gut movements and gastrointestinal fluids as it passes through the gut. The drug release mechanism is surface erosion, which is effected through water diffusion, polymer hydration, disentanglement and dissolution (Marvola et al., 2004). The entrapment in the Egalet® matrix also protects the active compounds from oxygen and humidity and therefore the technology is suited for chemically unstable substances and thus is able to increase shelf-life of the drug product (Marvola et al., 2004; Quinten et al., 2009).

An additional attribute of the erosion based system is its ability to deliver water-insoluble compounds in a controlled manner. The shell is biodegradable but with a disintegrating profile making the shell last longer than the matrix. By altering the composition of the shell and matrix, many drug formulations and ways of release can be achieved. The altering of the shape and surface area of the pill can also affect release times. The pills are made with injection molding, similar to plastic molding, in order to complete the creation process in one fluid step. They are the first company to manufacture pharmaceuticals using this technology (Bar-Shalom et al., 2003).

6.9.2 Manufacturing

The unique Egalet® formulation is produced using an injection moulding technology (Fischer, 2012). This technique ensures a higher uniformity of weight and content when compared with conventional compressed tablets or capsules and confers several benefits such as accuracy, reproducibility, fast drug development and low production cost.

The manufacturing process follows standard procedures for injection moulding of thermoplastic materials. This process allows manufacturers to vary the rate of production easily and to produce very high volumes with high standards of accuracy in a virtually automatic environment. This technique is not only relatively cheap but ensures that Egalet® tablets are reproducible with a minimum batch to batch variation. The Egalet® manufacturing facility in Denmark holds GMP approval (www.egalet.com/index.dsp?area=32).

Injection molding is accurate, easy to reproduce (for manufacturing large quantities), has a low cost of production, and allows for simple technology transfer. The process is actually quite simple. Initially the cavity is empty. The piston moves forward, creating the shape for the shell, and the coating material is injected. Next, the coat material hardens, and the matrix material that contains the drug is injected while the piston is recedes. Finally, the matrix hardens while the piston ejects the finished tablet. A schematic view of the Egalet® production flow is shown in Fig. 6.20.

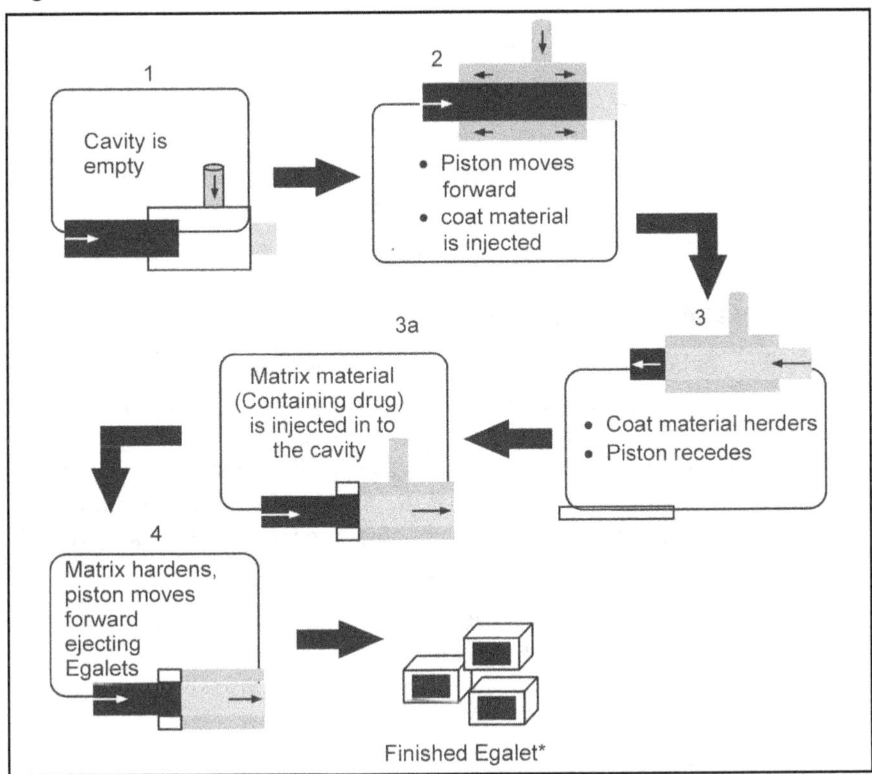

FIGURE 6.20 Production flow of an Egalet® tablet.

6.9.2.1　Egalet® Prolonged Release Tablets

The Egalet® prolonged release system consists of two components: shell (coat) and matrix. The drug is distributed evenly throughout the Egalet® matrix for constant release over time as the shell (coat) and matrix are eroded by body fluids as it travels through the gastrointestinal tract. The rate of release can be altered by adjusting the composition of the polyethylene glycol (PEG) carrier within the matrix. The Fig. 6.21 illustrates the mechanism of drug release of an Egalet® Prolonged Release tablet.

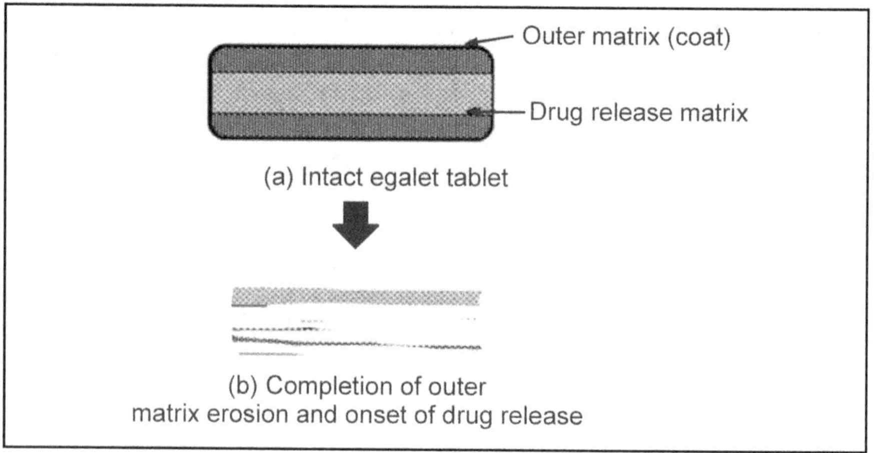

FIGURE 6.21 Mechanism of drug release of an Egalet® prolonged release tablet.

6.9.2.2　Egalet® Delayed Release

The Egalet® delayed release consists of three compartments: an outer matrix (coat), a drug release matrix and a lag component. The drug is contained in the inner (middle) layer of the matrix, with the outer layers providing a predetermined delay in release of the drug. By alteration of lag component polymer the release of the drug can be timed to mimic the natural rhythms of a disease such as the morning stiffness and pain experienced by arthritis patients on waking.

The mechanism of drug release through an Egalet® delayed release tablet is displayed in Fig. 6.22.

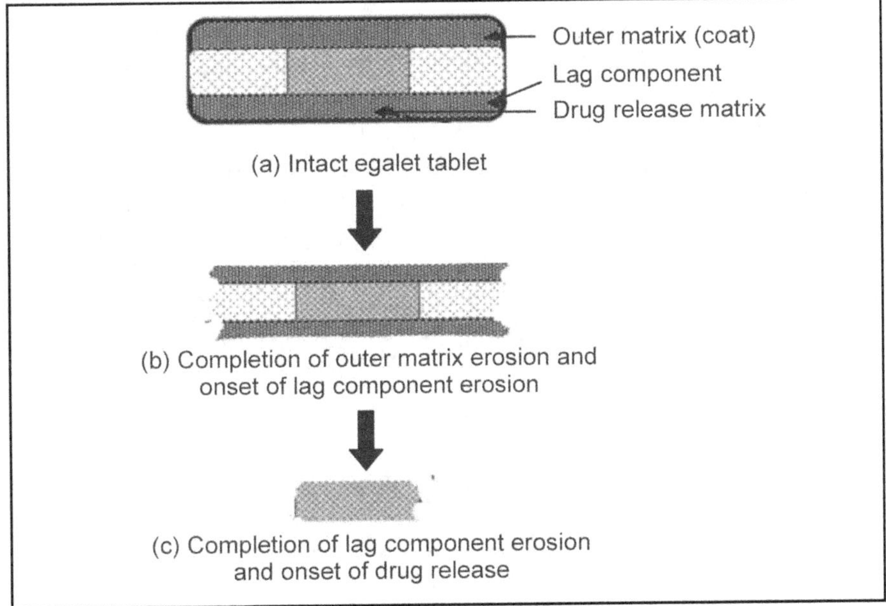

FIGURE 6.22 Mechanism of drug release of an Egalet® delayed release tablet.

6.9.3 Factors Affecting Drug Release from Egalet® Tablets

6.9.3.1 Erosion of Matrix

The desired mode of the erosion of matrix is such that at the point of initial matrix erosion, the water should not diffuse into the matrix until the point of release to avoid drug hydrolysis and diffusion and thereby reducing the effects of luminal enzymatic activity. So the objective is to select a balanced polymer which erodes as fast as the diffusion of water into the matrix.

PEO/PEGs can be used by melt and cast into solid shapes, as in suppositories. Low-molecular-weight PEGs (up to 6000) made into solid shapes do erode heterogeneously in water, but have low melting points, rendering them impractical for oral dosage forms. High-molecular-weight PEO/PEG solid shapes form gels in water and the gel will either reduce release of water-insoluble substances or will impede the release of water-soluble ones. Addition of poly (ethylene glycol) monostearate (PEG-MS) to the higher-molecular-weight PEO/PEGs in the right proportion results in solid shapes eroding heterogeneously. A possible explanation for this effect is that when molten PEO/PEG cools and solidifies, it assumes a structure that is partly crystalline and partly amorphous, with cracks or fissures. Water penetrates rapidly through the fissures and the surface and deeper layers begin to dissolve simultaneously, resulting in gel formation. PEG-MS melted together with PEO/PEG, when cooled, align so that the PEG portion will blend itself with the PEO/PEG and the MS part will tend to be left on the surface of the particles. It renders the fissures hydrophobic and impassable to water. This results in heterogeneous erosion, because the erosion proceeds layer by layer. This matrix (PEO/PEG, PEG-MS, an optional filler, and different drugs) shows zero-order release *in vitro* irrespective of pH but directly dependent upon rate of agitation.

6.9.3.2 Agitation

The rate of agitation is a factor which is directly related to the erosion of the tablet. Rate of erosion is directly proportional to the speed of rotation in the dissolution test. Use of cellulose derivative such as CAP, HPMC decreases the rate of erosion at the acidic pH but not at near-neutral or basic pH. This effect can be used to modify the relative rates of erosion at different agitations if the given agitation is associated with a particular pH, for example, in the stomach relative to the small intestine.

6.9.3.3 Surface Area of Tablet

The rate of erosion and thus rate of release is directly proportional to three dimensional surface area of the matrix. An eroding sphere loses surface at a rate proportional to the radius at the third potency (volume = $4/3 \times \pi \times r^3$) whereas a flat slab loses surface at a rate nearly proportional to the thickness or height of the slab (volume = length × width × height). All this is true if the whole surface of the matrix is exposed. By encasing the matrix in a tube which is open at one or both ends will expose the same area for erosion at all times and will result in controlled erosion and zero-order performance. Changing the area of the tube which is exposed will modify the erosion and release accordingly. By this method we can entrap two different drugs at both end and can get a controlled release of both the drugs.

6.9.3.4 Immediate Release Layer (Lag Compartment)

These types of tablets contain two types of plugs, the outer plug may contain an active substance which may or may not be different from the one in the internal section. By this we can achieve a two-step release of the same drug. By using two plugs method we can design formulations having following features: (Bar-Shalom et al., 2003)

(a) Different drug can be used in inner and outer matrix in order to deliver a drug combination.

(b) Same active substance in the outer and inner plug but at different concentration, to achieve a desired release profile.

(c) No drug in the outer plug to achieve a delay in the onset of the release to deliver chronotherapeticals.

6.10 Enterion Capsule Technology

There has been considerable growth in the number of molecules developed by various companies and research groups. However many of the molecules have challenged pharmaceutical (e.g. solubility) and biopharmaceutical (e.g., permeability) properties which restricts drug development process. The companies have to think many ways in order to solve these critical issues so that drugs can be released into the market. A wide variety of techniques are currently available to pursue such screening studies. The pharmaceutical companies are conducting human absorption studies in order to get a route map for drug development. These studies are conducted during early stages of drug development using a specialized capsule to provide targeted release of drug in various parts of gastrointestinal tract in a non-invasive manner. The most advanced technology in this area is enterion capsule (Phaeton Research, Nottingham, UK), which has emerged as the market leader. It is used for targeted delivery of a wide range of different drug formulations into any desired region of the gut. A lot of pharmaceutically relevant formulations can be loaded into the reservoir including active pharmaceutical ingredient, particulates, pellets, crushed tablets, solutions and suspensions (Prior et al., 2003).

6.10.1 Discription of Technology

Phaeton Research developed the Enterion capsule in collaboration with PA Consulting Group, Melbourn, Hertfordshire, UK. It is a 32 mm long, round-ended capsule and contains a drug reservoir with a volume capacity of approximately 1 ml. The capsule can be loaded with either a liquid formulation (e.g., solution, suspension) or a particulate formulation (e.g., powder, pellets) through an opening 9 mm in diameter, which is then sealed by inserting a push-on cap fitted with a silicone O-ring. The floor of the drug reservoir is the piston face, which is held back against a compressed spring by a high tensile strength polymer filament (Fig. 6.23) (Manoj Kumar, 2010; Wilding, 2001). The features of enterion capsule is depicted in Table 6.12. When the capsule arrives at the target site in the GI tract, it is remotely triggered by application of an oscillating electromagnetic field, which is generated over the abdominal cavity by an external radiofrequency (RF) generator. The frequency is low enough for negligible absorption of energy by the body tissues, but sufficiently high to induce usable power in a tuned coil receiver (pickup coil) embedded inside the wall of the capsule. The electric current induced by the magnetic field in the receiving coil is fed to a low-power heater resistor, which is situated within a sealed electronics compartment. The small size of the heater (< 1 mm^3) results in a rapid temperature rise in just a few seconds. The spring filament that anchors the piston is in direct contact with the heater. As rapid heat buildup occurs, the filament quickly reaches a critical temperature at which point it softens and immediately breaks under the tensile strain of the spring and the relatively low mass and friction coefficient of the piston produces a high acceleration. Therefore, once the spring is released, it drives the piston into the drug chamber. Under the continued forward motion of the spring-driven piston, the entire capsule contents are actively expelled into the surrounding GI environment within milliseconds (Wilding et al., 2000).

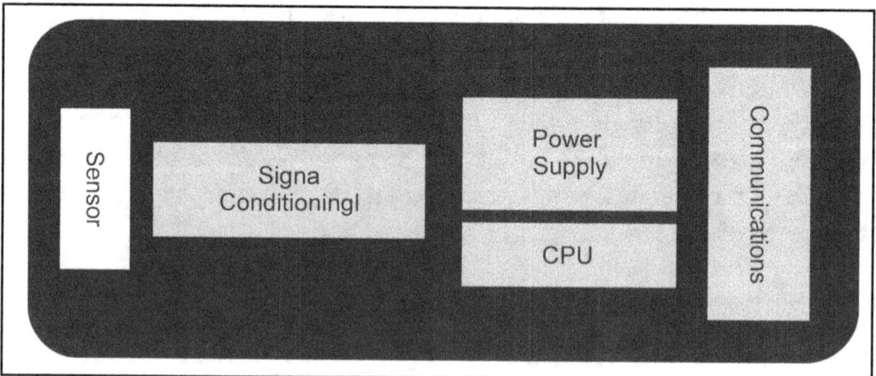

FIGURE 6.23 A block diagram of a swallowable capsule.

TABLE 6.12

Key design features of the Enterion capsules (Prior et al., 2003)

Essential attribute	Enterion design feature
Biocompatible	Medical grade plastics used for fabrication of all parts that come into contact with gastrointestinal luminal fluids
Readily swallowed by volunteers	Round-ended with overall dimensions (32 × 11 mm in diameter) comparable to 000 sized gelatin capsule
Easy tracking of capsule location	Short half-life radionuclide sealed inside a radiotracer port allows tracking via a gamma camera
Suitable for delivering a range of physical form	Spring-driven piston ensures rapid and complete delivery of particulate, semisolid and liquid formulations
High loading capacity	Drug chamber approximately 1 ml in volume
No drug leakage prior to activation	Compressed silicone O-ring provides a reliable closure system with high seal integrity
Reliable activation at all intestinal sites	Compressed spring provides an onboard energy source; radiofrequency pulse activation frequency selected to avoid absorption by human tissues; proprietary cap release mechanism based on a unique "rolling" O-ring design
Feedback signal to confirm drug delivery	Radiofrequency pulse signal generated on forward motion of the piston

6.10.2 Tracking the Enterion Capsule

To track of the Enterion capsule, a radioactive marker indium-111 (^{111}In) is placed inside a separate sealed tracer-port to allow real time visualization using the gamma scintigraphy. It is administered to a volunteer with a water drink containing technetium-99 m (^{99m}Tc). When the capsule reaches the target location, it is remotely triggered by an oscillating magnetic field. The capsule contents are then actively ejected rapidly. Upon activation the capsule emits a confirmatory radio frequency signal that is used as a positive indicator. Pharmacokinetic data generated in this way allows a direct relationship to be established between human drug absorption and the target site drug delivery. The radio labeled water provides an outline of the GI tract, and the ^{111}In radiolabel allows us to superimpose the Enterion capsule to map its location precisely. Such information can be extremely valuable, especially for complex molecules, when selecting appropriate drug development strategies and "enabling technologies (Allescher et al., 2001)."

6.10.3   Application of the Technology

The main application of this technology is assessment of bioavailability at various sites of gastrointestinal tract. Large number of new chemical entities is being developed and a large number of drugs have issues of poor solubility and permeability. On the basis of this technology we can decide strategy or type of modified release dosage forms which would be better for drug. It is also feasible using this technology to know whether there is small window of absorption in particular areas and the feasibility of formation of an oral modified release dosage form. Traditionally invasive techniques have been used for assessment of bioavailability in various segments of the gastrointestinal tract. This has issues with the patient convenience and consumption of large amount of time. With the use of enterion technology time and cost of drug development can be saved and it helps in design and development of appropriate formulation.

6.11 Hydrophilic Sandwich

Hydrophilic sandwich is one type of device which is based on time delayed release system. It consists of system within a system i.e., a capsule is contained within a capsule in order to provide the time dependent delay of the material placed within the internal capsule. The smaller capsule having intended material (may be a drug or some material) is placed inside a bigger capsule and the space between these two capsules is filled with a hydrophilic polymer, HPMC. The release of the material kept in the inner capsule is dependent on the degradation of the outer two layers holding the inner capsule in a protective environment. When the whole device comes in contact with aqueous media the outer gelatin layer ruptures leaving behind HPMC layer surrounded with aqueous media. The property of the HPMC is such that it forms a gel layer in presence of water or aqueous fluid and the gel layer is responsible for sustaining or delaying the release of trapped moiety. The swollen HPMC gel layer controls the release of drug from inner capsule until water or aqueous media enters and attacks the inner capsule shell. The release of the drug from the inner capsule is controlled by the thickness as well as the swelling and consequently the barrier property of sandwiched HPMC layer. The barrier property of this layer can be managed by varying the molecular weight and density of the gelling polymer. Moreover, various grades of HPMC are available in the market and using a judicious blend of these the release can be optimized to suit the requirement. The time delay can also be modified by incorporating some filler or other polymers with the HPMC. Two types of hydrophilic sandwich capsules are available; one having outer capsule 000 size and inner capsule 0 size while other known as "mini hydrophilic sandwich" consists of 0 size external capsule and size 4 internal capsule.

References

Abdelbary, G., Eouani, C., Prinderre, P., Joachim, J., Reynier, J., and Piccerelle, P. (2005). Determination of the in vitro disintegration profile of rapidly disintegrating tablets and correlation with oral disintegration. *Int J Pharm* **292,** 29-41.

Ahuja, A., Ali, J., Qureshi, J., Baboota, S., and Arora, S. (2006). Pulsatile drug delivery systems: An approach for controlled drug delivery. *Indian Journal of Pharmaceutical Sciences* **68,** 295-300.

Allescher, H.D., Teuffel, W., Wessels, G., and Feussner, H. (2001). Endoscopy within the network of diagnostic imaging. *Internist (Berl)* **42,** 297-304.

Aulton, M.E., and Taylor, K.M.G. (2013). Aulton's Pharmaceutics: The Design and Manufacture of Medicines (Churchill Livingstone/Elsevier).

Azarmi, S., Roa, W., and Lobenberg, R. (2007). Current perspectives in dissolution testing of conventional and novel dosage forms. *Int J Pharm* **328,** 12-21.

Bar-Shalom, D., Slot, L., Lee, W.W., and Wilson, C.G. (2003). Development of the Egalet Technology. In Modified-Release Drug Delivery Technology, M.J. Rathbone, J. Hadgraft, and M.S. Roberts, eds. (New York: Marcel Dekker, Inc. New York), p. 975.

Bussemer, T., Dashevsky, A., and Bodmeier, R. (2003). A pulsatile drug delivery system based on rupturable coated hard gelatin capsules. *Journal of Controlled Release* **93,** 331-339.

D.J., Z., M.J., G., D.G., B., W., M.S., G., S.P., and P., M. (2003). Method of making coated chewing gum products containing various antacids (US Patent).

Dodds, M.W., Hsieh, S.C., and Johnson, D.A. (1991). The effect of increased mastication by daily gum-chewing on salivary gland output and dental plaque acidogenicity. *J Dent Res* **70,** 1474-1478.

Eckenhoff, B., Theeuwes, F., and Urquhart, J. (1987). Osmotically actuated dosage forms for rate-controlled drug delivery. *Pharmaceutical Technology* **11,** 96-105.

European Pharmacopoeia (6th ed), Counsil of Europe Strabourg, France, 2007.

Fischer (2012). Matrix compositions for controlled delivery of drug substances (U.S: Egalet A/S (London, GB)).

Gadhavi, A.G., Patel, B.N., Patel, D.M., and Patel, C.N. (2011). medicated chewing gum - a 21st century drug delivery SYSYTEM. *International journal of pharmaceutical science and research* **2,** 15.

Gandhi, B.R., Mundada, A.S., and Gandhi, P.P. (2011). Chronopharmaceutics: as a clinically relevant drug delivery system. *Drug Deliv* **18,** 1-18.

Gavaskar, B., D, V.R., and Rao, Y.M. (2011). Medicated Chewing Gum – A Novel Approach to improve Patient Compliance. *International Journal of Research in Pharmaceutical and Biomedical Sciences* 2.

Ghosh, T.K., and Pfister, W.R. (2005). Drug Delivery to the Oral Cavity: Molecules to Market (Taylor & Francis).

Gupta, B.P., Thakur, N., Jain, N.P., Banweer, J., and Jain, S. (2010). Osmotically controlled drug delivery system with associated drugs. *J Pharm Pharm Sci* **13,** 571-588.

İkinci, G., Şenel, S., Wilson, C.G., and Şumnu, M. (2004). Development of a buccal bioadhesive nicotine tablet formulation for smoking cessation. *International Journal of Pharmaceutics* **277,** 173-178.

Imfeld, T. (1999). Chewing gum--facts and fiction: a review of gum-chewing and oral health. *Crit Rev Oral Biol Med* **10,** 405-419.

Jambhekar, S. (1990). Pharmaceutical dosage forms: Tablets. Vol. I. Edited by H. H. Lieberman, L. Lachman, and J. B. Schwartz. Marcel Dekker: New York. 1989. 592 pp.

K. Mochizuki and F. Yokomichi, Google Patents, (1976).

Krogel, I., and Bodmeier, R. (1999). Floating or pulsatile drug delivery systems based on coated effervescent cores. *Int J Pharm* **187,** 175-184.

Kvist, C., Andersson, S.B., Fors, S., Wennergren, B., and Berglund, J. (1999). Apparatus for studying in vitro drug release from medicated chewing gums. *Int J Pharm* **189,** 57-65.

Liu, L., Khang, G., Rhee, J.M., and Lee, H.B. (1999). Sandwiched osmotic tablet core for nifedipine controlled delivery. *Biomed Mater Eng* **9,** 297-310.

Liu, L., Ku, J., Khang, G., Lee, B., Rhee, J.M., and Lee, H.B. (2000). Nifedipine controlled delivery by sandwiched osmotic tablet system. *J Control Release* **68,** 145-156.

Madhav, N.V.S., Shakya, A.K., Shakya, P., and Singh, K. (2009). Orotransmucosal drug delivery systems: A review. *Journal of Controlled Release* **140,** 2-11.

Malaterre, V., Ogorka, J., Loggia, N., and Gurny, R. (2009). Oral osmotically driven systems: 30 years of development and clinical use. *European Journal of Pharmaceutics and Biopharmaceutics* **73,** 311-323.

Manoj Kumar, A.A., Prashant Kaldhone, Abhay Shirode and Vilasrao. J. Kadam (2010). Platform technologies for colon targeted drug delivery system : A Review Article. *Journal of Pharmacy Research* **3**, 5.

Marvola, J., Kanerva, H., Slot, L., Lipponen, M., Kekki, T., Hietanen, H., Mykkanen, S., Ariniemi, K., Lindevall, K., and Marvola, M. (2004). Neutron activation-based gamma scintigraphy in pharmacoscintigraphic evaluation of an Egalet constant-release drug delivery system. *Int J Pharm* **281**, 3-10.

Morales, J.O., and McConville, J.T. (2011). Manufacture and characterization of mucoadhesive buccal films. *European Journal of Pharmaceutics and Biopharmaceutics* **77**, 187-199.

Morjaria, Y., Irwin, W.J., Barnett, P.X., Chan, R.S., and Conway, B.R. (2004). In vitro Release of Nicotine From Chewing Gum Formulations. *Dissolution technologies* **11**, 4.

N.K., A., and A, G.S. (2001). Process for manufacturing a pharmaceutical chewing gum. , US, ed. (United state of america).

Nagai, T., and Konishi, R. (1987). Buccal/gingival drug delivery systems. *Journal of Controlled Release* **6**, 353-360.

Nair, A.B., Kumria, R., Harsha, S., Attimarad, M., Al-Dhubiab, B.E., and Alhaider, I.A. (2013). In vitro techniques to evaluate buccal films. *J Control Release* **166**, 10-21.

Pagare, P.K., Satpute, C.S., M, V., Jadhav, and Kadam, V. (2012). Medicated Chewing Gum: A Novel Drug Delivery System. *Journal of Applied Pharmaceutical Science* **02**, 14.

Patel, V.F., Liu, F., and Brown, M.B. (2012). Modeling the oral cavity: In vitro and in vivo evaluations of buccal drug delivery systems. *Journal of Controlled Release* **161**, 746-756.

Patra, C.N., Swain, S., Sruti, J., Patro, A.P., Panigrahi, K.C., Beg, S., and Rao, M.E. (2012). Osmotic Drug Delivery Systems: Basics and Design Approaches. Recent Pat Drug Deliv Formul.

Prior, D., Connor, A., and Wilding, I. (2003). The Enterion Capsule (New York: Marcel Dekker, Inc. New York).

Qiu, Y. (2009). Chapter 20 - Rational Design of Oral Modified-Release Drug Delivery Systems. In Developing Solid Oral Dosage Forms, Q. Yihong, C. Yisheng, G.Z.Z. Geoff, L. Lirong, Y.C.G.G.Z.Z.L.L. William R. PorterA2 - Yihong Qiu, and R.P. William, eds. (San Diego: Academic Press), pp. 469-499.

Quinten, T., Beer, T.D., Vervaet, C., and Remon, J.P. (2009). Evaluation of injection moulding as a pharmaceutical technology to produce matrix tablets. *European Journal of Pharmaceutics and Biopharmaceutics* **71**, 145-154.

Rachana Maheshwari, V.J., Rehana ansari, S.C. Mahajan, Garvita joshi (2013). A review on lozenges. *British biomedical bulletin* **1**, 10.

Rassing, M.R., and Jacobsen, J. (2002). Medicated Chewing Gum. In Modified-Release Drug Delivery Technology, M.J. Rathbone, J. Hadgraft, and M.S. Roberts, eds. (New York: Marcel Dekker).

Remington, J.P., and Osol, A. (1980). Remington's Pharmaceutical sciences (Mack).

Robinson, B.L.A.J.R. (2005). Preclinical Assessment of Oral Mucosal Drug Delivery Systems (United States of America: CRC Press).

Rømer Rassing, M. (1994). Chewing gum as a drug delivery system. *Advanced Drug Delivery Reviews* **13**, 89-121.

Ross, A.C., MacRae, R.J., Walther, M., and Stevens, H.N. (2000). Chrono pharmaceutical drug delivery from a pulsatile capsule device based on programmable erosion. *J Pharm Pharmacol* **52**, 903-909.

Salamat-Miller, N., Chittchang, M., and Johnston, T.P. (2005). The use of mucoadhesive polymers in buccal drug delivery. *Advanced Drug Delivery Reviews* **57**, 1666-1691.

Sastry Srikonda, P.K., Brian Barclay (2006). Osmotic Controlled Drug Delivery Systems (United States of America: McGraw-Hill Companies).

Sharma, G.S., Srikanth, M.V., Uhumwangho, M.U., Phani, K.K., and Ramana, K.M. (2011). Recent trends in pulsatile drug delivery systems - A review, Vol 2.

Smart, J.D. (1993). Drug delivery using buccal-adhesive systems. *Advanced Drug Delivery Reviews* **11**, 253-270.

Stefan, L., Claes, L., and Ove, F. (1974). Chewable smoking substitute composition (U.S.: Aktiebolaget Leo).

Stevens, H.E. (2003). Pulsincap and Hydrophilic Sandwich(HS) Capsules: Innovative Time-Delayed Oral Drug Delivery Technologies (New York: Marcel Dekker, Inc. New York).

Stevens, H.N.E. (1998). Chrono pharmaceutical drug delivery. *Journal of Pharmacy and Pharmacology* **50**, 5-5.

Stevens, H.N.E., Rashid, A., and Bakhshaee, M. (1994). Drug delivery devices, U.S. Patents, ed. (British Technology Group Limited).

Sudhakar, Y., Kuotsu, K., and Bandyopadhyay, A.K. (2006). Buccal bio-adhesive drug delivery — A promising option for orally less efficient drugs. *Journal of Controlled Release* **114**, 15-40.

Surana, A.S. (2010). Chewing Gum: A Friendly Oral Mucosal Drug Delivery System. *International Journal of Pharmaceutical Sciences Review and Research* **4**, 4.

Theeuwes, F. (1975). Elementary osmotic pump. *Journal of Pharmaceutical Sciences* **64,** 1987-1991.

Theeuwes; Felix , H.T. (1974). Osmotic dispensing device with maximum and minimum sizes for the passage way U.S. Patent, ed. (U.S.: Alza Corporation (Palo Alto, CA)).

Ueda, S., Ibuki, R., Kawamura, A., Murata, S., Takahashi, T., Kimura, S., and Hata, T. (1994). Development of a novel drug delivery system, time-controlled explosion system (TES). IV. In vivo drug release behavior. *J Drug Target* **2,** 133-140.

Verma, R.K., Arora, S., and Garg, S. (2004). Osmotic pumps in drug delivery. *Crit Rev Ther Drug Carrier Syst* **21,** 477-520.

Verma, R.K., Krishna, D.M., and Garg, S. (2002). Formulation aspects in the development of osmotically controlled oral drug delivery systems. *Journal of Controlled Release* **79,** 7-27.

Wilding, I. (2001). The Enterion Capsule: A Novel Technology for Understanding the Biopharmaceutical Complexity of New Molecular Entities (NMEs). *Drug development and delivary* **1.**

Wilding, I., Hirst, P., and Connor, A. (2000). Development of a new engineering-based capsule for human drug absorption studies. *Pharmaceutical Science & Technology Today* **3,** 385-392.

William, P.V., and Millind, T. (2012). A Comprehensive Review On Medicated Chewing Gum. *International Journal of Research in Pharmaceutical and Biomedical Sciences* **3,** 13.

Wong, P.S.L., Gupta, S.K., and Stewart, B. (2003). Osmotically Controlled Tablets (New York: Marcel Dekker, Inc. New York).

Woolfson, A., Garland, M., Shaikh, R., Donnelly, R., and Raj Singh, T. (2011). Mucoadhesive drug delivery systems. *Journal of Pharmacy and Bioallied Sciences* **3,** 89-100.

www.egalet.com/index.dsp?area=32, a.o.

Zema, L., Loreti, G., Melocchi, A., Maroni, A., and Gazzaniga, A. (2012). Injection Molding and its application to drug delivery. *Journal of Controlled Release* **159,** 324-331.

7   Coarse Dispersion

Sharad P. Pandey[1], Tripti Shukla[3], Vinod K. Dhote[1], Kanika Dhote[1] and Puneet Bhatnagar[2]

[1]Truba Institute of Pharmacy, Karond - Gandhi Nagar Bypass Road, Bhopal-462 038, India.

[2]Rishiraj College of Pharmacy. Bhavrasala, Behind SAIMS Hospital,. Sanwer Road, Indore- 453 331, India.

[3]School of Pharmacy, Peoples University, Bhanpur Bypass Road, Bhopal- 462 037, India.

7.1   Introduction

Insolubility of the number of compounds presents a prime hurdle in the development of a suitable formulation for oral administration. To overcome such hurdles, the development of a dosage form by employing newer techniques is of utmost important in context of the pharmaceutical industry.

Development of disperse system may be one of the better solutions for the oral administration of such poorly water soluble drugs. Disperse system may be defined as the heterogeneous system, which contains one phase as dispersed phase and second phase as dispersion medium. The dispersed phase is uniformly distributed in the dispersion medium (Solid, Liquid or Gas).

The Dispersion system may be classified as:

7.1.1 Molecular Dispersion

Molecular dispersion is a true solution containing solute as dispersed phase in form of separate molecules which are homogeneously

224

distributed throughout the solvent or dispersion medium. The molecule size is less than 1 nm (Banker et al., 1998).

7.1.2 Colloidal Dispersion

Colloids are micro-heterogeneous dispersed systems having the size of the dispersed phase particles within the range 1-1000 nm. The colloid system cannot be separated under gravity, centrifugal or other forces. Dispersed phase of colloids may be separated from the dispersion medium by micro-filtration (Banker et al., 1998; Banker et al., 2002a).

7.1.3 Coarse Dispersion

Coarse dispersions are characterized by relatively fast sedimentation of the dispersed phase caused by gravity or other forces (Wasan, 2007). Dispersed phase of coarse dispersions may be easily separated from the continuous phase by filtration. It is a heterogeneous dispersed system, in which the dispersed phase particles are larger than 1000 nm (Banker et al., 2002b; Florence and Siepmann, 2009). Basic details of various types of disperse systems and their size is mentioned in the Table 7.1.

TABLE 7.1

Different disperse systems with their size

Dispersed phase	Dispersion medium	Molecular dispersion	Colloidal dispersion	Coarse dispersion
		Dispersed Phase < 1 nm	Dispersed Phase 1.0 nm-0.5 µm	Dispersed Phase > 0.5 µm
Solid	Liquid	Nacl in water	Polymer in water	Suspension: calamine in water
Liquid	Liquid	Alcohol in Water	Liquid surfactant micelles	Emulsions: Milk
Gas	Liquid	Carbonated water	Foam	Foam
Solid	Solid	Solid dispersion	Colloidal gold in glass	Solid suspension
Liquid	Solid	Mineral oil in paraffin		Creams, solid emulsion
Gas	Solid	Hydrogen in palladium	Solid Foam	Solid Foam
Solid	Gas	Sublimed Idoine	Smoke	Dust
Liquid	Gas	Water vapour	Fog	spray
Gas	Gas	Air	N/A	N/A

Dispersed systems possess a wide range of application in pharmacy. Liquid dispersions such as emulsions and suspensions have an advantage of being easily administered and exhibit flexibility of dose as compared to solid dosage forms. This is important especially in case of infants, children and elderly patients, who have difficulty in swallowing solid dosage form.

Smaller particle size of drug present in dispersed system has large surface area which leads to a higher rate of drug dissolution for dispersions containing smaller particles as compared to solid dosage form which contain larger particles.

A suspension dosage form is often selected if the drug is insoluble in aqueous vehicle or when attempts to solubilize that drug through the use of surface-active agent or any other solubilizing agent are made which in turn compromise the stability and safety after oral administration. The unpleasant or bitter taste of dissolved drug molecule can often be improved by such formulations.

Colloidal systems have been used extensively in the pharmacy and colloids have been used in nuclear medicine as diagnostic aids. They may act as adjunct, enhance or promote the effects of various agents such as toxins adsorbed on a colloidal carrier or anti-cancer agents e.g., colloidal copper. Certain drugs have shown to improve their therapeutic activity or efficacy when formulated in a colloidal state. Colloidal silver chloride, silver iodide and silver protein are effective germicides and lack irritation that is the characteristic of ionic silver salts (Banker et al., 2002b).

On the other hand emulsions represent a group of popular oral and topical dosage forms. Oils and drugs with objectionable taste and texture can be developed for oral administration by formulating them in an emulsion form. As a result mixed oil based, laxatives, oil soluble vitamin, vegetable oils, and high fat nutritive preparations can be formulated and presented in wild variety of types. As far as quality of the dosage form is concerned some of the properties need to be controlled viz viscosity, appearance and the degree greasiness of in case of dermatological and cosmetic products.

All such types of the dosage forms which are categorized under the coarse dispersion along with their formulation considerations are described in this chapter.

7.2 Fundamentals of Suspension System

Suspension may be defined as biphasic system in which a finely divided solid (dispersed phase) is dispersed in a continuous phase (dispersion medium). The dispersion as such is thermodynamically unstable which is stabilized by using suspending agents (Banker et al., 2002a). Suspensions may be classified in various ways depending upon their mode of administration, size of the particles and their behavior (Table 7.2).

TABLE 7.2

Classification of suspensions

Basis for classifying suspension	Different classes of the suspension	
Routes of Administration	Oral Suspension	
	Parenteral suspension	
	Topical suspension	
Electro kinetic Nature	Flocculated	
	Deflocculated	
Size of the Particles	Colloidal Suspensions	< 1 µm
	Coarse suspension	> 1 µm
	Nano suspension	< 0.1 µm

7.2.1 Advantages and Disadvantages of Suspension

- Drug in suspension exhibits higher rate of bioavailability than other dosage forms. The bioavailability of different dosage forms is in the following order:

    Solution > Suspension > Capsule > Compressed Tablet > Coated tablet

- Efficient taste masking can be done by preparation of suspension of insoluble complexes of bitter drugs and resin or by the coated particles of bitter drugs viz. ornidazole suspension.

- Chemical stability of certain drugs can be improved by the suspension formulation e.g., Procaine penicillin G.

- Duration and onset of action can be improved and controlled.

Disadvantages of the suspension:

- Handling and transportation of such dosage forms.

- Physical changes as sedimentation and caking may arise serious concern.

- Preparation and stability may not be simple in some cases.
- Uniformity of dosing fluctuates because of rheological changes.

7.2.2 Properties of an Ideal Suspension

In spite of several drawbacks, suspension is one of the prime choices for the administration of water insoluble drugs in liquid dosage form. Settling of the dispersed particles on storage is a common problem for all type of suspensions effecting the product efficiency and efficacy (Jain and Sharma, 2010). Therefore it is of utmost importance to know the specific characteristic of a suspension so that a better formulation can be prepared. Some of the features of an ideal suspension are:

- The sedimentation of the suspended particles should be low as much as possible and should not produce a distinct layer.

- If settling of the particles occurs, cementing or caking should not occur and it should be easily redispersible.

- Rheological properties of the suspension should allow easy pour from the bottle in case of oral preparation. Similarly it should also possess syringe ability in case of parenteral formulation. While it should easily spread over the skin also the consistency should be maintained in case of dermal preparations (Jain and Sharma, 2010).

- Aesthetic value should be good along with its chemical and physical stability.

- In case of parenteral suspensions it should not lose its integrity and therapeutic significance if it is subjected to sterilization.

7.2.3 Theoretical Consideration of Stable Formulation

Sedimentation of the suspended particles in a suspension formulation is a biggest problem for its stability. Hence before development of a stable pharmaceutical suspension it is necessary to study the entire factors which contribute towards sedimentation. The word sedimentation may be defined as the settling of the particles, floccules or agglomerates under the gravity. It has been observed that the Brownian motion of the particle in applied dispersion medium limits to the chances of sedimentation. But such type of movement cannot be seen in the pharmaceutical suspension, due to larger particle size and viscosity of the dispersion medium

(Remington et al., 2006). The rate of the sedimentation of the particles may be described with the help of stokes law:

$$\text{Rate of sedimentation} = \frac{d^2(\rho_1 - \rho_2)g}{18\eta}$$

Where

> d = diameter of the particle, cm
> ρ_1 = density of the dispersed phase, g/cm^3
> ρ_2 = density of the dispersion medium, g/cm^3
> $\acute{\eta}$ = Viscosity of the dispersion medium, poise
> g = gravitational acceleration (9.87 m/sec^2)

The formula describes three major factors which can affect the rate of sedimentation as well as the stability of a suspension formulation.

7.2.4 Particle Size and its Distribution

It is a well-known fact that the larger particles will settle rapidly. So to prevent the chance of sedimentation it is better to reduce the particle size of the suspended material by milling (by colloidal mills or homogenizers). It has been noted that the sedimentation decreases approximately four times, if the particle size get decreased by half of its original size.

But at the similar time reduction of the particle size up to 50 µm may lead to the formation of agglomerates. Decreasing the particle size of any solid facilitates the liquid penetration because of increased surface area but the agglomerates oppose to the wetting of particle due to air entrapment inside behaving like a hydrophobic solid. Reduction in particle size or increase in surface area leads to the formation of agglomerates or coggules due to the change in electro-kinetic behavior of the particle (Subrahmanyam, 2000) and can be explained by the formula given below.

$$W = \Delta G = \gamma_{SL} . \Delta A$$

Where

> W = Work done to reduce the particle size
> ΔG = Increase in surface free energy
> γ_{SL} = interfacial tension at liquid-solid interface
> ΔA = increase in surface area at interface due to size reduction

From the above equation it can be easily understood that reduction in the particle size or increase in surface area will make the system thermodynamically unstable and this system will spontaneously try to be stable in order to reduce the surface free energy, which can best achieved firstly, by reducing the surface area i.e., regrouping of particles leading to formation of agglomerates, cogules or flocs. Secondly, the system can be made stable by reducing the interfacial tension (γ_{SL}) through addition of some surface active agents which may reduce the γ_{SL}.

According to stokes law another parameter which greatly effects the sedimentation of the particle is viscosity. The equation clearly states that if the viscosity of the system will be higher the settling of the particle will be lowered. But the viscosity should always be optimized properly, because a higher viscous dispersion medium may cause hindrance in redispersion after settling of the particle and on the other hands it may also lead to problems related to dispensing.

In general, suspensions can be classified in the different ways as mentioned above, but on the basis of nature and behavior of the solid as their electro kinetic property, suspension can be classified broadly in to two basic categories i.e., flocculated and deflocculated suspension.

7.2.5 Flocculated Suspensions

Flocculation may be referred as the formation of light fluffy, loose aggregates of discreet particles held together in a network like structure either because of adsorption of macromolecules or due to bridging during the precipitation or due to increased Van-der-wal forces rather than shorter range repulsive forces. Sometimes the term flocculation is confused with *agglomeration* and *coagulation*. While agglomeration is just the formation of closely bound aggregates of large number of particles and coagulation (over flocculation) refers to the aggregation of particles in liquid state alone and sometimes in the form of fluid gel structure (Hiestand, 1964). There are various factors which affect flocculation and can be outlined as follows:

- Effect of polymer dosage
- Effect of shear on the flocs
- Effect of particle size

- Effect of molecular weight
- Effect of pH
- Effect of temperature

Overflocculated or coagulated suspensions form a harder cake unlike to the flocculated suspensions. Overflocculation may occur due to the addition of excessive amount of flocculating agents or due to the prolonged exposure to the extreme thermal conditions.

Good pharmaceutical suspensions can be best achieved by formation of stable flocs which minimizes the chance of deflocculation and agglomeration (Hiestand, 1964). Stable flocs consist of rigid particles of suspended material which tend to cluster together in weak aggregates with minimum contact points. The number of contact point in a cluster increases the degree of flocculation (Garzon-Sanabria et al., 2013).

The major advantages of a stable flocs are:

- Aggregated particles may be separated easily with minimum shear stress and reform a network like structure after removing the stress.
- Stable flocs may be resuspended easily, while they get settled faster and achieve high volume of sediment rather than deflocculated system.
- The stable flocs may also be produced by aseptic techniques.

There are number of techniques which may be used to produce flocculated suspensions. The selection of method depends on the property of drug and class of suspension which has to be prepared. A brief discussion about such conditions which bring about flocculation is being provided below:

7.2.5.1 Inter-Particle Collision

It is well evident fact that if the solid particles are brought closer to less than 0.01 micron, the adhesive forces predominate over the repulsive forces. Agitation of a suspension causes particles to come close or even collision, allowing natural flocculation (Garzon-Sanabria et al., 2013). Fig. 7.1. illustrates formation of agglomerates in suspensions

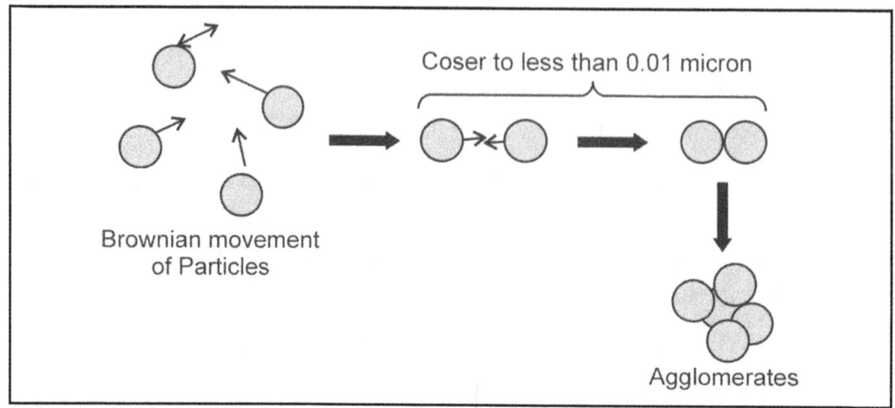

FIGURE 7.1 Formation of agglomerates in suspensions.

7.2.5.2 Reduction of Electrical Charge

Most dispersions in aqueous media carry an electric charge. Charge reduction lowers down electrical repulsion and enables coagulation to proceed to a further degree. Charge is neutralized by the addition of reagents giving rise to charged ions opposite in charge to that carried by the particles, e.g., inorganic salts such as $NaCl$, $CaCl_2$, $Al_2(SO_4)_3$, etc., which give rise to Na^+, Ca^{2+}, Al^{3+} (Fig. 7.2). The most highly charged cations are very much more effective, and in practice Al^{3+} and Fe^{3+} salts are mainly used (Garzon-Sanabria et al., 2013; Lachman et al., 1992).

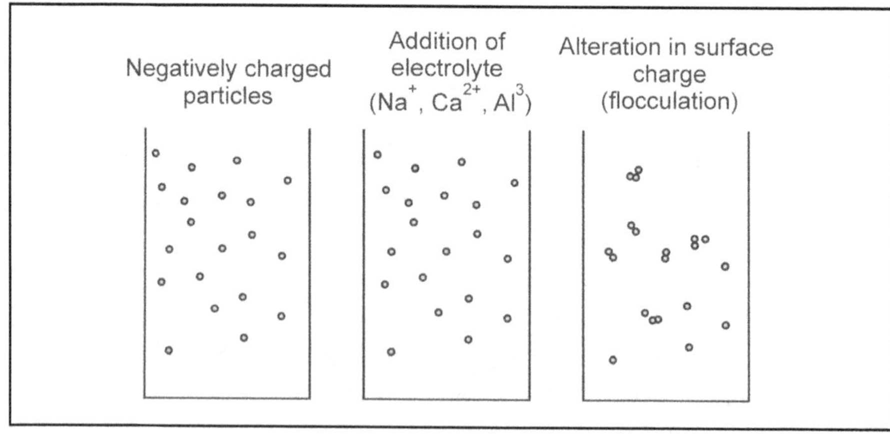

FIGURE 7.2 Effect of the charge of particles on flocculation.

7.2.5.3 Synthetic Bridging Flocculants

This system works on the principle that synthetic polymers of high molecular weight are long enough for one end to adsorb onto one particle and the other end onto second particles and by this way it leads to the formation of flocs as shown in Fig. 7.3 (Gregory and Barany, 2011; Zhou and Franks, 2006).

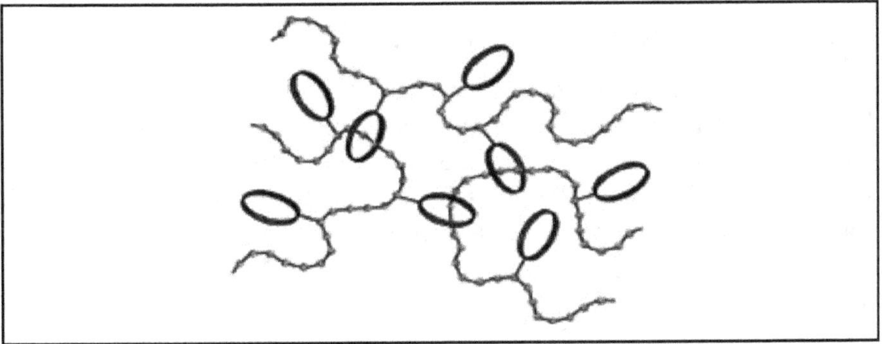

FIGURE 7.3 Representation of the formation of the bridge between the particles.

Most bridging flocculants carry either a positive (cationic) or a negative (anionic) charge serving the two basic purposes:

- They provide a means of adsorption onto the particle surface by electrostatic attraction.

- They cause the polymer molecule to extend and uncoil due to charge repulsion along the length of the polymer chain, so that the molecule is more nearly linear and can therefore accommodate more particles.

As most suspensions contain negatively charged particles it is expected that cationic polyelectrolytes would be most suitable. In general, the higher the molecular weight, the better the flocculation and the faster the sedimentation rate. With lower molecular weight flocculants, the flocs are small and have higher resistance to shear.

Natural bridging polymers

Natural polymers such as starch, gums, glues and alginates etc., function as bridging flocculants but are of a much lower molecular weight than synthetics and are only capable of a much lower degree of flocculation. Polysaccharides (starch, dextrin, etc.) are effective in neutral and slightly alkaline conditions, and organic colloids (glue, gelatin, albumen, casein, etc.), which, consists of aggregates of giant molecules, are effective in acid solution. Natural polymers are generally non-ionic, but may be rendered slightly anionic or cationic by chemical treatment. However, ionic character is of little importance since they have little effect on zeta potential and appear to function by hydrogen bonding (Zhou and Franks, 2006).

7.2.6 Deflocculated Suspension

Deflocculation is the absence of association which occurs when repulsive forces between particles predominate. Particles repel each other and remain as discrete, single particle. Repulsion forces prevail, the particles separate or deflocculate. Particles in these systems settle very slowly in stages, but ultimately form dense sediment which is considerably more compact than the corresponding sediment of a flocculated system and more difficult to redisperse.

Particle motion in such type of suspension is due to Brownian motion, convection currents, and sedimentation (gravity). When the particles settle, a dense mass is formed since there is no association between deflocculated particles. Downward movement due to gravity and the lateral motion due to Brownian movement facilitate tight packing of larger particles with the smaller particles filling the void spaces. Particles at the bottom of the cake are gradually pressed together by the weight of the ones above. Ostwald Ripening and Temperature Cycling effects cause particles to fuse together into a solid mass (Wasan, 2007).

In order to stabilize deflocculated systems, it is necessary to add a suspending and/or a gelling agent to retard settling and agglomeration of the particles by functioning as an energy barrier. Deflocculated suspension can be prepared by three major methods.

- Mutual repulsion to large zeta potential
- Adsorption of large or small hydrophilic or lyophilic colloid on larger suspended particles
- Steric hindrance due to absorbance of oriented non-ionic electrolyte or polyelectrolyte.

Flocculated and deflocculated suspension differs in their settling behavior (Nash et al., 2002) as well as other physical and rheological properties which have been summaried in Table 7.3.

TABLE 7.3

Differences in flocculated and deflocculated suspensions

S. No.	Flocculated suspension	Deflocculated suspension
1.	Contains light, fluffy group of particles which are held together by week vanderwal forces	Particles repel each other and remain as discrete, single particles
2.	Rate of sedimentation is high because of particle get settled in the form of flocs.	Because of minimal size of the single particles, sedimentation rate is compara-tively slow
3.	Sediment is formed slowly.	Sediment is formed rapidly
4.	Sediment is easy to disperse because of loosely packed aggregates do not form harder cake like structure	Redispersibility is very tough because of harder cake formation due to stronger attractive forces between the particles
5.	Shows pleasing appearance because of longer stability and uniformly dispersed particles	Shows unpleasant appearance due to faster settling of particles in form of flocks leading to clear supernatant fluid
6.	Flocs get generated because of change in surface charges	Sometimes faster sedimentation may occur due to formation of bigger particles due to Ostwald ripening

7.2.7 Formulation of Stable Suspension

Physical stability of a suspension can be controlled by two major techniques. The first technique utilizes the use of flocculating agents for enhancing the dispersibility of the particles and the second technique imparts the use of viscosity enhancing agents to reduce the sedimentation of the suspended particles. But still, developing a stable suspension formulation needs a number of components, which keep the solid particles in discrete form and suspended state.

1. Components of suspending system
   - (a) Wetting agent
   - (b) Deflocculating agent
   - (c) Flocculating agent
   - (d) Thickeners
2. Components of the suspending vehicles
   - (a) Buffering agents
   - (b) Osmotic agents
   - (c) Coloring and flavoring agents
   - (d) Preservatives

Wetting agent

The degree of wettability depends on the affinity of drugs for water and whether the solids are hydrophilic or hydrophobic. Hydrophilic solids are easily wetted by water and can increase the viscosity of aqueous suspensions. Hydrophobic solids repel water but can be wetted by non-polar liquids.

The rate of wetting is often determined by placing measured amount of powder on the undisturbed surface of water containing a given conc. of surfactant and measuring the time required to completely wet and sink the powder.

Wetting agents are surfactants that lower the interfacial tension and contact angle between solid particles and liquid vehicle. Non-ionic surfactants are most commonly used as wetting agents in pharmaceutical suspension. Non-ionic surfactants having HLB value between 7-10 are best as wetting agents although surfactants with HLB value 10 are often used for this purpose. Common type (Lachman et al., 1992) of wetting and surfactant includes

1. Anionic surfactants, e.g., SLS, Docusate sodium
2. Nonoionic surfactants e.g., Polyoxy sorbiton esters, sorbitan esters etc.

Polysorbate-80 is the most widely used surfactant for formulation of suspension because of its very low toxicity and compatibility with most formulation ingredients, whereas ionic surfactants are not generally used because they are not compatible with many adjuvants and cause change in pH. All surfactants are bitter except Pluronics and Poloxamers. Polysorbate 80 is most widely used surfactant both for parenteral and oral suspension formulation (Allen et al., 2002; Ludwig and Ooteghem, 1988). Polysorbate 80 gets adsorbed on drug particle and decreases its zeta potential which stabilizes the suspension but the same also gets adsorbed on plastic container decreasing its preservative action.

(Kuentz et al., 2006) have reported surfactant-free drug suspensions formulated using octenyl succinate-modified starches especially for toxicological, pharmacokinetic and pharmacodynamic studies.

(Deflocculated and dispersing agent): It is well evident that the dispersibilty of a suspension can be increased by altering the surface charge on the particle and their density. Deflocculating agents are the organic salt of sulfonic acid (different types) that can alter the surface charge of particle through physical adsorption. Generally, most of the

deflocculating agents are not considered safe for oral preparation but lecithin and their derivatives are acceptable.

Flocculating agent: Any substance which is capable of reducing the zeta potential of the suspension to zero may be used as flocculating agent. Small concentration (0.01-1%) of neutral electrolyte, such as sodium or potassium chloride is sufficient to induce flocculation. But this is only for the suspensions containing weekly charged particles such as steroids. In case of highly charged particles such as insoluble polymer or polyelectrolyte, similar concentrations (0.01-1%) of di or trivalent ions will be needed to induce flocculation. e.g., Potassium hydrogen phosphates, calcium sulfate, etc.

Thickening agents: This is a common term used for the substances which enhance the viscosity of a system when added. Some thickening agents are gelling agents, which form a gel. It is assumed that these materials get adsorbed and increase the strength of hydration layer formed around the suspended particle by hydrogen bonding and molecular interaction (N.K and S.N, 2010; Nash et al., 2002). Typically, the concentrations used range from 0.5% to 5%, but the viscosity will depend on the suspended particle's tendency to settle.

- Natural hydrocolloids: Acacia, tragacanth, alginic acid, carrageenan, locust bean gum, guar gum, gelatin.
- Semisynthetic hydrocolloids: Methylcellulose, sodium carboxy-methylcellulose, HPMC etc.
- Synthetic hydrocolloids: Carbopol
- Clays: Bentonite, Veegum etc.

Majority of these agents are protective colloids in their lower concentration (<0.1%) and viscosity enhancers in their high concentration (> 0.1%).

Buffering agents: Buffers are employed within pharmaceutical solutions or suspensions to control the pH of the formulated product. Especially the formulation which contains drugs with ionizable group should always have a buffering agent to avoid any change in pH. But use of such agents should be done with utmost care because a minor change may lead to the change of pattern in flocculation leading to instability of suspensions. Generally pH of suspension should be kept between 7.0-9.5, preferably between 7.4-8.4. Most commonly used buffers (Nash et al., 2002; regulation, 2009) are salts of week acids such as carbonates, citrates, gluconates, phosphate and tartrates. Among all the above mentioned agents Na phosphate is most widely used buffer in pharmaceutical suspension system while Citric acid is preferred to stabilize pH of the suspension between 3.5 to 5.0.

***Colouring and flavouring agents*:** Flavoring and coloring agents are added to increase patient acceptance. Only sweetening agent is not capable of complete taste masking of unpleasant drugs therefore, flavoring agents are incorporated. The selection of color should be based on the type of flavor being used e.g., green with mint-flavored, red for strawberry-flavoured formulations. Color aids in identification of the product. The color used should be acceptable by the regulatory agency of that region/country.

The four basic taste sensations are salty, sweet, bitter and sour. It has been proposed that certain flavors should be used to mask these specific taste sensations. Most widely used flavoring agents include fennel oil, peppermint, vanilla, raspberry, glycyrrhizin, cinnamon and lemon oil. Sometimes a combination of flavors is used to achieve the optimal taste-masking property.

Colors are obtained from natural or synthetic sources. Natural colors are obtained from mineral, plant and animal sources. Mineral colors (also called as pigments) are used to color lotions, cosmetics, and other external preparations. Plant colors are most widely used for oral suspensions. The synthetic dyes should be used within range of 0.0005% to 0.001% depending on the depth of color required.

Most widely used colors are mentioned as follows (regulation, 2009):

- White   :   Titanium dioxide
- Blue   :   Brilliant blue, Indigo carmine, Indigo
- Red   :   Amaranth, Carmine
- Yellow   :   Tartarazine, Sunset yellow, Carrots, Saffron, etc.
- Green   :   Chlorophyll
- Brown   :   Caramel (brown)

7.2.8   Stability of a Suspension

Assessment of stability of developed dosage form is an important aspect. This is specifically more important in case of dispersed system including suspension. Stability of a suspension can be studied in below described three different ways; chemical stability, physical stability and crystal growth.

7.2.8.1 Chemical Stability

In suspension dosage forms, it has been observed that suspended drug gradually degrades as the solid phase gradually dissolves in vehicle. Generally this degradation follows the zero order kinetics, with the rate constant solely dependent on the saturation solubility of the drug in solution (N.K and S.N, 2010). This degradation may be minimized by decreasing the solubility of suspended drug. So, during the formulation of suspension this fact should be kept in mind that the selection of pH of the formulation should be in such a way that minimizes the degradation of the drug. Sometimes this degradation may also be attributed to catalysis initiated due to the environmental factors such as oxygen, light and trace elements (Sinko et al., 2004).

7.2.8.2 Physical Stability

Physical stability is the major concern in almost all suspension systems because of separation upon standing. This may lead to the unequal dispensing of the dose to be poured out and administered. Hence settling of the particles in a suspension system should be minimal and if settled it should be easily redispersible. The sedimentation of the particles is favored because of floc formation, agglomeration or coagulation due to the presence of charges on their surfaces. The extent of the sedimentation is quantitatively expressed by two major parameters which are applicable to the flocculated suspension; sedimentation volume and degree of flocculation.

Sedimentation volume is defined as the ratio of ultimate volume of the sediment to the initial volume of the suspension. While, the degree of flocculation may be defined as the ratio of sedimentation volume of flocculated suspension to that of deflocculated suspension.

For better stability it is always desired that the solid particles must remain unchanged in size and form. Crystal growth can lead to changes in particle size while, solid-to-solid, polymorphic, amorphous-to-crystalline, and degree of hydration transformations can change the form of the particles. The effect of size of the particles and their properties on the settling of the particles (Stoke's law) has been discussed earlier in this chapter.

7.2.8.3 Crystal Growth

Crystal growth is potentially the most serious problem that can occur in a suspension. It may cause caking, changes in sedimentation, and alter bioavailability. If a metastable drug form is used to manufacture a suspension, the saturated solution which exists in suspension is supersaturated relative to a more stable form. The drug crystallizes as the more stable form and more metastable drug dissolves in order to re-establish the saturated metastable solution. This continues until the transformation is complete.

At the similar time Ostwald ripening is a phenomenon of concern leading to the crystal growth due to high surface free energy of small particles. The small particles have a greater ratio of surface area to particle mass than large particles. The greater solubility of the smaller particles, produces solutions which are supersaturated relative to the larger particles therefore, dissolved molecules tend to crystallize on the surface of the large particles thereby extending the lattices and causing growth of the surface upon which they crystallize.

7.2.9 Evaluation of Suspension

Stability as well as acceptance of suspension formulation depends on several parameters, so it is necessary to evaluate it for various attributes described below:

7.2.9.1 Appearance

Appearance is one of the most prominent characteristics for the better product acceptability. During the study three major things i.e., colour distribution, presence of air flocs and floc formation (adhered on the wall) is studied primarily. The particle size distribution, clarity of formulation, the viscosity of gum dispersion, quality control of water is monitored to keep an eye on the product quality.

7.2.9.2 Photomicroscopic Examination

Particle size and crystal shape play very important role in the stability of a formulation, so it is significant to study the particle size and crystal behavior using microscope and other different particle size analyzing techniques. Average particle size can be used to check out whether the system is flocculated or deflocculated. Flocculated system consists of flocs and hence would display higher average particle size as compared to the other deflocculated system.

7.2.9.3 Organoleptic Properties (color, taste, odor)

Change in colour, odour and taste is a major criteria to assess the stability of an oral suspension. Variation in colour indicates poor particle size distribution or differences in size of particles. Variation in taste also indicates change in particle size distribution or change in crystal habit.

7.2.9.4 Sedimentation Rate, Volume, Resuspendability

Lower sedimentation and easy redispersion of the suspended particle is first and foremost important criterion for an ideal suspension formulation. A simple graduated measuring cylinder may be used to study the rate of sedimentation, sedimentation volume and degree of flocculation which are the major parameters to be tested to investigate the physical stability of a suspension. Sedimentation volume (F) may be defined as the ratio of ultimate volume of the sediment (Vu) to initial volume of the suspension (Vi).

$$\text{Sedimentation volume (F)} = \frac{\text{Ultimate volume of the sediment (Vu)}}{\text{Initial volume of the suspension (Vi)}}$$

Similarly, the degree of flocculation (β) may be defined as the ratio of sedimentation volume of flocculated system (F) to the sedimentation volume of deflocculated system (Fd).

$$\text{Degree of flocculation } (\beta) = \frac{\text{Sedimentation volume of flocculated system (F)}}{\text{Sedimentation volume of deflocculated system (Fd)}}$$

During the study, sufficient wide cylinder should be used to overcome the wall effect which is attributed to the interaction of the suspended particles with that of the walls of the container and leads to the change in concentration as well as viscosity near the walls of the tube/container. Small and narrow cylinders favor the suspension because of the adhesive forces acting between the inner surface of the container and the suspended particle.

For checking the redispersibility, a mechanical stirrer simulating the human arm motion can be used to achieve reproducible results under controlled condition. Alternatively, the cylinder containing suspension may be rotated through 360°C completing circular motion. The time taken to redisperse total sediment or number of revolutions is taken as endpoint for the study.

7.2.9.5 Viscosity

Stability of a suspension is solely dependent on the sedimentation rate of dispersed phase, which is in part dependent on the viscosity of the dispersion medium. The viscosity of the dispersion medium is measured before mixing with dispersed phase as well as after formulation of suspension.

7.2.9.6 pH Value

pH also effects the stability of a aqueous suspension. Naseer and co-workers have reported that the floc size and rheological behavior of kaolinite suspensions change significantly with change in both electrolyte concentration and solution pH (Nasser and James, 2009).

7.2.9.7 Zeta Potential Measurement

Zeta potential is a physical property which is exhibited by any particle in suspension. Zeta potential is the electric potential in the interfacial double layer at the location of the slipping plane versus a point in the bulk fluid away from the interface. In other words, zeta potential is the potential difference between the dispersion medium and the stationary layer of fluid attached to the dispersed particle (Nash et al., 2002; Sinko et al., 2004).

It is a well known phenomenon that when a particulate matter is dispersed in water, the development of a net charge at the particle surface takes place and this largely affects the distribution of ions in the surrounding interfacial region, resulting in an increased concentration of counter ions (ions of opposite charge to that of the particle) close to the surface resulting in the formation of double layer around each particle. The liquid layer surrounding the particle may be considered in two parts; the first, an inner region where the ions are strongly bound, called the Stern layer, and the second an outer region where the ions are loosely attached, called diffused layer (Fig. 7.4). Within the diffused layer there is a notional boundary inside which the ions and particles form a stable entity. When a particle moves (e.g., due to gravity), ions within the boundary move with it, but any ions beyond the boundary do not travel with the particle. This boundary is called the surface of hydrodynamic shear or slipping plane. The potential that exists at this boundary is known as the zeta potential. Value of zeta potential reflects the future stability of suspensions so it monitored time to time to ensure optimum zeta potential (Sinko et al., 2004).

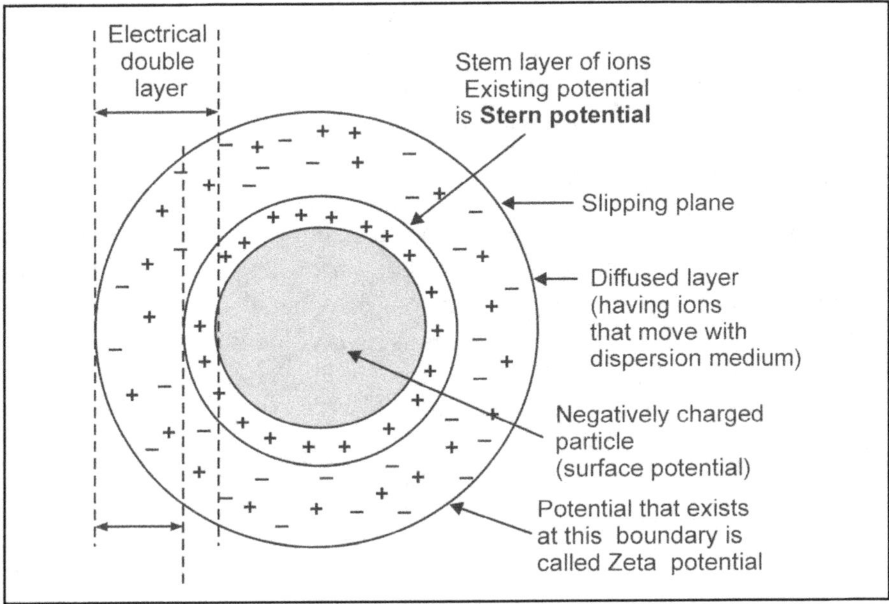

FIGURE 7.4 Graphical representation showing the basic understanding of zeta potential.

It has been noted that the zeta potential values lower (less negative) than −15 mV usually represent the onset of agglomeration. The threshold region of either coagulation or dispersion exists from about −14 mV to −30 mV. Values more electronegative than −30 mV generally represent sufficient mutual repulsion to result in stability (i.e., no agglomeration), similarly the Zeta potential value more the +30 also shows better stability. Zeta potential is measured by either Zeta meter or micro-electrophoresis.

7.2.9.8 Freeze Thaw Cycling

Freeze-thaw cycle testing is a part of stability testing, in which the product is exposed to the series of extreme rapid changes of temperature to determine the stability of the formulation. (Carless and Foster, 1966; Carless et al., 1968) had investigated various crystal forms of cortisone acetate and reported acceleration of sulfathiazole crystal growth in suspension that underwent temperature cycling. Sometimes it has also been noted that some of the suspension component have greater effect during freeze thaw cycling (e.g., preservative, protective colloid).

7.2.9.9 Drug Content Uniformity

Drug content can be checked by withdrawing specific volume of suspension and analyzing the drug contained in that sample using appropriate analytical technique i.e., UV spectroscopy or HPLC or some other techniques. Samples from the upper middle and lower portion are taken from a well-mixed suspension.

7.2.9.10 Dissolution Testing

In general, the rotating paddle method utilizing an aqueous dissolution medium is the recommended method for dissolution testing of suspension. For low viscosity suspensions an accurate dose can be placed at the bottom of the dissolution vessel using a volumetric pipette. A slow agitation rate of 25 rpm is generally recommended for less viscous suspensions (Abdou et al., 2000) (Fig. 7.5).

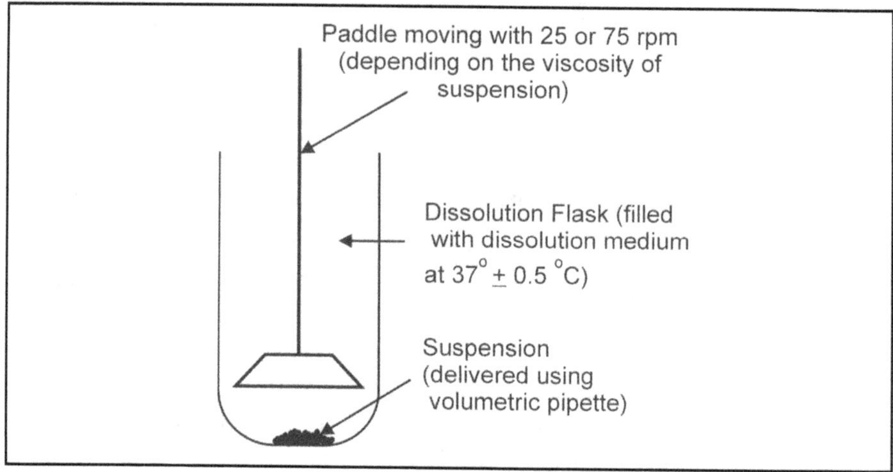

FIGURE 7.5 Representation of dissolution testing for suspension.

For high viscosity suspensions, the dose to be tested for dissolution study is need to be weighed followed by quantitative sample transfer to the dissolution vessel to ensure accuracy of the sample size introduced. High viscosity suspensions may also require a faster agitation rate such as 50 or 75 rpm to prevent sample mounding at the bottom of the vessel (da Fonseca et al., 2009).

Ideally, sample weight/volume should reflect a typical dose of the product. However testing a partial dose e.g., ≥ 10– 20 % of the usual product dose, is recommended in case of drugs where use of surfactant is required to obtain and maintain sink condition.

USP dissolution apparatus 4 can be used for the release study of the colloidal dispersions by adding a medication in the sample holder system. An adapter covered with the dialysis membrane is placed in the sample holder for retaining the sample to be studied for *in-vitro* release as shown in Fig. 7.6 (Bhardwaj and Burgess, 2010). Gao and Westenberger, 2012 used the flow-through method with and without the dialysis adapter to observe the release of an acetaminophen suspension.

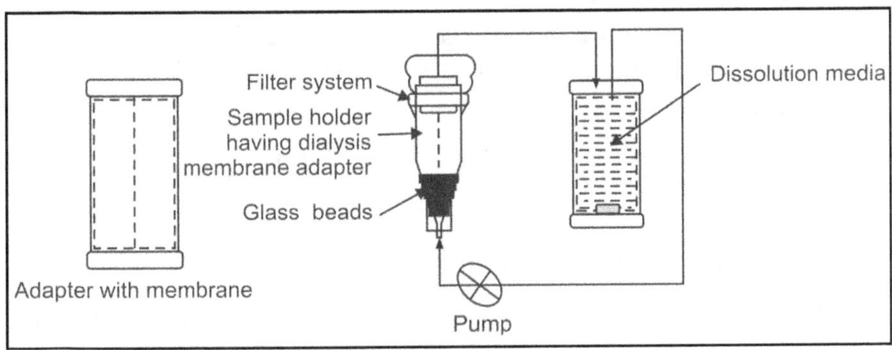

FIGURE 7.6 Modified dissolution apparatus for suspensions.

7.3 Pharmaceutical Emulsions

Emulsion may be defined as thermodynamically unstable biphasic system of two immiscible liquids, in which one liquid is dispersed as fine droplets (dispersed phase) throughout another liquid (dispersion medium) in form of small droplets and the whole system is stabilized with the help of an emulsifying agent. The globules are usually opaque and white and size ranges from 0.25 to 10 micron.

The emulsion system may be classified in following types:

- Oil in water emulsion (O/W)
- Water in oil emulsion (W/O)
- Multiple emulsion
- Microemulsion/nanoemulsion

All the emulsion systems are stabilized with the help of an emulsifying agent also known as emulsifier. They act by reducing the interfacial tension at the oil-water interface. The emulsifying agent gets concentrated at liquid-liquid interface, providing a physical barrier to avoid coalescence. Emulsifying agents may be classified into three basic groups as mentioned below (Sinko et al., 2004):

1. **Surface active agents**

    These agents get adsorbed leading to the formation of mono-molecular layer at the liquid-liquid interface and reduce the interfacial tension.

2. **Hydrophilic colloids**

    These form a multi-molecular layer around the dispersed oil droplets in O/W emulsion and grant stability to the formulation.

3. **Finely divided solid particles**

    The finely divided solid particles become adsorbed at the liquid-liquid interface of two immiscible liquids

7.3.1 Advantages of Emulsions

- Taste masking of bitter drug can be accomplished by incorporating the drug in the inner core of the emulsion (dispersed phase) e.g., vitamin containing emulsion.

- It is always economical to prepare an emulsion of poorly water soluble drug rather than to solubilize it using expensive solvents.

- Bioavailability of certain drugs like acyclovir can be improved by enhanced absorption when incorporated in emulsion.

- The system may also be prepared for the sustained release of drugs as in case of some depot injections. Multiple emulsions may also serve better for this purpose.

- Radio-opaque emulsions are used as diagnostic material in X-ray examination.

- Majority of topical creams are emulsion, sometime the emulsion is also used as base in certain semisolid preparations.

- Emulsion prepared after dissolving the fat soluble nutrient in oil phase and water soluble nutrient in water phase may serve better and fulfill the nutrition requirement in terminally ill patient.

7.3.2 Theory of Emulsification

There are several theories proposed to explain the action of emulsifying agents in stabilizing emulsions. A theory describing emulsification process should fulfill the two basic criteria; stability of the emulsion and type of the emulsion to be prepared. Some of the theories are being explained here.

7.3.2.1 Mono-Molecular Adsorption

This theory states that the emulsifying agents used get adsorbed on the interface between two immiscible liquids leading to reduction of interfacial tension and likewise reduction of surface free energy which in turn leads to emulsification of one immiscible liquid into the other one as globules (Fig. 7.7). This minimization of surface free energy reduces the tendency of coalescence of globules (Sinko et al., 2004). This reduction in coalescence is also attributed to the formation of monolayer by surfactant/emulsifying agent at the interface.

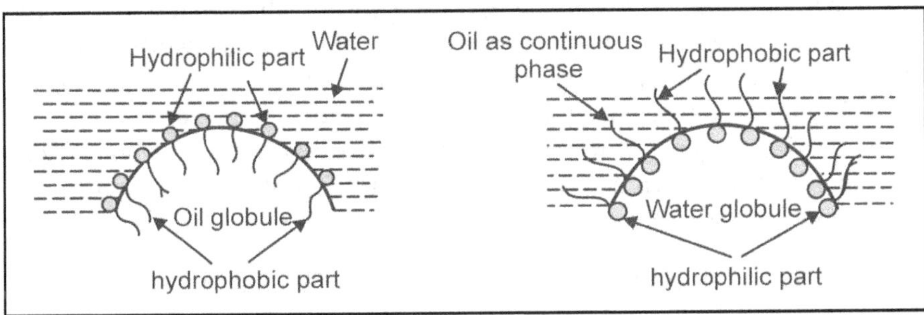

FIGURE 7.7 Diagrammatic representation of behavior of water/oil molecules in opposite medium.

Recently it has been noted that combination of emulsifiers rather than use of single one is more beneficial for emulsion formation. Some important combinations include sodium cetyl sulphate and cholesterol, cetyl alcohol and sodium oleate.

7.3.2.2 Multi-Molecular Adsorption

Some agents like hydrated lyophilic colloids are used for several years as emulsifying agents. They form a multimolecular layer at the liquid-liquid interface (Fig. 7.8) but do not reduce the interfacial tension. At the same time such agents also increase the viscosity of the system and produce auxiliary effect of promoting stability. Since the agents forming layer around the droplets are invariably hydrophilic, they tend to promote the formation of O/W emulsion.

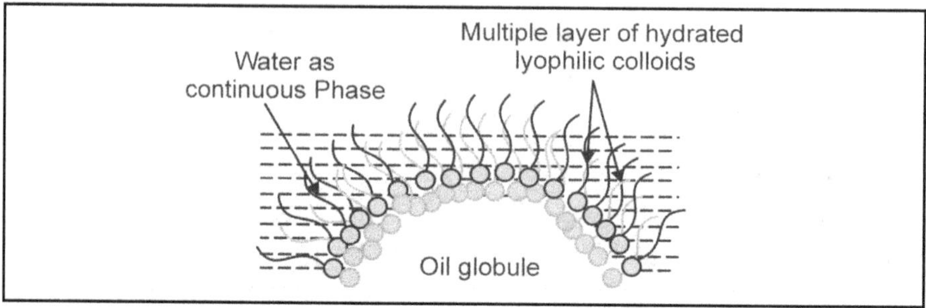

FIGURE 7.8 Diagrammatic representation of integral part of emulsion formed through colloids.

7.3.2.3 Solid Particle Adsorption Theory

Small solid particles like bentonite ($Al_2O_3.4SiO_2.H_2O$), veegum (magnesium, aluminum and silicate), hectorite, magnesium hydroxide, aluminum hydroxide and magnesium trisilicate, that are wetted to some degree by both oil, and water can act as emulsifying agents. These particles form a particulate film around the dispersed droplets as shown in Fig. 7.9. The agent which is wetted preferentially by oil form W/O emulsion and those which are wetted by water form O/W emulsion.

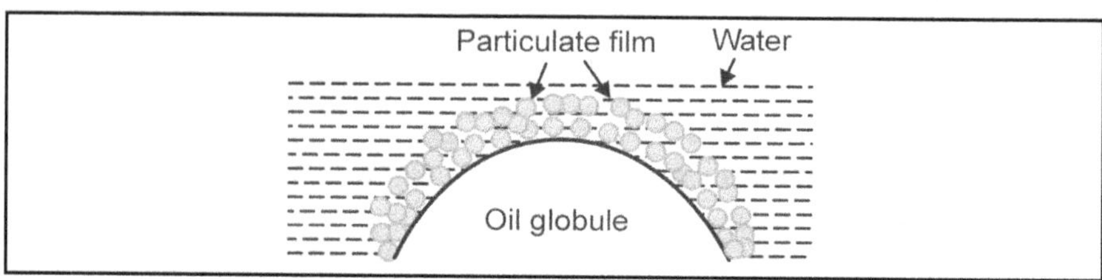

FIGURE 7.9 Wetting action of an   emulsifying agent.

7.3.3 Emulsion Type and Means of Detection

Differentiating an emulsion between o/w or w/o with naked eye is almost impossible. Some techniques are available which can be used to identify the type of emulsion formed. These techniques are discussed below in brief:

7.3.3.1 Dilution Test

The basic principal behind the dilution test is that if the continuous phase (dispersion medium) is added to the emulsion system it will lead to dilution without cracking or phase separation of the emulsion while addition of dispersed phase will lead to cracking of the emulsion (Fig. 7.10). O/W emulsion can be diluted with the water without cracking and similarly w/o emulsion can be diluted with oil without phase separation.

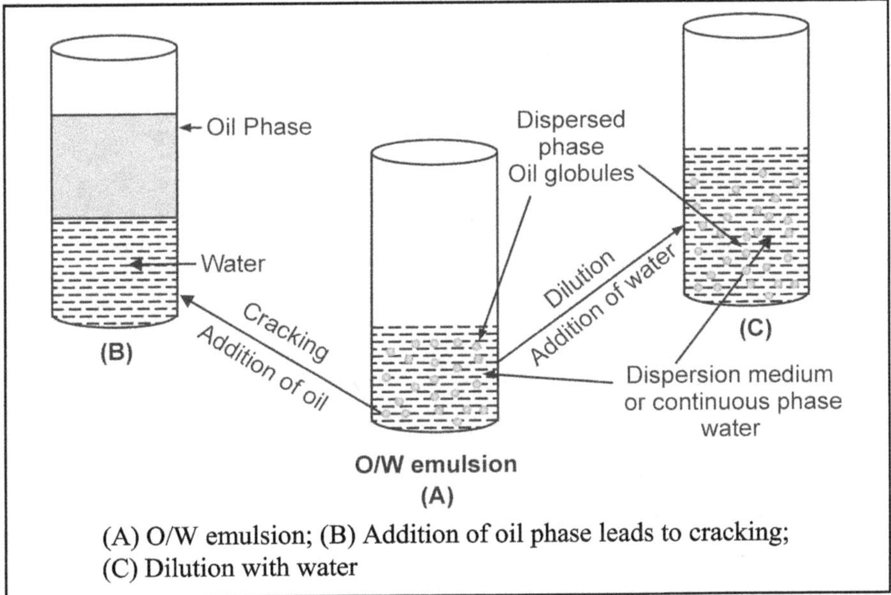

FIGURE 7.10 Schematic representation of dilution test.

7.3.3.2 Conductivity Test

Water is a good conductor of electricity whereas oil does not facilitate conduction of electrical current. Therefore, when a circuit connected to a bulb is placed in the emulsion it leads to the glowing of the bulb in case the continuous phase is water as shown in Fig. 7.11. If the continuous phase is replaced with oil, the bulb does not glow.

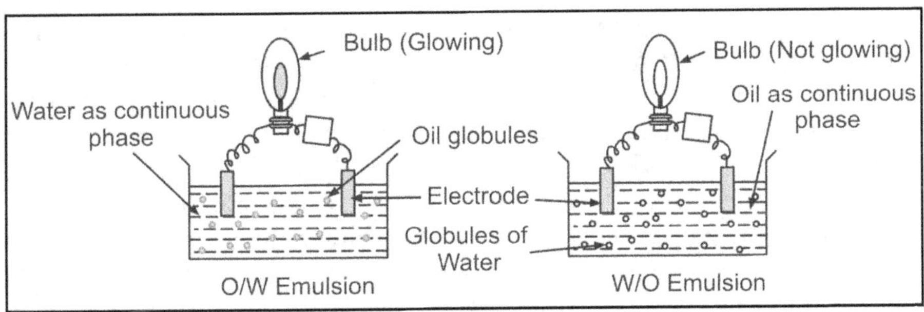

FIGURE 7.11 Illustration of the conductivity test for emulsions.

7.3.3.3 Dye-Solubility Test

In this test, a water soluble dye such as methylene blue is added in minute amount, to the emulsion. The dye dissolves uniformly throughout the system if water is the continuous phase (O/W emulsion), whereas the dye will form a cluster on the surface if oil forms the continuous phase in case of W/O emulsion (Fig. 7.12).

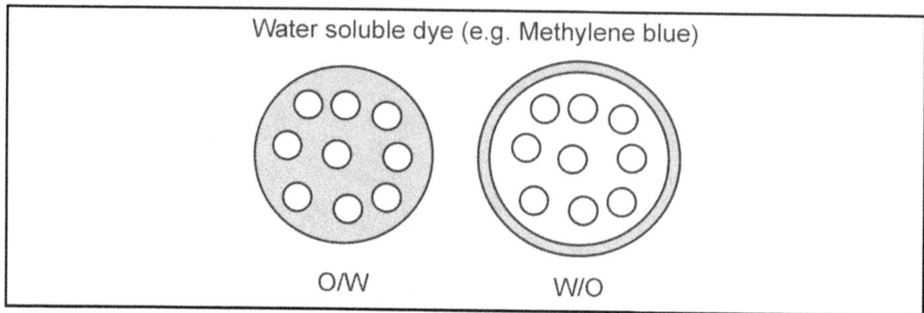

FIGURE 7.12 Diagrammatic illustration of the dye test.

7.3.3.4 Fluorescence Test

Oils produce fluorescence under UV light, while water does not give rise to fluorescence. Therefore, O/W emulsion shows dot pattern and W/O emulsion fluorescence throughout the system.

7.3.3.5 CoCl$_2$/Filter Paper Test

When a dried filter paper impregnated with CoCl$_2$ (Blue) is dipped into the O/W type of emulsion it changes to pink colour. But the same test may not work if the emulsion is unstable or breaks in presence of electrolyte (N.K and S.N, 2010).

7.3.4 Stability of Pharmaceutical Emulsions

Stability is the first and foremost criteria during the development of any pharmaceutical formulation. The major concern with reference to the stability of the emulsion is phase separation of emulsion in constituent phases i.e., water and oil phase. This phase separation may occur due to coalescence of globules, creaming or flocculation. Secondly, it should maintain its elegance, taste, odour etc., for the entire product life. The other phenomenon which is of utmost importance is phase inversion i.e., change of emulsion type o/w to w/o because of change in temperature. The instability of emulsion may be classified as follows:

7.3.4.1 Chemical Instability

Sometimes it has been observed that the catalysis in micellar system may lead to decomposition of the drugs e.g., hydrolysis of alkyl sulfate. While on the other hand some lipid materials are also prone to the oxidative degradation (rancidity). This problem can be eliminated with the help of proper type and concentration of anti-oxidant selection. However the best way is to avoid the use of such lipid material as far as possible.

7.3.4.2 Physical Instability

It has already been discussed earlier that the emulsion is thermodynamically unstable system. The physical instability can be divided in to three basic segments; flocculation or creaming, coalescence or breaking and phase inversion.

7.3.4.2.1 Flocculation or Creaming

Flocculation of emulsion may be defined as the association of smaller neighboring globules to form a colony like structure in the external phase. Flocculation is considered as the precursor of coalescence. This association of globules basically depends on size and size distribution of the globules, charges on the globule surface and viscosity of the medium.

Such flocculation of the globules (usually more than 1 mm) leads their movement, either in upward or downward direction depending upon the densities of two liquids, used to formulate the emulsion (Eccleston, 2007; Khan et al., 2011). The rate of movement of globules in the upward or downward direction can be best interpreted with the help of stokes law described in section 2.3. The limitations of this equation are similar, as that described in case of suspension.

It has been noted that if the density of the dispersed phase is less than that of dispersion medium as in case of o/w emulsion, the velocity of sedimentation will be negative leading to the creaming in upward direction whereas downward creaming occurs if the internal phase is heavier than the external phase as in case of w/o emulsion (Carter, 2000).

In practice, use of viscosity enhancing agents, and minimization of globuler size can minimize the chances of creaming.

7.3.4.2.2 Coalescence and Breaking

It may be defined as the merging process of two or more droplets, bubbles or particles to form a single larger daughter droplet, bubble or particle. As it has been already mentioned in the previous section of this chapter that flocculation is precursor of coalescence and therefore it can be understood that coalescence is an irreversible process whereas flocculation can be reversed and globules can be dispersed with gentle shaking at initial stages. When the breaking of emulsion occurs because of coalescence, it cannot be re-dispersed, since the film of emulsifier, surrounding the globule is destroyed. The major factors which prevent the coalescence in a flocculated emulsion is mechanical strength of the interfacial layer (Eccleston, 2007). Some basic reasons of coalescence include insufficient amount of emulsifying agent, altered partitioning of emulsifying agent and incompatibility of emulsifying agent.

7.3.4.2.3 Phase Inversion

Phase inversion is the phenomenon whereby the phases of liquid-liquid dispersion interchange such that the dispersed phase spontaneously inverts to become the continuous phase and vice versa as shown in Fig. 7.13.

It can produce finer emulsion if controlled properly, but changes generally occur due to uncontrolled phase inversion which usually leads to breaking of the system. An o/w emulsion stabilized by sodium stearate can be inverted to w/o type by addition of calcium chloride with the formation of calcium stearate. Phase inversion is also favored by change in phase volume ratio.

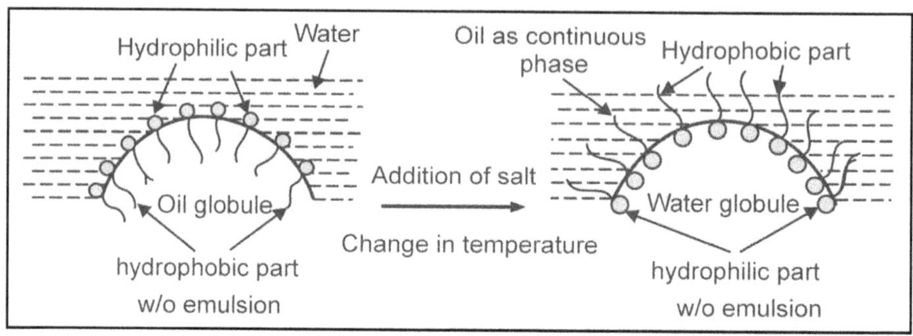

FIGURE 7.13 Phase inversion in the emulsion.

Based on the Bancroft's rule, it is possible to change an emulsion from O/W type to W/O type by inducing changes in surfactant HLB. Some common reasons of phase inversion include:

- The order of addition of the phases
- Nature of emulsifier
- Phase volume ratio
- Temperature of the system
- Addition of electrolytes and other additives

Change in temperature is very important phenomenon which may lead to phase inversion. It has been observed that as the temperature increases, the water solubility of ethoxylated nonionic emulsifiers becomes poorer leading to chances of phase inversion (Carter, 2000). The temperature at which the inversion occurs is called as phase inversion temperature. Phase inversion temperature is generally considered as the temperature at which the hydrophilic and lipophilic properties of an emulsifying agent is in balance and therefore also called HLB temperature.

7.3.5 Formulation of Emulsion

Emulsion formulation contains different materials which provide desirable property, increase its stability and acceptance. The basic entities which are necessary for a stable and universally accepted emulsion are listed below:

7.3.5.1 Immiscible Phases

These are the most important component because the definition of emulsion itself says that it is the system of two immiscible liquids and therefore without immiscible liquids the existence of emulsions cannot be thought of. Some materials which are commonly used in pharmaceutical or cosmetic emulsion system are:

- Polyols (butylenes glycol, glycerin, polyethylene glycol etc) and water: polar materials
- Ester (Fats, lanolin vegetative oil etc), fatty acids and alcohols, hydrocarbons (butane, propane, mineral oil, and petroleum products): non polar materials
- Miscellaneous (halohydrocarbons, plant and animal waxes, silicon fluid etc): non polar materials

7.3.5.2 Emulsifiers

These are the agents which stabilize the emulsion system either by reducing the interfacial tension or by forming the barrier layers at the liquid-liquid interface. These materials possess certain degree of affinity to both polar and nonpolar liquids. The detail mechanism has already been discussed in the earlier section on the theory of emulsification. There are two types of emulsifying agents on the basis of effect they produce. First category is primary agents (true emulsifying agents) which can form and stabilize emulsions by themselves. The second category is auxiliary agents (stabilizers) which alone do not form fine emulsions but assist the primary emulsifying agents in forming stable emulsion.

For a stable emulsion it is very important to choose the right emulsifier which has optimum and desired HLB value. A general classification has been mentioned in the Table 7.4 with examples (Banker et al., 1998; Carter, 2000). In 1984, Griffin has developed a method for calculating the balanced mixture of emulsifier which could produce a specific type of emulsion, known as emulsifier HLB scale. Higher number indicates hydrophilic property and lower number indicates hydrophobic nature as indicated schematically in Fig. 7.14. Emulsifier with higher number produces o/w emulsion while the emulsifier with lower value results in w/o type emulsion.

TABLE 7.4

Common examples of surfactants used as emulsifier

S. No.	Type	Examples	HLB value/ Range
1.	Non ionic	Sorbitan alkyl esters: Spans	2-9
		Polysorbates (Tween)	
		Polyoxyethylene glycol alkyl ethers (Brij)	10-17
		Poloxamers	7-19
2.	Anionic	Alkyl sulfates e.g. sodium lauryl sulfate	30-40
		Soaps	12-30
3.	Cationic	Quaternary ammonium compounds	
4.	amphiphiles	Difatty alkyl triethanolamine derivatives	16-17
5.	Zwitterionic	Alkyl betain derivative	-

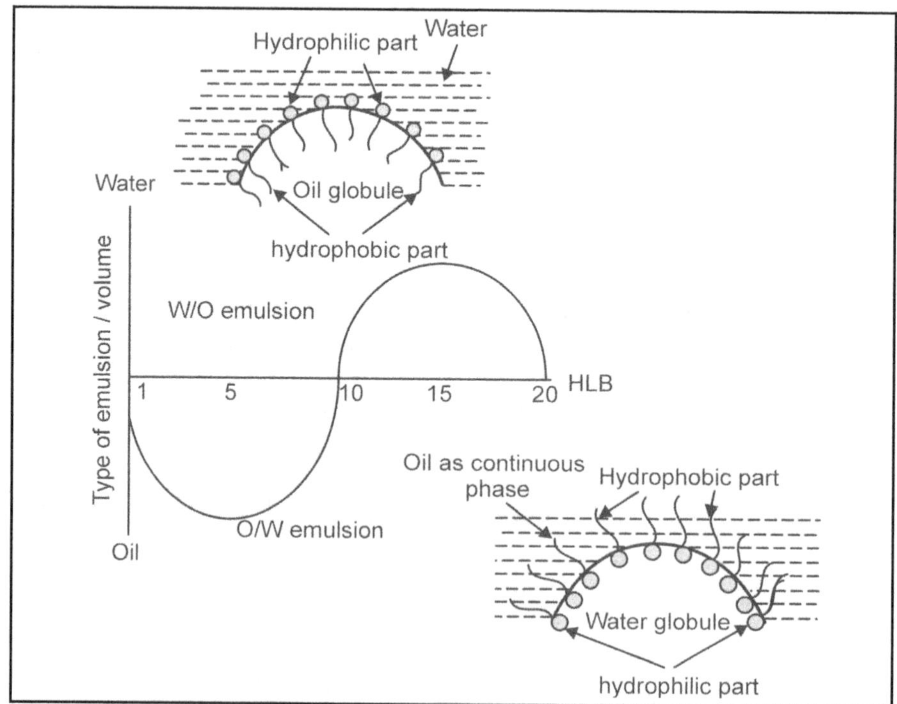

FIGURE 7.14 Representation of the HLB scale.

In spite of single surfactant, it has been observed that a combination of emulsifier (oil and water soluble both) produces better stability to the system. The required blend of emulsifier to achieve specific HLB can be calculated using following formula (Block et al., 1989):

$$HLB_{blend} = f\,HLB_A + (1\text{-}f)\,HLB_B$$

where f is the fraction of surfactant A in the surfactant mixture of surfactant A and surfactant B having different HLB values.

The type of emulsion to be formed entirely depends on the selection of emulsifier. This relation can be easily understood by Bancroft's rule which states that if the phase in which an emulsifier is more soluble constitutes the continuous phase e.g., if the surfactant is more soluble in the water system then the water will be continuous phase leading to the formation of O/W emulsion.

Though, the Bancroft's rule and HLB scale have provided a better principle to get a stable emulsion system exceptions still exist (Tadros et al., 2004).

7.3.5.3 Auxiliary Agents (Emulsion Stabilizers)

Auxiliary agents or emulsion stabilizers (Banker et al., 1998; Block et al., 1989) are emulsifiers, which are obtained from natural sources and are able to form hydrated lyophilic colloids (called hydrocolloids) that form multimolecular layers around emulsion droplets. As already discussed previously in this chapter, these types of emulsifiers have little or no effect on interfacial tension, but exert a protective colloid effect, reducing the chances of coalescence they act by providing a protective sheath around the droplets or imparting a charge to the dispersed droplets (so that they repel each other) or swell to increase the viscosity of the system (so that droplets are less likely to merge).

Hydrocolloid emulsifiers may be classified as:

- Vegetable derivatives, e.g., acacia, tragacanth, agar, pectin, carrageenan, lecithin
- Animal derivatives, e.g., gelatin, lanolin, cholesterol
- Semi-synthetic agents, e.g., methylcellulose, carboxymethylcellulose
- Synthetic agents, e.g., carbopols®

Naturally occurring plant hydrocolloids are inexpensive, easy to handle, and nontoxic, but they are very prone to microbial growth and thus their formulations require a preservative. Vegetable derivatives are generally limited to be used in o/w emulsion.

The animal derivatives generally form w/o emulsions. Lecithin and cholesterol form a monomolecular layer around the emulsion droplet instead of the typical multimolecular layers. Cholesterol is a major constituent of wool alcohols and it gives lanolin the capacity to absorb water and form a w/o emulsion but the allergic reactions and microbial growth are two major limiting factors for the use of such emulsifiers.

A variety of fatty acids (e.g., stearic acid), fatty alcohols (e.g., stearyl or cetyl alcohol), and fatty esters (e.g., glyceryl monostearate) serve to stabilize emulsions through their ability to thicken the emulsion. Because these agents have only weak emulsifying properties, they are always used in combination with other emulsifiers and hence fall in the category of auxiliary emulsifier.

7.3.5.4 Preservatives

An emulsion may have a natural material as a constituent, which will enhance the probability of microbial growth. Even in absence of any natural material, the mixture of lipid and water itself is sufficient for the microbial growth. Such microbial growth may lead to foul smelling due to rancidity of lipid material, breaking of the emulsion system, degradation of drug components etc. So it is necessary to include preservative in the formulation. These are the substances which prevents the spoilage of food materials and pharmaceutical preparation by inhibiting the growth of microorganism.

There are number of possibilities which lead to microbial contamination ranging from employing natural emulsifiers and other raw materials, containers & equipment, processing conditions & environment and personnel involved in manufacturing. Preservation of emulsion dosage form is somewhat different from other formulations. In general a single preservative is enough to protect the dosage form from physical or chemical degradation. However, in case of emulsion combination of preservative is preferred rather than a single agent. The reason being in the presence of two phases and which are equally susceptible to be attacked. Two preservatives, one having affinity towards aqueous phase and other for oily phase can be employed. A single preservative can also be employed if that has the desirable attribute to preserve both the phases of emulsion. This can be explained on the basis of partitioning behavior of the agents employed. Material which has optimum portioning between aqueous and oily phases can be employed alone to guard the emulsion. However, before employing such material, the partitioning performance should be assessed quantitatively in the preformulation stage. Some common types of preservatives that are used to protect emulsions are listed Table 7.5.

TABLE 7.5

List of common preservatives used in the emulsions

Type of preservative	Examples	Characteristic and utility
Alcohols	Chlorbutanol, phenoxy-2 ethanol	Used in ophthalmic formulations
Aldehydes	Formaldehyde, gluteraldehyde	
Phenolic compounds	Phenol, cresol, chlorothymol, chlorometaxylenol etc.	
Quaternary compounds	Chlorhexidine and salts, benzalkonium and benzethonium chloride, cetyl pyridinium chloride etc.	Broad spectrum
Mercurials	Phenyl mercuric acetate Sodium ethylthimercuricsalicylate	
Acids and their derivatives	Benzoic acid, sorbic acid and dehydroacetic acid etc.	Antifungal agents
Miscellaneous	Imidazolidinyl urea compound, 2,4,4' trichloro 2'-hydroxy diphenylether	Broad spectrum but specific against gram positive bacteria

Apart from the above properties, there are some characteristics which should be fulfilled by a preservative:

- It should have low toxicity.
- It should be stable to heat.
- It should be bactericidal rather than a bacteriostatic.
- A good preservative should kill all the bacteria in the formulation within specified period of time i.e., rapid action is required.
- It should be effective against wide range of micro-organisms e.g., bacteria, fungi, yeast etc.
- It should be compatible with the other components of the emulsion and should not react with any of the additives since it has been found that certain preservatives like phenols and ester of

parahydroxybenzoic acid lose their activity in presence of non-ionic emulsifiers due to formation of complex or get solubilized in the micelles formed due to use of excess emulsifying agents.

7.3.5.5 Antioxidants

Exposure of any formulation or product which contains organic materials, especially lipid may degrade due to auto oxidation. The oxidation of lipid material or oil especially unsaturated oils may cause the rancidity of the oil or lipid present in formulation leading to foul smell. On the same line, there are some drugs which may degrade due to oxidation process.

Auto-oxidation may be inhibited by checking the presence of oxygen. This can be done with the help of antioxidants. The selection of antioxidants depends on its safety, efficacy, acceptability and its specific use. Antioxidants work on either of the several mechanisms outlines below:

- Some antioxidant get oxidized itself in place of drug or oil and in this way protect the required component. These materials are termed as reducing agents e.g., sodium sulfate, sodium metabisulfite etc.

- Some agents block the oxidative chain reaction e.g., butyl hydroxyl anisole (BHA) and butyl hydroxyl toluene (BHT).

- Some agents enhance the effectiveness of blocking agents e.g., ascorbic acid, citric acid, tartaric acid etc.

- There are some agents which form complex with the catalyst promoting the oxidative reaction e.g., EDTA.

In place of using a single chemical, it is advisable to use the combination of two or three compounds with different mechanisms to achieve pronounced action. Some common anti-oxidants which are frequently used in emulsions include gallic acid, propyl gallate, ascorbic acid, ascorbyl palmitate, L-tocoferol, BHA and BHT etc. Most of the antioxidants are used in the concentration range of 0.001% to 1%. BHT, BHA, propyl gallate and L-tocopherol are very popular in cosmetic and pharmaceutical industry. However, the use of BHT, BHA, and propyl gallate in oral formulatios is limited because of their unpleasant odour and bitter taste. L- tocopherol is one the most suitable antioxidants for pharmaceutical preparations.

7.3.6 Method of Preparation of Emulsion

The formation of emulsion requires the breakup of dispersed phase in to the fine globules. There are different types of instruments which can be used to promote such breakup and emulsification either in lab or for large scale production. Emulsions may be prepared using a porcelain mortar and pestle, a mechanical blender or mixer or by a hand homogenizer. Basically three major methods are used to prepare the emulsion on small scale in a laboratory. These are:

- Continental or dry gum method

- English or wet gum method, and

- Bottle or Forbes bottle method

In the first two methods, initially the primary emulsion is prepared by using the specific ratio of oil, water and gum for different types of oils as mentioned in the Table 7.6 (Carter, 2000).

TABLE 7.6

Different ratio of oil, water and gum for preparation of primary emulsion

Type of oil	Example	Quantity for preparing primary emulsion		
		Oil	Water	Gum
Fixed oil	Almond oil, arachis oil, castor oil etc.	4	2	1
Mineral oil	Paraffin oil	3	2	1
Volatile oil	Cinnamon oil, peppermint oil etc.	2	2	1
Oleo-resin	Male fern extract	1	2	1

7.3.6.1 Dry Gum Method

In dry gum method for the preparation of primary emulsion, the emulsifying agent (usually acacia) is mixed with the oil before the addition of water in the above mentioned ratio. During the preparation of emulsion great care should be taken for selecting the system which has to be used for the trituration. Generally, a rough surface should be used in place of smooth one for preparing a better emulsion. Solid substances such as preservatives, stabilizers, colorants, and any flavoring material are usually dissolved in a suitable volume of water (assuming water is the external phase) and added as a solution to the primary emulsion to produce the final formulation.

7.3.6.2 Wet Gum Method

In the wet gum method, the emulsifying agent is added to water to form mucilage, and then the oil is slowly added to form the emulsion. In this method, the proportions of oil, water, and gum are same as in the dry gum method, but the order of mixing is different. Mucilage of the gum is prepared by triturating granular gum in a mortar with twice its weight of water. The oil is then added slowly with trituration to emulsify the oil.

7.3.6.3 Bottle or Forbes Bottle Method

Bottle method is another form of dry gum method and mainly used for preparing the emulsions containing volatile oils or less viscous oils. The method is useful for the extemporaneous preparation of emulsions from volatile oils or oleaginous substances of low viscosities. Powdered acacia is placed in a dry bottle followed by addition of two parts of oil, and the mixture is thoroughly shaken in the capped container. A volume of water approximately equal to that of the oil is then added in portions and the mixture is thoroughly shaken after each addition. When all of the water has been added, the primary emulsion thus formed may be diluted to the proper volume with water. For viscous oil, this method is not suitable because it cannot be agitated properly in the bottle when mixed with the emulsifying agent.

7.3.7 Preparation of Emulsion at Industrial Scale

At the industrial scale, proper agitation to prepare an emulsion is provided using specific equipment or instruments, which can be divided into four basic categories:

    A. Mechanical stirrer;
    B. Homogenizers;
    C. Ultrasonicators;
    D. Colloid mills

Shear stress is amongst the crucial factors which need to be optimized in order to formulate an emulsion of desired parameters. The shear stress can be varied by changing the mode and degree of agitation required for dispersing one phase into other. This in turn depends on some factors which can be outlined as following:

- Total volume of liquid to be mixed,
- The viscosity of the system,
- Interfacial tension at oil-water interface.

The last two factors are influenced by the emulsion type, phase ratio and the type and concentration of emulsifier.

7.3.7.1 Agitators/Mechanical Stirrers

An emulsion may be prepared by using various impellers mounted on shafts by placing it directly into the system to be emulsified. For a low viscosity fluid a simple propeller can be used while turbine type system will be needed to agitate a viscous system.

The rotational speed of impeller controls the degree and intensity of agitation. The resultant efficiency of mixing is controlled by the type of impeller, its position in the container, the presence of baffles, and the general shape of the container. Agitators are used particularly for the emulsification of easily dispersed, low-viscosity oils.

7.3.7.2 Colloid Mill

When a high speed rotor approximately at speeds of 2000 to 18,000 rpm, rotates on a stator, it produces high degree of shear leading to the production very fine globules of dispersed phase.

The proximity of the rotor and the stator can be adjusted. When a mixture (for preparing emulsion) is passed between the rotor and the stator, because of the high shear a fine dispersion of uniform size can be obtained. The shearing forces applied in the colloid mill usually raise the temperature within the emulsion. Hence, a coolant is used to absorb excess heat. Particularly this technique is applied to prepare suspensions containing poorly wetted solids but may be very useful for preparing, relatively viscous emulsions.

7.3.7.3 Homogenizers

Mechanical stirrers with a proper propeller, frequently produce a satisfactory emulsion at laboratory scale. But, for further reduction in particle size, homogenizers may be employed.

Homogenizers may be used in one of the two ways:

(i) The ingredients in the emulsion are mixed and then passed through the homogenizer to produce the final product.

(ii) A coarse emulsion is prepared (one of the different ways reported) and then passed through a homogenizer for the purpose of decreasing the particle size and obtaining a greater degree of uniformity and stability.

The coarse emulsion (basic product) enters the valve seat at high pressure (1000 to 5000 psi), flows through the region between the valve and the seat at high velocity with a rapid pressure drop, causing cavitation; subsequently the mixture hits the impact ring causing further disruption and then is discharged as a homogenized product. It is postulated that circulation and turbulence are responsible mainly for the homogenization that takes place (Allen Jr et al., 2005).

Sometimes a single homogenization may produce an emulsion which, although possess lower particle size but has a tendency to clump/form clusters. Emulsions of this type exhibit increased creaming tendencies. This is corrected by passing the emulsion through the first stage of homogenization at a high pressure (e.g., 3000 to 5000 psi) and then through the second stage at reduced pressure (e.g., 1000 psi). This breaks down any clusters formed in the first step (two stage homogenization).

7.3.7.4 Ultrasonic Devices

There are many laboratory size ultrasonicators which can be used for the preparation of emulsions by the use of ultrasonic vibrations. An oscillator of high frequency (100 to 500 kHz) is connected to two electrodes between which a piezoelectric quartz plate is placed. The quartz plate and electrodes are immersed in an oil bath and, when the oscillator operates, high-frequency waves flow through the fluid. Emulsification is accomplished by simply immersing a tube containing the emulsion ingredients into this oil bath (Khar R. K et al., 2013).

7.3.8 Evaluation of Emulsions

A pharmaceutical emulsion can be evaluated for the different below mentioned parameters:

- Physical examination: Visual observation for creaming, coalescence and oil separation
- Chemical analysis
    - Determination and characterization of drug substance, oil and other excipients
    - Determination and characterization of free fatty acids and oxidative degradation product
    - Determination of pH
- Pharmaceutical Characterization
    - Globule size and its distribution
    - Electro-kinetic behavior

- Viscosity
- Drug content
- Release of drug

7.3.8.1 Globule Size and its Distribution

Size and size distribution of globules in the emulsion are important for both the stability as well as for biopharmaceutical consideration. It has been noted that the larger particles show more tendency towards coalescence and increase in droplet size. While the improper size distribution may interfere with absorption of drug leading to either inadequate response or toxic effects (Khan et al., 2011). Hence it is of prime importance to find out the size and size distribution of the dispersed globules. Some methods which can be used to predict the size and its distribution are:

- Microscopic measurement of apparent diameter
- Use of some electronic counting devices such as coulter counter
- By checking the light scattering behavior and related reflectance relationship
- Use of some sophisticated instruments like particle size analyzer.

7.3.8.2 Electro-Kinetic Behavior

The electro-kinetic behavior of the emulsion can be measured either by moving boundary method or by observing the movement of particles under the influence of electric current. Sophisticated instruments like zetasizer can be used to measure the zeta potential of emulsions.

7.3.8.3 Drug Release Behavior

There are several methods reported in the literature which can be used to assess the release behavior of the dispersed systems. Instruments like modified USP dissolution apparatus-1, modified USP dissolution apparatus-4 or dialysis membrane diffusion technique can be employed to measure the release behavior.

7.3.8.3.1 Modified USP Dissolution Apparatus

Drug release study from the disperse system such as emulsion, liposome, nanoparticles etc., can be done by making a modification to the USP dissolution apparatus 1 (as mentioned in the Fig. 7.15). The basket of the USP dissolution apparatus 1 is replaced with glass cylinder closed at the lower end by dialysis membrane (Abdel-Mottaleb and Lamprecht, 2011).

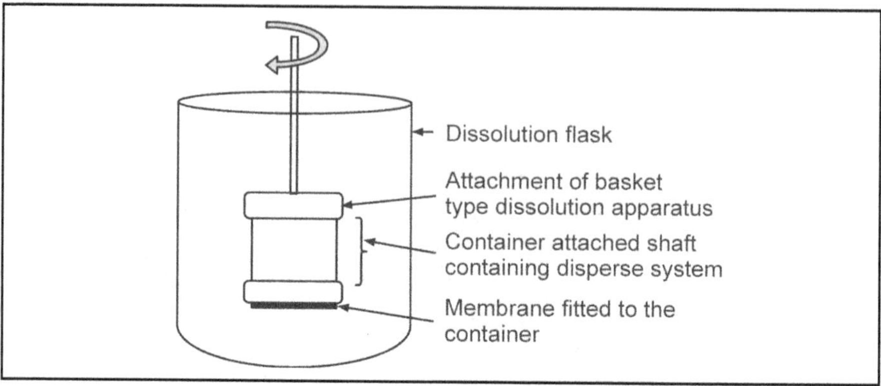

Figure 7.15 Modified dissolution apparatus for emulsions.

7.3.8.3.2 Dialysis Sac Method

Drug release study by the dialysis sac method can be done by placing the dialysis sac containing disperse system in a suitable release media as mentioned in the individual monographs. The graphical representation is mentioned in Fig. 7.16. If the drug in not soluble in the media of drug release experiment; a small percentage of some surfactant or co-solvent is added to facilitate the dissolution of released drug to maintain sink conditions.

The pore size of the dialysis membrane can limit diffusion across the membrane. So during the release study selection of the membrane should be done as per the requirement. (Bhardwaj and Burgess, 2010) have reported the use of 50 kDa MWCO dialysis membrane for the study of release behavior of dexamethasone loaded liposomal preparation and (Üstündag-Okur et al., 2014) reported the use of dialysis bag for studying the release behaviour of ofloxacin loaded microemulsion.

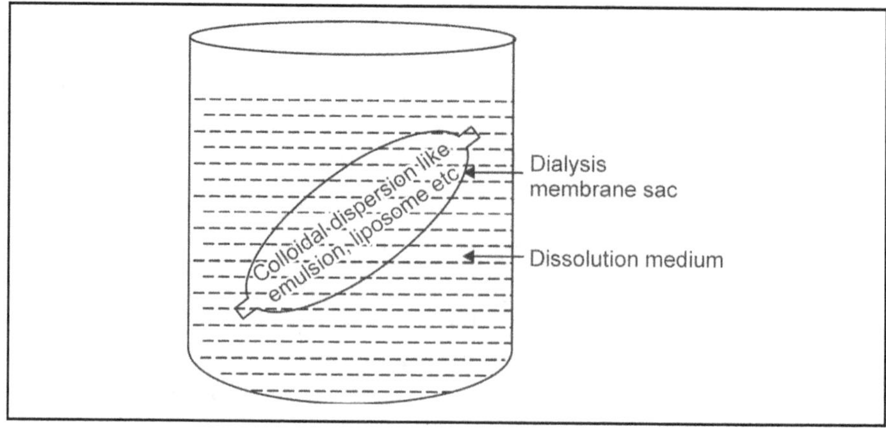

FIGURE 7.16 Dialysis sac method.

7.3.8.3.3 Modified USP Dissolution Apparatus 4

USP dissolution apparatus 4 can be used for the release study of the dispersions systems like suspension, emulsions, etc. The release study can be performed by placing formulation in the sample holder of the apparatus. An adapter covered with the dialysis membrane is placed in the sample holder for retaining the sample to be studied as shown in Fig. 7.16.

7.4 Sustained Release Suspensions

In the current scenario of cut throat competition, it is very difficult to maintain the therapeutic and pharamcoeconomic value of a product. Selection of suitable drug, excipients, and a suitable drug delivery system is a cumbersome task. During last few decades the world has witnessed the tremendous advancements in the field of pharmaceutical drug delivery technology and most of the dosage forms have undergone changes to incorporate such features which have increased their efficacy in terms of drug delivery. In case of problem of dysphasia (difficulty in swallowing) the liquid dosage forms including suspensions, emulsions, solutions, mixtures, syrups, etc., are best choices.

The conventional liquid dosage forms provide a significant release. But in order to maintain the desired therapeutic concentration of drug for effective treatment of acute and chronic illness; it becomes necessary to design a sustained release dosage form. This demand of providing drug release for a prolonged tenure can be promisingly justified by 'Sustained Release Suspensions' (SRS). In suspension the higher surface area of drug particles may facilitates their faster dissolution and hence may provoke faster drug absorption. They may be administered via oral, parenteral, ocular and topical route depending upon the severity of disease or on demand of therapy. The rationale behind designing of a SRS is summarized in Fig. 7.17.

There are certain demerits of SRS like dose dumping, poor *in vitro-in vivo* correlation, sometimes poor systemic availability of drug, cost of production, and stability concern. Therefore a logistic approach for manufacturing of SRS is required. The logistic approach may include buffering agents (like salts, sugar, polymer and antioxidants); elegancy imparting agents (like coloring agents, opacifiers etc.); viscosity imparting agents (like gelling agents, cross linking agents etc); stabilizers (like osmolarity agents, antimicrobial preservatives etc.); and taste enhancers (like sweeteners, flavoring agents etc.).

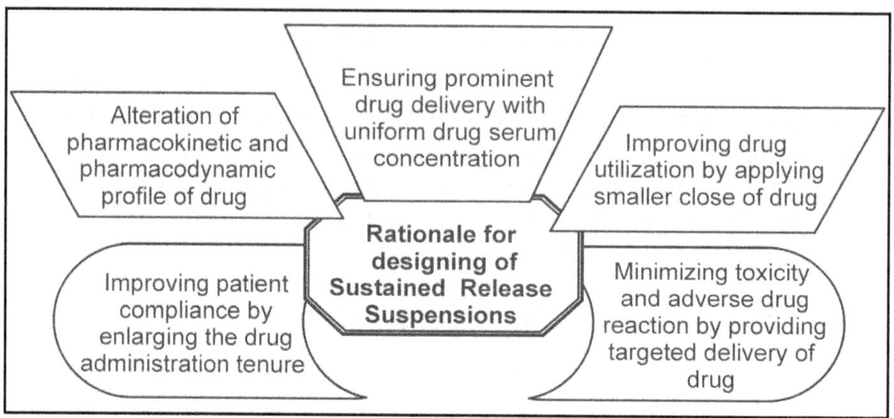

FIGURE 7.17 Rationale for designing of sustained release suspension.

These days, we are equipped with multifarious microparticulate and nanoparticulate systems like microcapsules, microparticles, nanoparticles, liposomes, solid lipid nanoparticles, nanowires, nanoshells, carbon nanotubes, nanocapsules, micelles, and hybrid nanoparticles which can be effectively used to produce SRS. These novel particles can be prepared various method presented in Fig. 7.18.

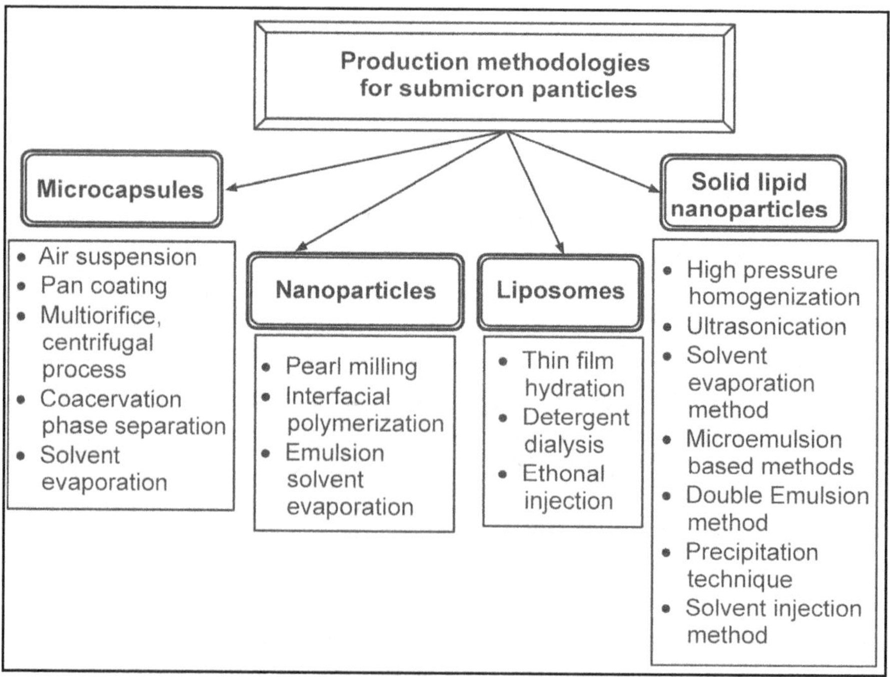

FIGURE 7.18 Production methodologies for submicron particles.

This sub-micron drug loaded particles may be transformed into SRS by various methods which can be explained as follows:

Ion exchange resins: This involves the mixing of the drug solution with resins which is then suspended in liquid carrier for oral administrations.

In-situ gelling system: This process involves the preparation of two solutions viz. water insoluble polymer solution in organic solvent and drug solution. When the above mixture is added in body it transformed into gel.

Poorly water soluble API: The method is generally taken into account for poorly soluble drugs. In this method microencapsulated drugs are suspended in vehicle and administered to patients.

The prepared SRS can be evaluated for various physicochemical attributes as has been discussed with dispersed systems.

7.5   Conclusion

Coarse dispersions viz. suspensions and emulsions represent conventional dosage forms which are known for their versatility and flexibility in the adjustment of the dose size. These have been pioneering dosage forms specifically in the pediatric medications and constitute major volume of the segment (pediatric division) which is because of the ease of administration, palatability and simpler methods to formulate the system. However the dosage forms suffer from stability concerns but with the advent of some modern excipients and recent advancements in the formulation technology such issues have become evitable. Sustained release suspensions have been newer form of suspensions which either consist of novel drug delivery systems or are formulated to achieve specific drug release to sustain the action of drug for better results. However the same holds great potential and much can be achieved to aid in drug delivery through research in this field.

References

Abdel-Mottaleb, M.M., and Lamprecht, A. (2011). Standardized *in vitro* drug release test for colloidal drug carriers using modified USP dissolution apparatus I. *Drug development and industrial pharmacy* **37**, 178-184.

Abdou, H., Hanna, S., MUHAMMAD, N., and Genaro, A. (2000). Remington: the science and practice of pharmacy, Vol 20.

Allen Jr, L.V., Popovich, N.G., and Ansel, H.C. (2005). Ansel's Pharmaceutical Dosage Forms and Drug Delivery Systems, 8 edn (Lippincott Williams and Wilkins, Philadelphia).

Allen, L., Popovich, N.G., and Ansel, H. (2002). Pharmaceutical dosage forms and drug delivery systems (Lippincott Williams and Wilkins).

Banker, G.S., Lieberman, H.A., and Rieger, M.M. (1998). Pharmaceutical Dosage Forms: Disperse Systems (Marcel Dekker).

Banker, G.S., Siepmann, J., and Rhodes, C. (2002a). Modern pharmaceutics (CRC Press).

Banker, G.S., Siepmann, J., and Rhodes, C. (2002b). Modern pharmaceutics (CRC Press).

Bhardwaj, U., and Burgess, D.J. (2010). A novel USP apparatus 4 based release testing method for dispersed systems. *International journal of pharmaceutics* **388,** 287-294.

Block, L., Lieberman, H., Rieger, M., and Banker, G. (1989). Pharmaceutical Dosage Forms-Disperse Systems. Emulsions and microemulsions, Lieberman, HA, Rieger, MM, Banker, GS, Editors, 335-378.

Carless, J.E., and Foster, A.A. (1966). Accelerated crystal growth of sulphathiazole by temperature cycling. Journal of Pharmacy and Pharmacology 18, 697-708.

Carless, J.E., Moustafa, M.A., and Rapson, H.D. (1968). Dissolution and crystal growth in aqueous suspensions of cortisone acetate. *The Journal of pharmacy and pharmacology* **20,** 630-638.

Carter, S. (2000). Disperse system In: Cooper and Gunn's Tutorial Pharmacy. In (New Delhi: CBS Publishers and Distributors), pp. 77-84.

da Fonseca, L.B., Labastie, M., de Sousa, V.P., and Volpato, N.M. (2009). Development and validation of a discriminative dissolution test for nimesulide suspensions. *AAPS Pharm Sci Tech* **10,** 1145-1152.

Florence, A.T., and Siepmann, J. (2009). Modern Pharmaceutics, Volume 2: Applications and Advances, Fifth Edition (CRC Press).

Gao, Z., and Westenberger, B. (2012). Dissolution testing of acetaminophen suspension using dialysis adapter in flow-through apparatus: a technical note. *AAPS Pharm Sci Tech* B 944-948.

Garzon-Sanabria, A.J., Ramirez-Caballero, S.S., Moss, F.E.P., and Nikolov, Z.L. (2013). Effect of algogenic organic matter (AOM) and sodium chloride on Nannochloropsis salina flocculation efficiency. *Bioresource Technology* **143,** 231-237.

Eccleston, GM, E. (2007). Emulsions and microemulsions. In Encyclopedia of pharmaceutical technology, S. J, ed. (USA: New York: Informa Healthcare USA), pp. 1561–1565.

Gregory, J., and Barany, S. (2011). Adsorption and flocculation by polymers and polymer mixtures. *Advances in colloid and interface science* **169,** 1-12.

Hiestand, E.N. (1964). Theory of coarse suspension formulation. *Journal of pharmaceutical sciences* **53,** 1-18.

Khan, B.A., Akhtar, N., Khan, H.M.S., Waseem, K., Mahmood, T., Rasul, A., Iqbal, M., and Khan, H. (2011). Basics of pharmaceutical emulsions: A review. *African Journal of Pharmacy and Pharmacology* **5,** 2715-2725.

Khar R. K, Vyas S. P, Ahmed F. J, and K, J.G. (2013). Biphasic liquids In The Theory and Practice of Industrial Pharmacy, Khar R. K, Vyas S. P, Ahmed F. J, and J.G. K, eds. (CBS publishers & distributers), pp. 653-715.

Kuentz, M., Egloff, P., and Röthlisberger, D. (2006). A technical feasibility study of surfactant-free drug suspensions using octenyl succinate-modified starches. *European journal of pharmaceutics and biopharmaceutics* **63,** 37-43.

Lachman, L., Lieberman, H.A., and Kanig, J.L. (1992). The theory and practice of industrial pharmacy, 3 edn.

Ludwig, A., and Ooteghem, M.V. (1988). Influence of the viscosity and the surface tension of ophthalmic vehicles on the retention of a tracer in the precorneal area of human eyes. *Drug development and industrial pharmacy* **14,** 2267-2284.

N.K, J., and S.N, S. (2010). A text book of professional pharmacy, 5 edn (Vallabh Prakashan).

Nash, R.A., Swarbrick, J., and Boylan, J. (2002). Encyclopedia of pharmaceutical technology.

Nasser, M., and James, A. (2009). The effect of electrolyte concentration and pH on the flocculation and rheological behaviour of kaolinite suspensions.

regulation, F. (2009). Food Safety and Standards Regulations, T.F.S.a.S.A.o. India, ed. (FDA).

Remington, J.P., Troy, D.B., and Beringer, P. (2006). Remington: The science and practice of pharmacy, Vol 1 (Lippincott Williams & Wilkins).

Sinko, P.J., Allen Jr, L.V., Popovich, N.G., and Ansel, H.C. (2004). 1: 1. Martin's Physical Pharmacy and Pharmaceutical Sciences.

Subrahmanyam, C. (2000). Textbook of physical pharmaceutics (Vallabh Prakashan).

Tadros, T.F., Vandamme, A., Levecke, B., Booten, K., and Stevens, C. (2004). Stabilization of emulsions using polymeric surfactants based on inulin. *Advances in colloid and interface science* **108,** 207-226.

Üstündag-Okur, N., Gökçe, E.H., Eğrilmez, S., Özer, Ö., and Ertan, G. (2014). Novel ofloxacin-loaded microemulsion formulations for ocular delivery. *Journal of Ocular Pharmacology and Therapeutics* **30,** 319-332.

Wasan, K.M. (2007). Role of Lipid Excipients in Modifying Oral and Parenteral Drug Delivery: Basic Principles and Biological Examples (John Wiley & Sons).

Zhou, Y., and Franks, G.V. (2006). Flocculation mechanism induced by cationic polymers investigated by light scattering. *Langmuir* **22,** 6775-6786.

Modified Release Drug Delivery Systems for Oral Route

Sharad P. Pandey[1], Vinod Dhote[1], Tripti Shukla[2] and M.S. Sudheesh[3]

[1]Truba Institute of Pharmacy, Karond - Gandhi Nagar Bypass Road, Bhopal-462 038, India.

[2]School of Pharmacy, Peoples University, Bhanpur Bypass Road, Bhopal-462 037, India.

[3]Faculty of Pharmacy, VNS Group of Institutions, Neelbud, Bhopal-462 044, India.

8.1 Introduction

Immediate release dosage forms for oral drug delivery such as tablets, capsules, suspensions etc., have been first and foremost choice of majority of practitioners. It has been a major part of the prescription against variety of clinical manifestations. In spite of a bunch of advantages that these formulations extend, they do possess some disadvantages such as high dose and dosing frequency, adamant release of drug, lower bioavailability for some category of drugs etc. Considering these issues, modified release drug delivery system (MRDDS) has been developed to achieve some premeditated and desired therapeutic objective by making deliberate change in rate of drug absorption at the site of absorption. MRDDS are mainly developed to achieve certain clinical benefits such as enhanced efficacy, patient compliance, improved bioavailability, optimized performance and selectivity for a specific activity (Singh B N, 2000). Clinically proven MRDDS can be very much commercially advantageous in terms of maximized drug potential, cost effectiveness and market expansion.

270

Basically, the modified release drug delivery systems are developed to deliberately alter the absorption by changing the release pattern of any drug in comparison to the conventional systems, according to the need i.e., time dependent or site specific. MRDDS can be broadly classified in to several types mentioned below (Qiu.Y, 2009):

1. Extended release drug products (ER)
2. Delayed-release drug products (DR)
3. Targeted-release drug products (TR)
4. Orally disintegrating tablets (ODT)

Extended release (ER) drug delivery systems are developed in such a way so as to release the active drug for an extended period of time after ingestion, decreasing dosing frequency of the drug in comparison to the conventional dosage forms. ER delivery systems are synonymously called as controlled drug delivery or sustained drug delivery systems (Qiu Y, 2011; Singh B N, 2000).

Delayed release delivery systems (DR) are basically designed to delay the release of any drug for a specific period of time or to avoid the release of drug to any specific site. The most common example of this system may be considered as enteric coated tablets (Qiu Y, 2011).

Targeted released drug delivery systems (TR) are designed to deliver the drug to any specific site. Osmotic pump is a perfect example which is specifically designed to administer the drug to the colon.

Orally disintegrating products (ODT) are basically developed for quick absorption of any drug to systemic circulation and it also enhances the patient compliance because it get easily dissolved in the volume of saliva and can be administered without water (Qiu Y, 2011).

It is a well-known fact that some of the diseases follow the circadian rhythm such as asthmatic episode, secretion of hormones etc. The modulation of the drug release in such a way so as to obtain therapeutic plasma concentration of drug at specific timing may be greatly helpful in case of certain diseases like asthma, angina pectoris, and morning arthritic pain. A general release pattern for modified release delivery systems can be explained through Fig. 8.1.

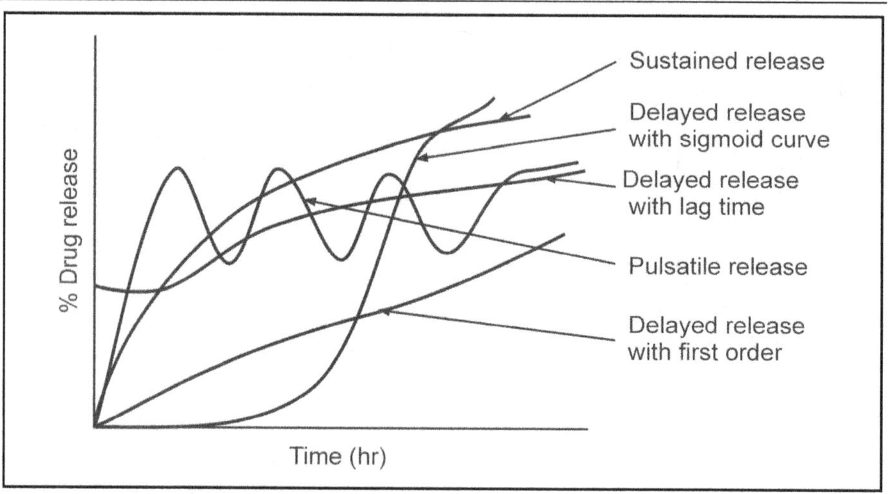

FIGURE 8.1 General release pattern for modified release delivery systems.

Modulation of release in majority of delivery systems has been done by using specific polymer or a blend of individual polymers. Apart from polymer characteristics, *in-vitro* and *in-vivo* release of the drug also depends on several other factors. Some common factors are dose, physiochemical behavior, pharmacokinetic behavior, biopharmaceutical and pharmacodynamic properties of the drug. On the other hand designing of dosage from also affects the release behavior of the drug. Each drug possesses some specific intrinsic properties that should be taken in to consideration during the designing of MR products. Some basic thoughtfulness which must be considered during designing of MR products are explained below (Qiu.Y, 2009; Singh B N, 2000):

1. The relationship between the pharmacological and toxicological response with exposure of drug should be clearly understood.

2. A basic understanding and feasibility assessment in terms of absorption behavior of drug through entire GIT should be well developed. As the absorption characteristics of a compound from a particular region in the GIT and residence time of dosage forms are the most important parameters which should be assessed during the development of an oral modified release delivery system.

3. The study of physicochemical properties of drug is one of the most critical steps during designing of any delivery system. Dose and solubility are the two most important factors to be given due

credit before selecting any technique for the development of modified release product.

4. The factors which may affect the release behavior of the drug such as drug loading, effect of excipient etc., should be clearly analyzed.

It has already been mentioned that polymer acts as a keychain in the modulation of drug release. There are number of different polymers belonging to different categories which are being extensively utilized for the similar purpose. Hydroxypropyl methyl cellulose, poly (methacrylic acid), natural gums etc., are some common examples, which modify the drug release by the formation of hydrophilic matrix. Whereas, the polymers for the formation of hydrophobic system is few with common example of fatty acid and their ester. Eudragit RL RS, cellulose acetate phthalate etc., are also being used for the purpose of formation of hydrophobic matrix. Some common polymers which are being extensively used are depicted in Fig. 8.2.

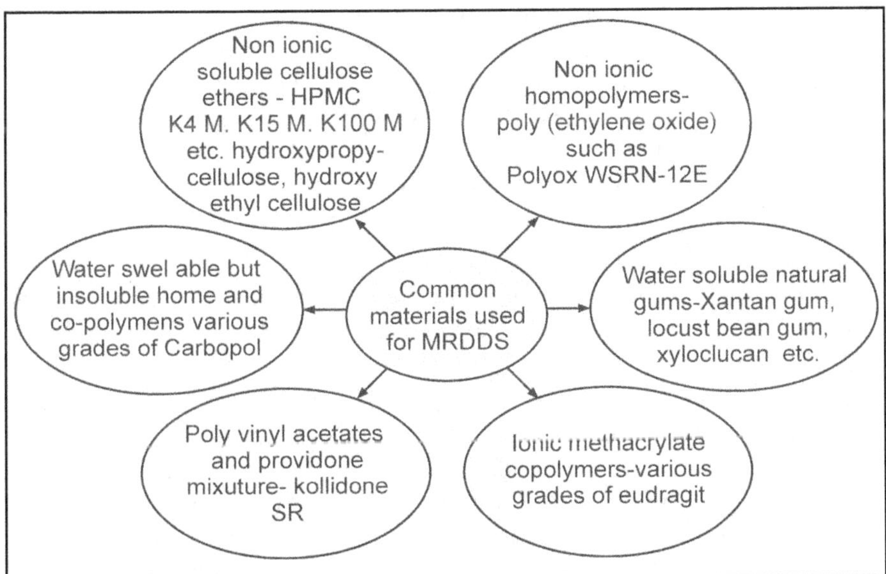

FIGURE 8.2 Polymers used to design MRDDS.

The basic approaches to develop modified release delivery systems have remained unchanged from decades such as development of swellable or erodible matrix or modifying the release by coating of tablets, granules and pellets or development of osmotic drug delivery system or use of combination of various traditional approaches used for modifying the drug release. As discussed earlier in this chapter, MRDDS presents an effective means to optimize the bioavailability and resulting blood concentration-time profiles of drugs. Recently, matrix based MRDDS have drawn the attention of researchers with significant advancements. Matrix systems generally consist of dissolved or dispersed drug within a swelling or slowly eroding polymer matrix and drug release occurs due to penetration of water into the system followed by diffusion of the drug. As an advancement hydrophilic gums have gained tremendous popularity in last few years leading to the development of various new MRDSS technologies viz. TIMERx technology, COSRx technology, MASRx technology etc.

8.2   TIMERx Technology

TIMERx technology was developed by Penwest Pharmaceuticals containing a pregranulated blend of synergistic heterodisperse polysaccharides to address the limitation of other oral drug delivery systems. There are several dugs which have been successfully incorporated in to the TIMERx drug delivery systems such as Cystrin CR (Oxybutynin) Opana ER, Nalbuphine ER. Till date, various drug formulations utilizing TIMERx technology have received regulatory approval in the United States, United Kingdom, Italy and Finland e.g., Nifedipine XL, a generic version of Pfizer's Procardia® XL for the treatment of hypertension and angina developed with Mylan (Staniforth and Baichwal, 2005).

The system consists of xanthan gum and locust bean gum and dextrose. Xanthan gum is a heteropolysachharide which gets easily dissolved in water leading to the formation of very viscous fluid. This occurs due to the formation of hydrogen bonding between two molecules of xanthan gum to form a helical structure which gets dispersed in to the medium providing thickness to solution and less movement for water (Fig. 8.3A) resulting in a controlled release (CR) matrix. In absence of any interlinking the xanthan gum cannot achieve the gel like structure. The locust bean gum is a homopolysacharide and more complex than xanthan gum. The locust bean gum fibers get attached to each other by several hydrogen bonds leading to a complex interlocked structure. The same has been represented vide Fig. 8.3B. In case of locust bean gum the gel forms at −60°C and hence cannot be used as CR material (Troy et al., 2002). But an unusual phenomenon occurs when the Xanthan gum is mixed with locust bean gum, the fiber of Xanthan gum gets entangled in the highly interlocked fiber structure of locust bean gum and a highly viscous matrix system is evolved due to synergism as shown in Fig. 8.4. This combination works as better CR material (Staniforth and Baichwal, 2005; Troy et al., 2002).

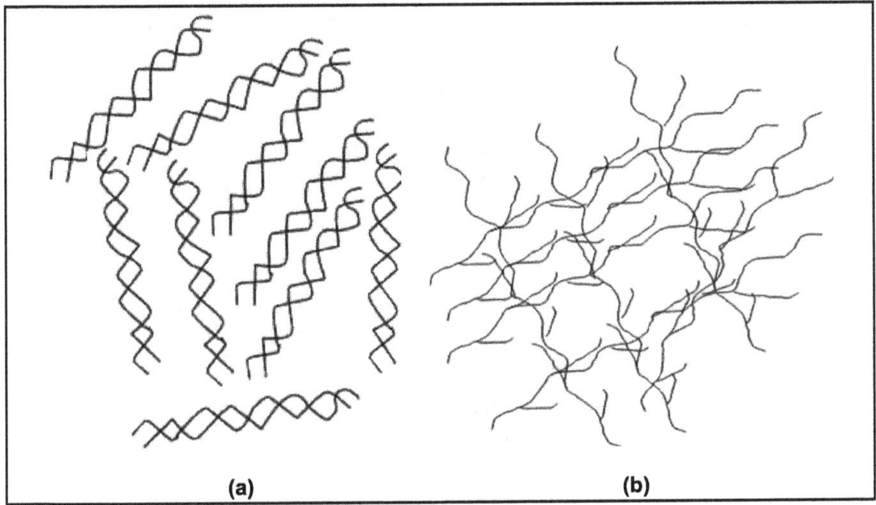

FIGURE 8.3 Schematic representation of xanthan gum in solution (a) and locust bean gum fiber in solution (b).

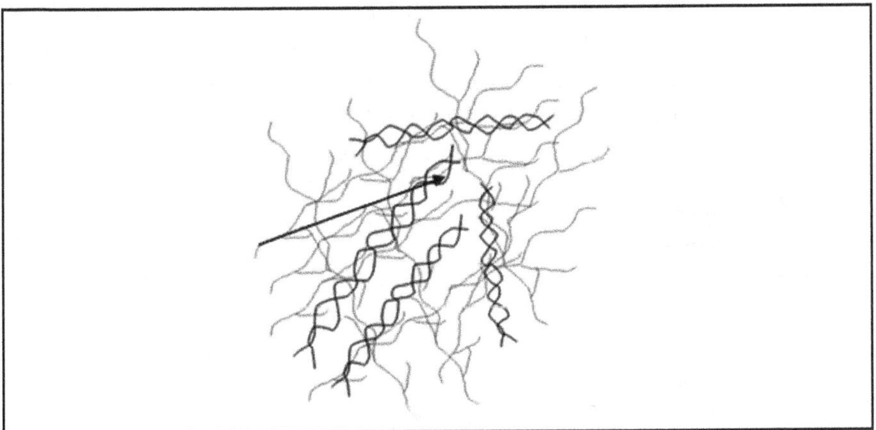

FIGURE 8.4 Interlocking of xanthan gum and locust bean gum fiber leading to high viscous solution.

During the formation of matrix system smooth regions of locust bean gum get associated with the helical part of xanthan gum leading to the formation of sufficiently hard gel like structure favored by cations and dextrose through hydrogen bond formation.

As discussed in the earlier section of this chapter, there are several factors which play role in designing of MRDDS. Similarly the release behavior in TIMERx technology is affected by certain factors such as dose of the incorporated drug, solubility of the drug, drug- polymer ratio, polymer ratio (Xanthan gum: Locust bean gum) and other excipients.

8.2.1 Advantages of the System

1. By using some other materials except polysaccharides, release of the matrix could be modified providing single order and multi order release profile viz. dextrose and cations (Staniforth and Baichwal, 2005).

2. The technology is very flexible i.e., wide range of drugs (poorly soluble to highly soluble) can be formulated with the system. Similarly, a wide range of dose can also be incorporated along with attainment of different types of release profiles e.g., first-order (Fig. 8.5A), zero-order (Fig. 8.5B), and pulsatile release (Troy et al., 2002).

3. Studies show that the better *In vitro-In vitro* correlation could be achieved.

4. In comparison to others, TIMERx technology is comparatively very easy to apply for development of dosage forms with simple steps like blending, compression and may overcome the deficiencies associated with conventional hydrophilic matrices.

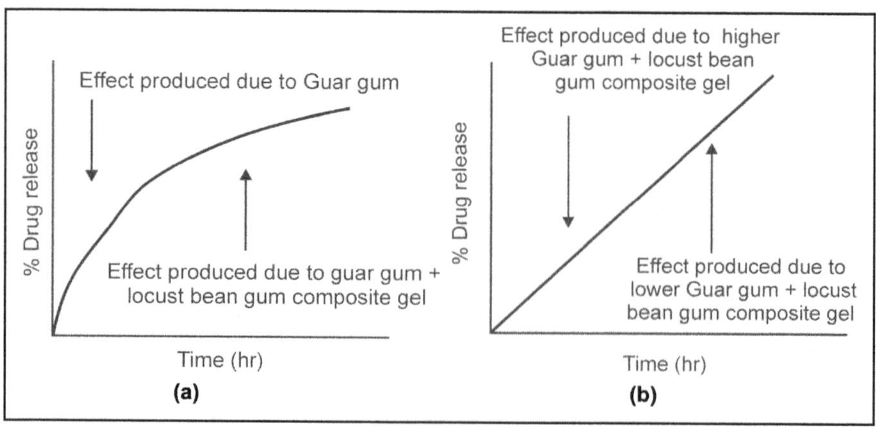

FIGURE 8.5 (a) Schematic presentation of first order release by TIMERx (b) Schematic presentation of zero order release by TIMERx.

8.2.2 Problems Associated with the Formulation

The major problem with this type of formulation is that both the major components of the system are of herbal origin and the quality of it may vary with the different crops as well as crop grown in different geographical conditions. At the similar time it will also be difficult to maintain the quality level of both the gums for a longer time because being natural in origin these polymers are also prone to microbial degradation (Staniforth and Baichwal, 2005).

8.2.3 Advancement

Geminex® and Synchrodose™ may be regarded as the advancement in the series of TIMERx technology. Geminex is controlled release form of TIMERx technology which allows the biphasic delivery of the same drug at different rate. At the same time different drugs can also be delivered by using Geminex. Similar to TIMERx system, it also has xanthan gum and locust bean gum as rate controlling polymer but two different formulations are incorporated in the same tablet using these polymers to achieve bi-modal drug delivery. The Synchrodose™ is a chronotherapeutic release of TIMERx technology containing drug entirely separated from the heterodisperse polysaccharide which is placed in a shell like structure that completely blocks the drug diffusion till desired time (Staniforth and Baichwal, 2005).

8.3 MASRx and COSRx: Modified Release Providing Systems

Development of the sustained release matrix based delivery system can be prepared by using hydrocolloids [polysaccharides, gums]. But the common problem which arises during the use of high viscosity water soluble hydrocolloids [alginates, locust bean gum etc.] is very fast hydration especially in compressed form. The issue which arises during the development of such formulation is the limitation to get hydrated after a certain extent. Natural hydrocolloids like natural gums may be better alternative considering the above two problems and this behavior of such polymers have fascinated the scientist to develop matrix based drug delivery system for modulating release behavior of any drug. Some common examples are xyloglucan, xanthan gum, and guar gum (Gao et al., 2011). MASRx and COSRx are two of the related technologies which were developed using guar gum. Guar gum is a naturally occurring high viscosity polymer, previously being used as disintegrating agent and binding agent in formulation of compressed tablet (David and Syed, 2002).

8.3.1 MASRx Technology

Guar-gum-based once-daily matrix sustained-release formulation (MASRx) releases the drug in a sustained manner by the drug polymer matrix after the swelling of gum when placed in the dissolution medium. The same has been depicted in Fig. 8.6.

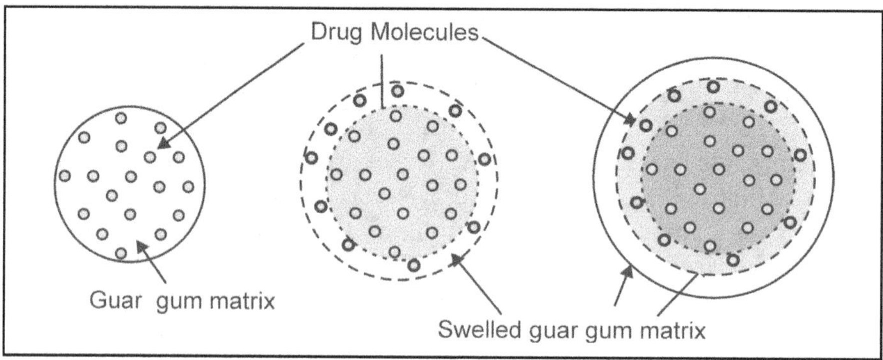

FIGURE 8.6 Schematic diagram showing swelling of guar gum in MASRx system.

Altaf and fellow workers prepared the MASRx delivery system for diltiazem using the guar gum obtained from different crops of different season to study the variability in release behavior. They reported that if the fines are used to prepare the tablet, the release of the system gets increased, probably because of high degree of hydration. The clinical evaluation of guar gum based formulation of diltiazem has shown a fair similarity with the marketed formulation releasing the drug up to 24 hr (David and Syed, 2002).

8.3.2 COSRx Technology

Constant sustained-release matrix (COSRx) can be developed by using high viscosity natural polysaccharide as rate controlling polymer. Initially, xanthan gum was used as rate controlling material followed by a combination of water-soluble and water-insoluble polymeric tablet coat to develop COSRx technology. Different viscosity grades of the polymers can be used for the development of COSRx delivery systems for low, moderate or high soluble drugs. When such formulations are placed in the dissolution medium, the medium starts to penetrate the polymeric membrane leading to swelling of the gum and drug release until the membrane gets ruptured because of hydrodynamic pressure developed due to swelling of gum (Fig. 8.7). Primarily, the release of drug starts from the sides of the tablet when it passes through the GIT providing nearly zero order drug release. Variations in the drug release could be obtained by varying the coating thickness.

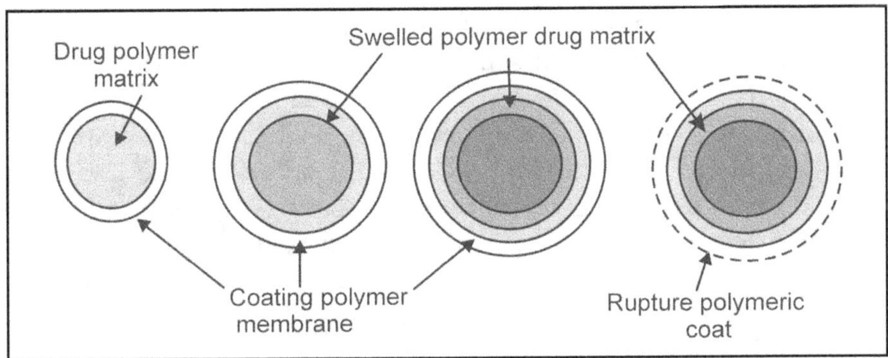

FIGURE 8.7 Schematic diagram showing swelling behavior of COSRx.

Altaf and Friend have developed the zero-order sustained release formulation of poorly water soluble drug nifedipine using low molecular weight guar gum, lactose monohydrate as porosity enhancer and 2% solution of RLPO & RSPO in 1:9 ratio as coating agent. The developed formulation displayed similar lag time of 2 hr as compared to marketed formulation procardia XL. They used low-viscosity carboxyvinyl polymer (Carbopol 974 P, NF) to maintain the nearly constant zero-order nifedipine release (David and Syed, 2002). Further studies have shown that other naturally occurring polymeric polysaccharides such as xanthan gum, xyloglucan, okra gum may also provide a better alternative with new coating materials like ethyl cellulose, cellulose acetate, and other esters to achieve desired release similar to COSRx and MASRx technology. Similarly, lactose monohydrate could also be replaced with micro-crystalline cellulose and other materials with similar properties.

8.4   Smartrix® Technology

Matrix formulation for MRDDS are prepared in such a way that their release behavior could be predicted better by Higuchi's square root law, which assumes that the surface area remains unchanged for the release of the drug. Different researchers have tried to modify the release behavior by modifying the surface area of the dosage form (Bayomi, 1994; Horst and Markus, 2002). McMullen and Bayomi described a geometric approach for zero-order release of drugs dispersed in an inert matrix accomplishing a quasilinear release profile by an erosion-controlled increase of the surface area (Bayomi, 1994; McMullen, 1989).

The concept of modification of release behavior by using geometric multilayer formulation was first developed by Cremer and Asmusen. The Smartrix® tablet technology is a multilayered tablet (Fig. 8.8) that was developed by LTS Lohmann Therapie-Systeme aiming towards the release of active component for an extended period of time leading to more patient compliance by reducing the dosing frequency and peak plasma concentration. These systems have different layers of different geometrical shapes following both diffusion and erosion based drug release. This type of release behavior is obtained by varying the surface area of different geometrical shapes (Moodley et al., 2012 and Zerbe and Krumme, 2002).

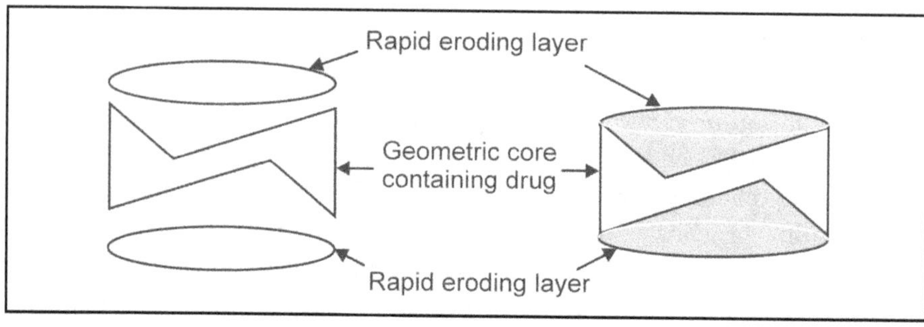

FIGURE 8.8 Schematic diagram of Smartrix® formulation.

As shown in the Fig. 8.8 the formulation constitutes three layers, the middle layer or core of specific shape having drug and the other two are the outer rapidly erodible layers. The middle layer having biconcave shape is tightly bound with two outer layers which after compression display convex structure. The thickness of the outer layers and the shape of the drug core control the release of drug usually in a linear fashion. Release of drug in this manner occurs due the geometric design of the core containing drug coupled with slowly eroding cover layers, providing quasi-linear release of the drug. The controlled erosion of outer layers causes a steady increase of the surface area available for the release of the drug leading to linear drug release (Fig. 8.9) (Horst and Markus, 2002; Moodley et al., 2012).

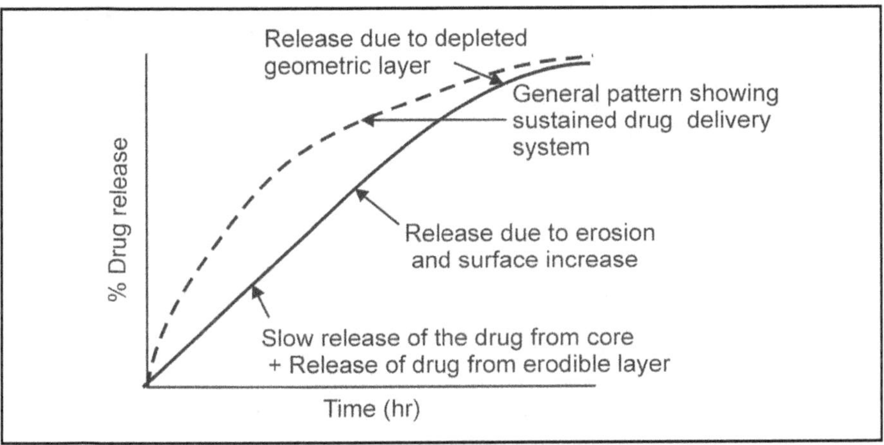

Figure 8.9 Schematic presentation of release behavior from Smartrix®

8.5   Geometrically Modified Core Containing Formulation: Procise Technology

Procise technology was developed by Glaxo and got patented in US and Europe. It contains geometrically modified core and a hole in the centre. The drug is mixed homogenously within the polymer core and coated with slowly permeable polymer (Fig. 8.10) surrounding entire core except hole (Chopra, 2002; Moodley et al., 2012). This type of formulation is prepared by direct compression of the core followed by compression coating using some special tooling.

This technology has been developed to have a view that the release pattern of the formulation can be changed by changing the geometry of core from zero order to first order. The release behavior of the drug from Procise technology, as dissolution based release or diffusion based release may be varied and achieved by changing the geometry of core (Moodley et al., 2012).

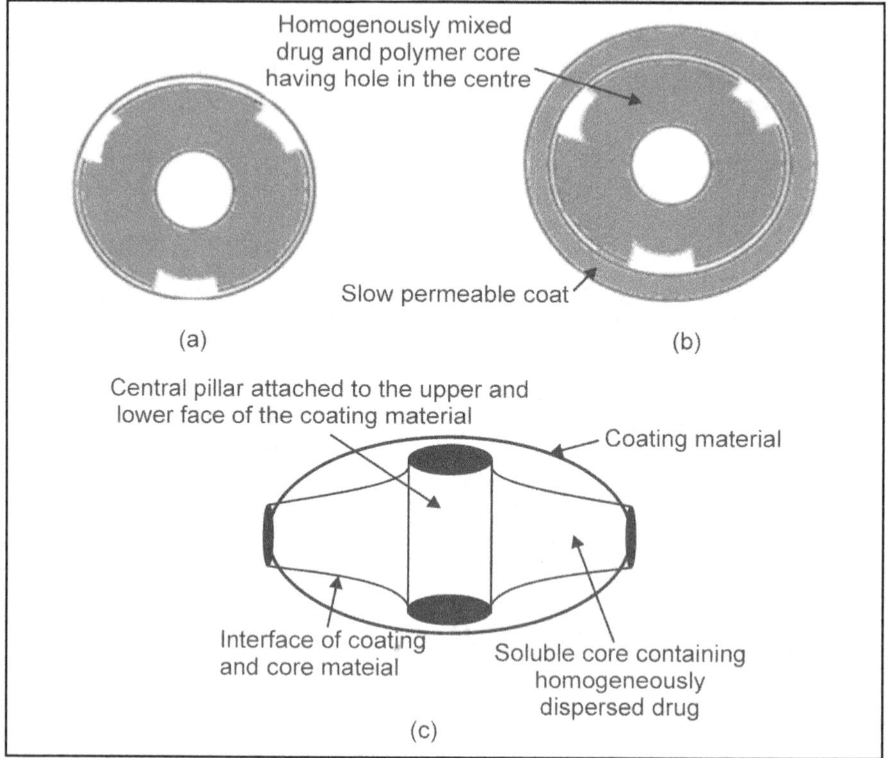

FIGURE 8.10 Schematic diagram of Procise (a) Aerial view of the core (b) Coated core (c) Cross sectional view.

8.5.1 Advantages of Procise Technology

1. Procise has advantage over many oral controlled drug delivery system (CDDS) in terms of the predicted release which can be better achieved in this system due to geometric configuration of the core.

2. Generally it has been observed that majority of CDDS formulation based on the diffusion control mechanism have lag time before the drug is released and some material is left out as residue even after complete release of the drug, while Procise system has no lag time as well as it does not leave any ghost residue.

3. Dose dumping can be avoided, as the core is itself very slowly dissolving unlike other CDDS formulations.

4. This type of formulation does not require any solvent due to compression coating leading to easy manufacturing (Chopra, 2002).

8.6   Ring Cap Technology

Ring cap technology is based on the formulation of capsule shaped modified matrix tablet formulation having strips in form of coating of insoluble polymer as shown in the Fig. 8.11. It has been designed in such a way that these strips modify the release of formulation by controlling the release of drug from coated surface area. The desired modification in the release from this formulation is achieved by increasing or decreasing the width and number of strips with their place. Dickason and co-workers have studied the effect of numbers and widths of bands on the release of acetaminophen and they found that the release of the drug decreases with increasing number and width of bands. They also proposed that the placement of band also influences release of the drug (Dickason D. A., 2002).

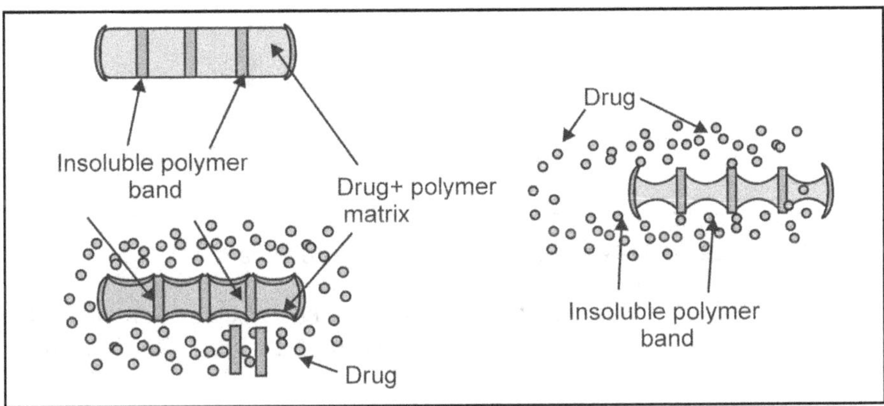

Figure 8.11 Schematic diagram representing Ringcap technology and release of the drug from Ringcap system.

8.6.1 Advantages

Ringcap technology has an advantage of having proprietary mathematical model to predict the release of drug in comparison of other CDDS formulation. This system can be developed for variety of drugs having wide range of solubility and concentration. The Ringcap system uses conventional matrix tablet excipients, offering a cost effective technology.

8.7   Pulsincap Technology

Pulsincap technology was developed by R.P. Scherer Corporation's setting a mile stone in the development of chronopharmaceutical delivery system (Garg. T., 2012). The research studies show that the time dependent triggering of the release of drug from a system is not an easy task but the pulsatile drug delivery system containing drug and hydrophilic polymer in a capsule like structure placed in different geometric conditions has provided a better alternate to get specific desired release of the drug from the system (Fig. 8.12).

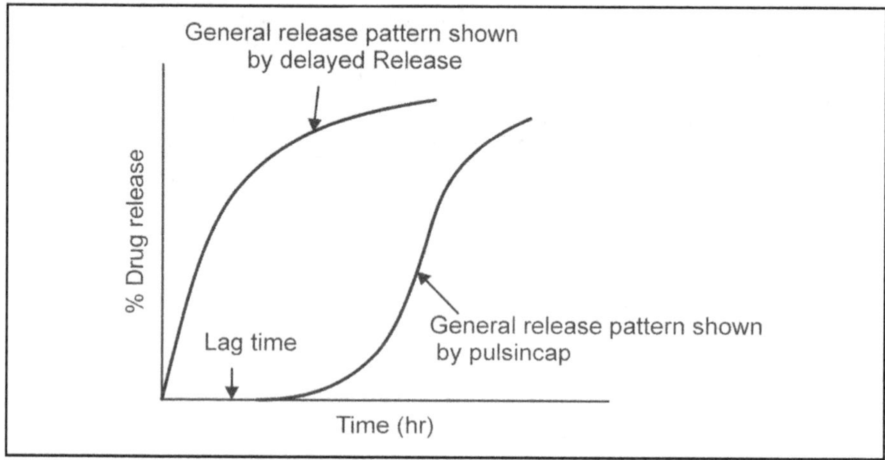

FIGURE 8.12 General release pattern exhibited by Pulsincap.

On the basis of drug and hydrophilic polymer arrangement in the capsular structure the Pulsincap technology, broadly classified in to three main categories:

8.7.1 Polymeric Hydrogel Capsule

Polymeric Hydrogel Capsule (made up of water permeable crossed linked polymers in place of conventional gelatin capsule bearing drug in its core having a cap of erodible polymer.)

This system was generated by using crossed linked polymers which form hydrogel like structure when placed in the dissolution fluid containing drug core and a material which works to propel the drug from hydrogel capsule fitted with a highly swellable and erodible polymeric plug (Fig. 8.13). The drug release from this system or time taken to start the release (Fig. 8.12) from such systems (lag time) can be regulated by using the concentration and thickness of polymeric layer forming the capsule which limits to the entry of water into the capsular system (Stevens, 2002; Stevens, 1999).

Once the water enters into the system it leads to rapid swelling of internal polymeric material placed beneath the drug/or mixed with drug leading to ejection of the polymeric plug from the top.

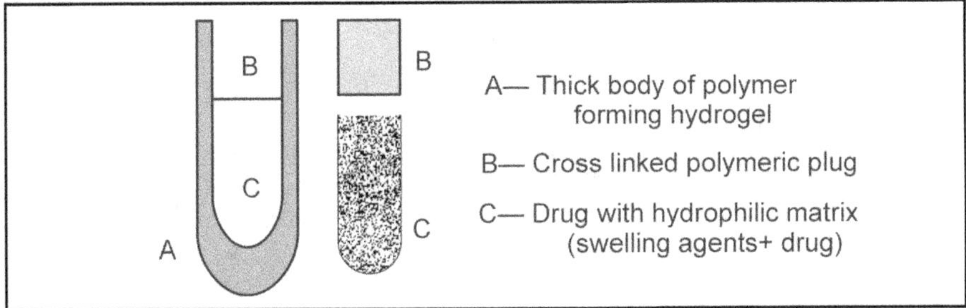

FIGURE 8.13 Schematic diagram of Pulsincap system having polymeric hydrogel capsule.

8.7.2 Gelatin Capsule having Impermeable Coating

Gelatin Capsule having Impermeable Coating (containing drug in the core having hydrogel plug at top inside the capsule)

The Pulsincap system prepared by using Gelatin capsule (A & B in Fig. 8.14) in place of polymeric hydrogel capsule consists of half of the system coated with impermeable polymer like ethyl cellulose filled with drug core (A) capped with swellable hydrogel cap; (B) which swells upon contact with gastrointestinal fluid and ejects out leading to complete release of the drug. The system in this category contains a capsule coated with semi-permeable polymer membrane having an osmogen (2) beneath the drug core (1) followed by hydrogel cap (3). The hydrogel plug gets ejected out due to hydrodynamic pressure built because of movement of water in presence of osmogen. (Stevens, 2002; Stevens, 1999).

8.7.3 Hydrophilic Polymer Sandwiched in between the Layers of two Capsules

This system can also be said capsule within the capsule (Fig. 8.15), in which the inner capsule (2) containing the drug and the hydrophilic polymer (3), is filled within the space of inner and outer capsule shell (1) forming a sandwich like structure. The release of the drug is delayed by the gel formation by the hydrophilic polymer after the dissolution of outer layer of the capsule. The molecular weight and concentration of the polymer as well as the inclusion of water soluble molecules like lactose, MCC etc., can affect the lag time (Stevens H.N.E., 1999).

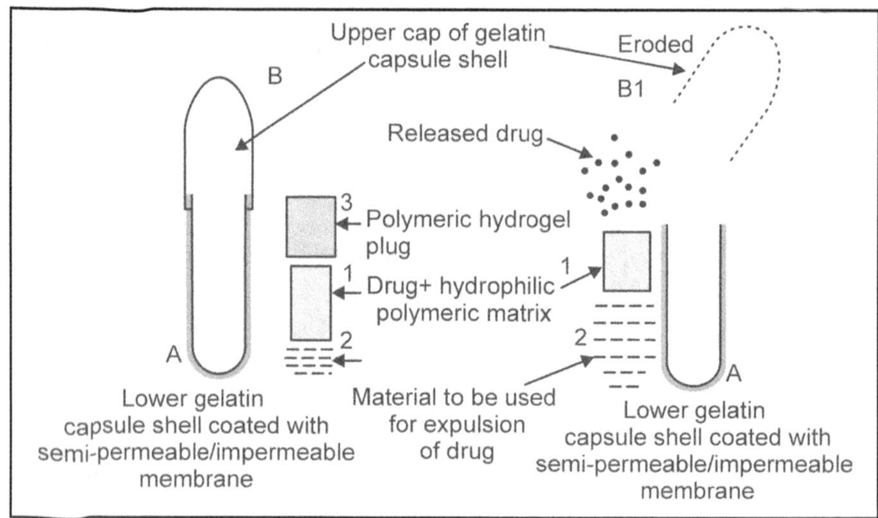

FIGURE 8.14 Schematic diagram showing various components of Pulsincap system gelatin capsule with impermeable coating.

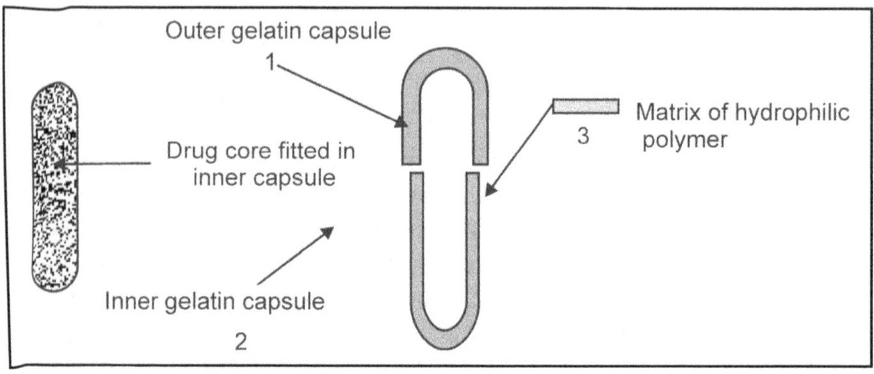

FIGURE 8.15 Schematic diagram showing various components of Pulsincap system containing sandwiched hydrophilic polymer in two capsule layers.

Pulsatile drug delivery using Pulsincap may be a better alternative in its category. As the clinical studies have shown promising results and better confidence in this system, the future studies and modification in this delivery system may prove its efficacy and utility in a better way.

8.8 Spheroidal Oral Drug Absorption System

Spheroidal Oral Drug Absorption System (SODAS) are a multi-particulate delivery system developed by Elan Corporation. This system is based on the production of controlled release bead which is being used to design the system. The technology encompasses multilayered system containing drug and various polymeric layers for the modification of release of drug. SODAS can provide delayed release, controlled release or immediate release followed by sustained release by using different polymers as coatings as shown in Fig. 8.16 (Moodley et al., 2012; Prajapati B, 2008).

SODAS technology can be used to deliver the drug to targeted regions of GIT in a controlled release manner. Combination of drugs can also be delivered without causing incompatibility as the two drugs can be separated by an inert polymeric layer. Elan Drug Technologies have developed the twice or once a day release dosage form of various drugs using SODAS technology including verapamil, diclofenac, fluvoxamine maleate etc. (Prajapati B, 2008).

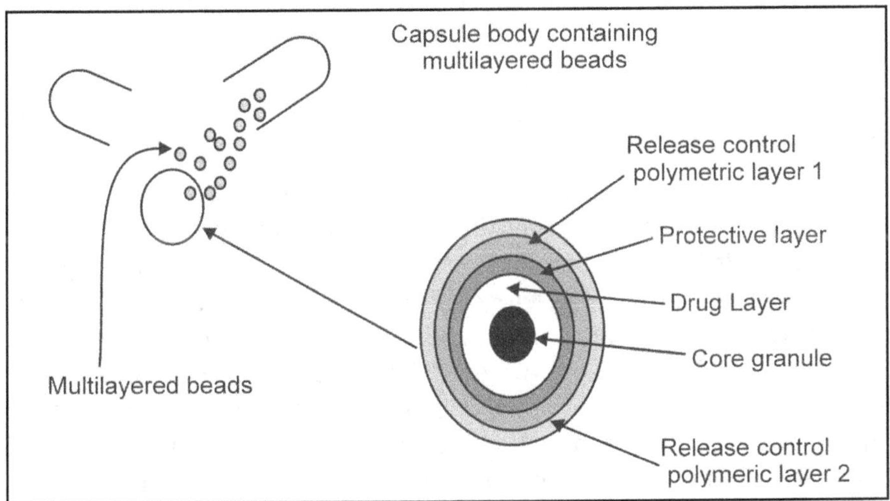

FIGURE 8.16 Schematic diagram showing cross section of SODAS technique.

SODAS can provide immediate release of the drug followed by sustained release of drug leading to the better patient compliance especially in case of management of pain. The ease and flexibility of such system can be understood through the fact that it could be even sprinkled on food for easy administration (Moodley et al., 2012; Prajapati B, 2008).

Sometimes the immediate release of the drug is not desirable and action of drug for the longer time is needed which can be achieved by chronotherapy using specially designed prolonged release dosage form.

Chronotherapeutic Oral Drug Absorption System (CODAS) was developed by Elan Corporation to accomplish the prolonged release of the drug. Some more systems which are developed (Prajapati B, 2008) on the similar principle are:

- Intestinal Protective Drug Absorption System (IPDAS® Technology) developed to avoid gastric irritancy.

- Time Multiple Action Delivery system (TMDS) utilizes time dependent release polymer for coating.

- Programmable Oral Drug Absorption System (PRODAS® Technology) consisting of different release pattern mini tablets in a capsule

- Programmed Multiple-action Delivery System (PMDS) especially designed to provide the multi-phasic drug delivery

8.9   Egalet Technology

Egalet technology was developed by Egalet Ltd. by injection molding technique for preparing controlled released products for series of compounds. It consists of erodible matrix (commonly polyethylene glycol monostearates and polyethylene oxides) containing drug partly covered with water impermeable coating (cetostearyl alcohol and ethylcellulose). The coating is done in such a way that the two ends of the cylinder should be non-coated and fitted with erodible plug as shown in Fig. 8.17. Time of release can be modified by changing the length/thickness and composition of the plugs (Daniel et al., 2002) while the release rate can be controlled by defining and fixing the size and area of erosion at one or both the ends resulting in approximate zero order release (Hemmingsen et al., 2011; Khan et al., 2009). The designing of this system should always be done in such a way that the gastric fluid should not permeate the impermeable coating while the plugs at one or both the ends should erode with exposure to gastric fluid (Daniel et al., 2002).

The major limitation of the technology is that the active content should not be more than 50% of the matrix and that there are several materials like phenols which are incompatible with PEG/PEO system leading to lowering of its melting point.

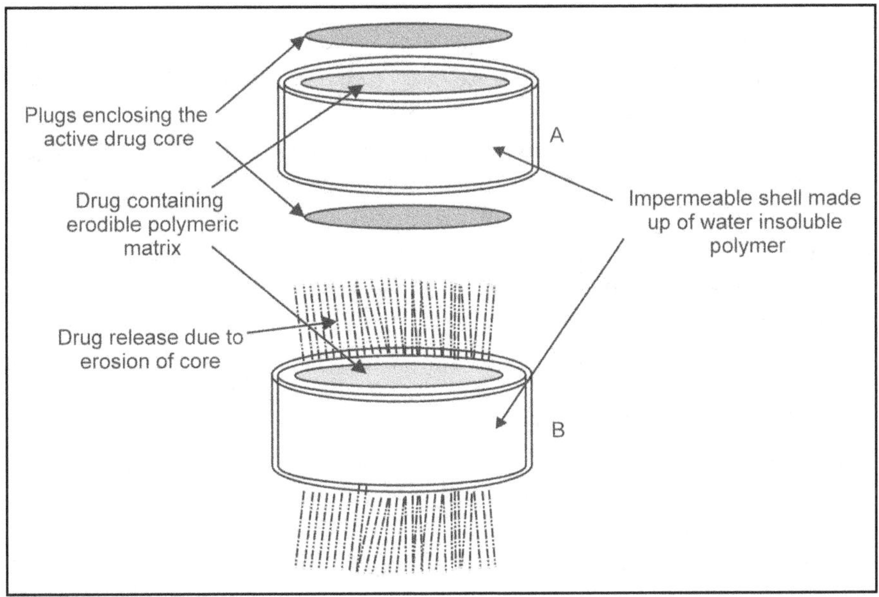

FIGURE 8.17 Schematic diagram showing components and release from the Egalet system.

8.10 Conclusion

It has been mentioned by a number of researchers that the oral drug delivery is the most convenient and highly sought mode for administration of drugs. Recent era has witnessed high end research to design and develop efficient drug carrier systems known as novel drug delivery systems but still much remains to be achieved. Advancement in the existing conventional dosage forms have been tried upon with the objective of keeping the original form but with enhanced efficacy and development per one's need. Such efforts have resulted in conventional dosage forms with reforms viz. formulation of tablets as dosage form displaying release pattern to cater the need. A number of technologies have been discussed in the chapter regarding the same but more research and correlation is needed before each of the technology is utilized to its maximum for the benefit of the healthcare.

References

Bayomi, M.A. (1994). Geometric approach for zero-order release of drugs dispersed in an inert matrix. *Pharmaceutical research* **11**, 914-916.

Chopra, S.K. (2002). Procise: Drug delivery systems based on geometric configuration. In Modified-Release Drug Delivery Technology, J.H. Michael J. Rathbone, ed. (CRC Press), pp. 35-48.

Daniel, B.-S., Lillian, S., Wang Wang, L., and Clive, G.W. (2002). Development of the Egalet Technology. In Modified-Release Drug Delivery Technology (Informa Healthcare), pp. 263-271.

David, R.F., and Syed, A.A. (2002). MASRx and COSRx Sustained-Release Technology. In Modified-Release Drug Delivery Technology (Informa Healthcare), pp. 21-33.

Dickason D. A., G.G.P. (2002). RingCap Technology. In Modified-Release Drug Delivery Technology, J.H. Michael J. Rathbone, Michael S. Roberts, ed. (U.S.A: CRC press), pp. 49-57.

Gao, P., Nie, X., Zou, M., Shi, Y., and Cheng, G. (2011). Recent advances in materials for extended-release antibiotic delivery system. *The Journal of antibiotics* **64,** 625-634.

Garg.T., C.A., Gupta. A., Khatri. N., Sharma. G (2012). Pulsatile drug delivery systems: Pulsincap system. *IOSR Journal of Pharmacy* **2,** 338-339.

Hemmingsen, P.H., Haahr, A.M., Gunnergaard, C., and Cardot, J.M. (2011). Development of a New Type of Prolonged Release Hydrocodone Formulation Based on Egalet(R) ADPREM Technology Using *In vitro-In vitro* Correlation. *Pharmaceutics* **3,** 73-87.

Horst, G.Z., and Markus, K. (2002). Smartrix System. In Modified-Release Drug Delivery Technology (Informa Healthcare), pp. 59-76.

Khan, Z., Pillay, V., Choonara, Y.E., and du Toit, L.C. (2009). Drug delivery technologies for chronotherapeutic applications. *Pharmaceutical development and technology* **14,** 602-612.

McMullen, J.N. (1989). Controlled release tablet, U.S.P. office, ed.

Moodley, K., Pillay, V., Choonara, Y.E., du Toit, L.C., Ndesendo, V.M., Kumar, P., Cooppan, S., and Bawa, P. (2012). Oral drug delivery systems comprising altered geometric configurations for controlled drug delivery. *International journal of molecular sciences* **13,** 18-43.

Prajapati B, S.H. (2008). Recent Techniques For Oral Time Controlled Pulsatile Technology. *The Internet Journal of Third World Medicine* **8,** 14-18.

Qiu Y, Z.D. (2011). Understanding Design and Development of Modified Release Solid Oral Dosage Forms. *Journal of Validation Technology* **17.**

Qiu.Y (2009). Rational designing of oral modified release drug delivery system. In Developing Solid Oral Dosage Forms: Pharmaceutical Theory & Practice, C.Y. Qiu Y, Zhang G.Z, Liu L, Porter W, ed. (U.S.A: Academic Press), pp. 469-496.

Singh B N, K.K.H. (2000). Drug delivery: oral route In Encyclopedia of Pharmaceutical Technology: Volume 20-Supplement 3, J. Swarbrick, and J.C. Boylan, eds. (CRC Press), pp. 1242-1262.

Staniforth, J.N., and Baichwal, A.R. (2005). TIMERx: novel polysaccharide composites for controlled/programmed release of drugs in the gastrointestinal tract. *Expert opinion on drug delivery* **2,** 587-595.

Stevens H.N.E., R.A., Bakhshaee M, Binns J.S., Miller C.J (1999). Expulsion of material from a delivery device, U.S.P. office, ed. (U.S.A: R.P. Scherer corporation, Troy, Mich).

Stevens, H.N.E, S. (2002). Pulsincap and Hydrophilic Sandwich (HS) Capsules. In Modified-Release Drug Delivery Technology (Informa Healthcare), pp. 257-262.

Troy, W.M., John, N.S., and Anand, R.B. (2002). TIMERx Oral Controlled-Release Drug Delivery System. In Modified-Release Drug Delivery Technology (Informa Healthcare), pp. 11-19.

9 Designing of Modulated Release Drug Delivery Systems by Pelletization Techniques

Vinod K. Dhote[1], Kanika Dhote[1], Sharad. P. Pandey[1], Tripti Shukl a[2] and Vandana Soni[3]

[1]Truba Institute of Pharmacy, Karond - Gandhi Nagar Bypass Road, Bhopal-462 038, India.

[2]School of Pharmacy, Peoples University, Bhanpur Bypass Road, Bhopal-462 037, India.

[3]Department of Pharmaceutical Sciences, Dr. H.S Gour Central University, Sagar-470 003, India.

9.1 Introduction

The word pellet is used to describe a variety of systematically product geometrically defined agglomerates obtained from diverse starting material. It consists of small discrete unit and exhibits some derived characteristics produced by agglomeration of fine powder with binder solution. Pelletization can be defined as an agglomeration (size-enlargement) process that converts fine powders or particles of bulk drugs and excipients into small, free-flowing, more or less spherical units (Palmieri et al., 2000; Sövgren, 1992). These pellets can eventually be coated and very often used in controlled-release dosage forms (Rubinstein, 2000).

Pellets typically ranges in size from about 0.5 mm to 1.5 mm, and are intended usually for oral administration (Kristensen H. G., 1993; Melia C.D., 1994). Pellets offer several advantages over a single unit dosage form.

Following desirable attributes can be achieved with the use of pellets in pharmaceutical field:

1. Improve aesthetic appearance of products.
2. Achieve control release rate of drugs when coated with polymers.

3. Improve flow properties and flexibility in formulation development and manufacturing.

4. It has less variance in transient time through the gastro intestinal tract (GI tract) than a single unit dosage form like tablet.

The pelletized products can improve the safety and efficacy of the active agent. These multiple-unit doses are usually formulated in the form of suspensions, capsules or disintegrating tablets, showing a number of advantages over the single-unit dosage system (Sellassie G., 2000).

9.1.1 History of Pelletization

The term pellet has been used by a number of industries to describe a variety of agglomerates produced from diverse raw materials, using different pieces of manufacturing equipment. These agglomerates include fertilizers, animal feeds, iron ores, and pharmaceutical dosage units and thus do not only differ in composition but also encompass different sizes and shapes. As a result, pellets meant different things for different industries. When it comes to pharmaceutical industry, it was only in the early 1950's, in response to a desire to sustain the release of drugs over an extended period of time, that the pharmaceutical industry developed a keen interest in the technology (Cimicata, 1951; Wong T.W., 2005). And it's been since the late 1970's, the advantages of pellets over single-unit dosage forms have been realized. In time, extensive research was conducted to develop pelletization techniques and major resources were allocated towards exploring methods that were faster, cheaper and more efficient, both in terms of formulation and processing equipment.

9.1.2 Advantages and Limitations

Pellets offer a significant number of advantages over conventional unit-dose systems.

9.1.2.1 Technological Advantages

Uniformity of dose can be achieved with the use of pellets. Layering techniques and extrusion spheronization technique offers great accuracy with uniform drug delivery.

1. Spheres have excellent flow properties. This becomes very useful in automated processes or in processes where exact dosing is required, e.g., tableting, moulding operations, capsule filling and packaging (Jones, 1989).

2. Prevention of dust formation, resulting in an improvement of the process safety, as fine powders can cause dust explosions and the respiration of fines can cause health problems.

3. Pellets can efficiently be used to achieve controlled release applications due to the ideal low surface area to volume ratio that provides an ideal shape for the application of film coating (Hincal A., 1994).

4. They can be blended to deliver incompatible bioactive agents simultaneously and/or to provide different release profiles at the same or different sites in the GI tract (Villar-Lopez et al., 1999).

9.1.2.2 Therapeutic Advantages

Pellets can disperse freely throughout the GI tract after administration and consequently the drug absorption is maximized.

1. The wide distribution of spherical particles in the GI tract limits localized build-up of the drug, avoiding the irritant effect of some drugs on the gastric mucosa.

2. Reduce inter- and intra-patient variability.

3. Modified-release multiparticulate delivery systems are less susceptible to dose dumping than single-unit dosage forms.

9.1.2.3 Limitations of Pelletization

1. It is difficult to compress pellets into tablets as they are too rigid. Therefore, they are often to be delivered encapsulated in hard gelatin capsule shells (Rubinstein, 2000).

2. Pelletization demands highly sophisticated and specialized equipment, thereby increasing the cost of manufacturing.

3. The control of manufacturing process is complicated with too many process variables as well as formulation variables (Chambliss, 1989).

9.1.3 Rationale of using Pelletization

The pharmaceutical industry has developed a great interest in pelletization due to a variety of reasons:

- Prevention of segregation of co-agglomerated components, resulting in an improvement of the uniformity of the content.

- Prevention of dust formation, resulting in an improvement of the process safety, as fine powders can cause dust explosions and the respiration of fines can cause health problems (Hincal, 1996).

- Increase in bulk density leads to reduction of bulk volume.

- The defined shape and weight improves the appearance of the product (Rahman et al., 2009).

- Improvement of the handling properties due to the free-flowing attribute of the pellets.

- Due to improvement in hardness of the pellets, the friability is reduced.

- Formation of pellets facilitates formulation of controlled release products (Heng et al., 1999).

9.2   Pelletization Techniques

The most commonly used and intensively investigated pelletization techniques include extrusion-spheronization, powder layering and solution/suspension layering. There are other methods available which can also be used for preparing pellets. Fig. 9.1 represents various techniques used for formulation of pellets. However, practical applicability of some of the methods is often very limited (Rahman et al., 2009; Shettigar and Damle, 1996).

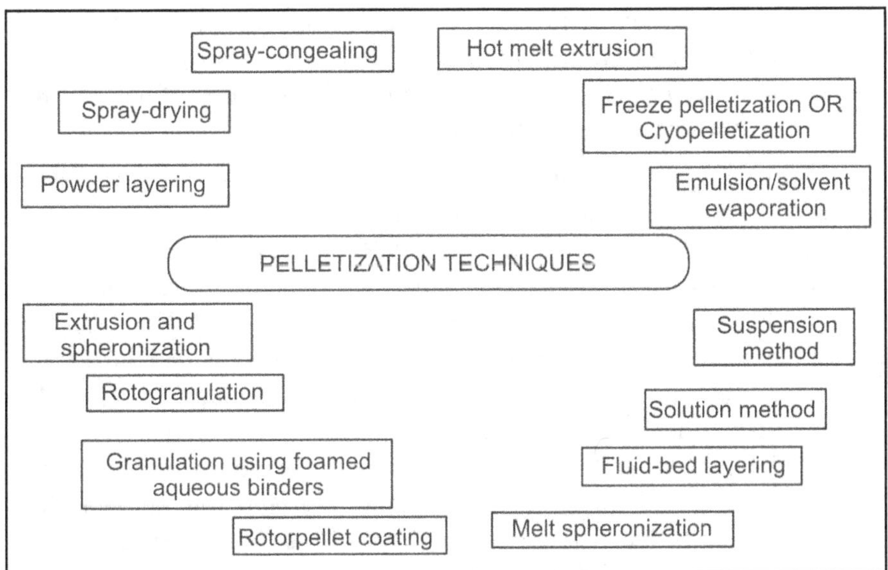

FIGURE 9.1 Classification of various techniques in pelletization.

9.2.1 Extrusion/Spheronization

Extrusion/spheronization is a multistage process for obtaining pellets with uniform size from wet granulates (extrudates). The method involves following steps (Mehta K, 2005):

- The dry mixing of the ingredients, in order to achieve homogenous powder dispersions.

- Wet massing, in which the powders are wet mixed to form a sufficiently plastic mass.

- An extrusion stage, in which the wet mass is shaped into cylindrical segments with uniform diameter.

- The spheronization stage, in which the small cylinders are rolled into solid spheres (spheroids).

- The drying of the spheroids, in order to achieve the desired final moisture content.

- Screening (optional), to achieve the desired narrow size distribution.

Extrusion consists in applying pressure to a wet mass until it passes through the calibrated openings of a screen or die plate of the extruder and further shaped into small extrudate segments. The extrudates must have enough plasticity in order to deform, but an excessive plasticity may lead to extrudates which stick to each other. The diameter of the segments and the final size of the spheroids depend on the diameter of the openings in the extruder screen (Mehta K, 2005).

"Extruder" is the equipment which carries out the process of extrusion; extruders are generally classified on the basis of the mechanism as: RAM type extruders, SCREW type extruders and Gear pelletizer. RAM type Extruders are not frequently used nowadays because high power consumption, but these are used only for very specialized extrusions. SCREW type extruders are most popular form of extruders; are suitable for heavy duty continuous runs and requires low power consumption. Gear pelletizer very commonly used extruder offers improved handling and metering properties; dust free operation; high pellet stability; suitable for batch/continuous process and provides smooth surface pellets (Fielden et al., 1992a). Fig. 9.2 represents various type of extruders used for formulation of pellets.

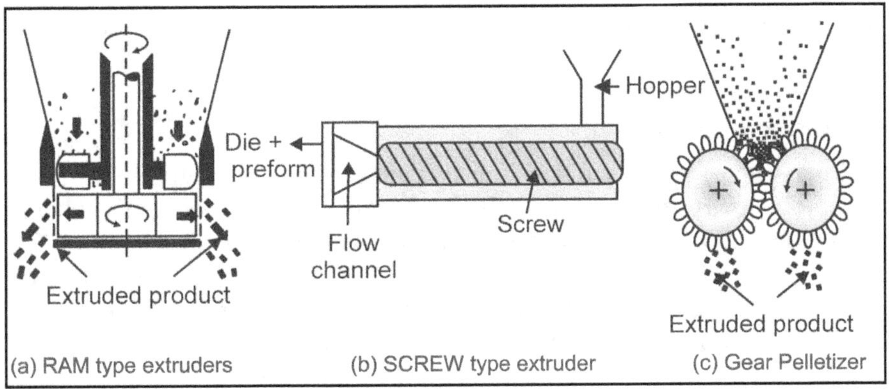

FIGURE 9.2 Types of extruders.

9.2.1.1 Advantages of Spheronization

- The flow characteristics of spheres make them suitable for transportation by most systems found in the pharmaceutical industry, including vacuum transfer.

- The packing of small spheres into small containers, such as hard gelatine capsules, or larger packages is much more convenient than other dry forms such as powders or granules (O'connor and Schwartz, 1985).

- Spheres are a dense material and provide the lowest surface area to volume ratio and thus can be coated with a minimum of amount of coating material.

- Coating can provide controlled and targeted release at different locations within the body (intestine, colonic regions etc).

- Spheres decreases production of fines and dust during transportation, handling and packaging.

- Depending on adhesive forces and surface characteristics, spheronization increases the hardness and reduces friability of granules.

Extrusion spheronization is a multi-step compaction process comprising of following steps,

9.2.1.2 Dry Mixing

Dry mixing of all ingredients is done to get homogeneous powder dispersion with the help of different types of mixers like twin shell blender, high shear mixer, tumbler mixer and planetary mixer (Mehta K, 2005).

9.2.1.3 Wet Massing

Wet massing of powder dispersion is done to produce a sufficient plastic mass for extrusion. This granulation is similar to a conventional wet granulation with the exception of the granulation endpoint. The granulation endpoint is determined by the behaviour of the wet mass during the extrusion operation. The most commonly used granulator is planetary mixer or sigma blade mixer or high shear mixer and Hobart mixer. Typically, planetary mixer is used routinely for both blending and granulation operation. High shear mixer introduces a high amount of energy into the wet mass which is transformed into heat and induces evaporation of granulation fluid due to which extrusion behaviour of the wet mass changes, to overcome this problem granulation bowl must be cooled (Fielden et al., 1992b; Hicks D., 1989).

9.2.1.4 Extrusion

The extrusion operation can be considered to be a specialized wet granulation technique as well as an integral part of the overall spheronization process. Extrusion is a method of applying pressure to wet mass until it flows through an opening to get converted into extruded product of uniform diameter (Crowley et al., 2007). The extrudate must have enough plasticity to deform but not so much that the extrudate particles adheres to other particles when rolled during spheronization process to convert into pellets. **Fig. 9.3 illustrates the formation of pellets in extrusion process.** The granulation solvent serves as the binding agent to form the granules and as lubricant during the extrusion operation (Mehta K, 2005).

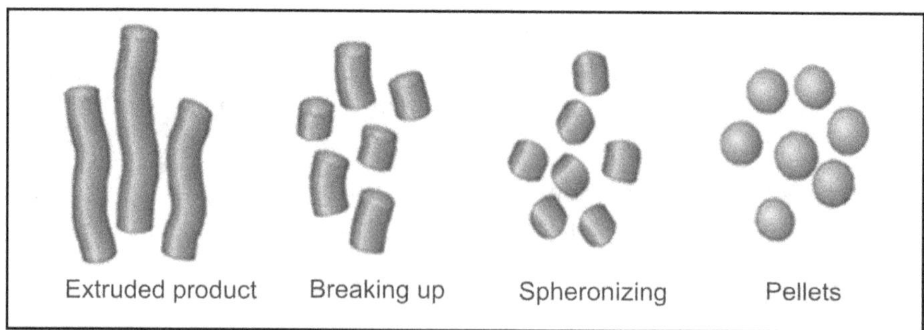

FIGURE 9.3 Formation of pellets by extrusion process.

9.2.2 Roto Granulation

Roto granulation is one of the most recent methods for the production of spheroids. The single-unit spheronizing system can be described using terms like centrifugal granulator, rotary fluidized-bed granulator, rotary fluid bed, rotary processor or rotor granulator (Summers M., 2002).

Regardless the name of the equipment, they all have the same main piece, a rotating disc. When the equipment is operating, this disk provides a centrifugal force which throws the pellets towards the wall of the processing chamber. Air via a slit between the disc and the wall of the chamber moves the particles in a vertical direction (Nakahara, 1964). As the fluidizing force decreases with the distance above the slit, the pellets fall towards the bottom of the disc. The centrifugal force is in relation with the rotation speed of the disc, while the vertical distance for which the particles move is dependent on the air velocity and volume (Hirjau M., 2011). Fig. 9.4 Shows schematic diagram of a Rota granulator.

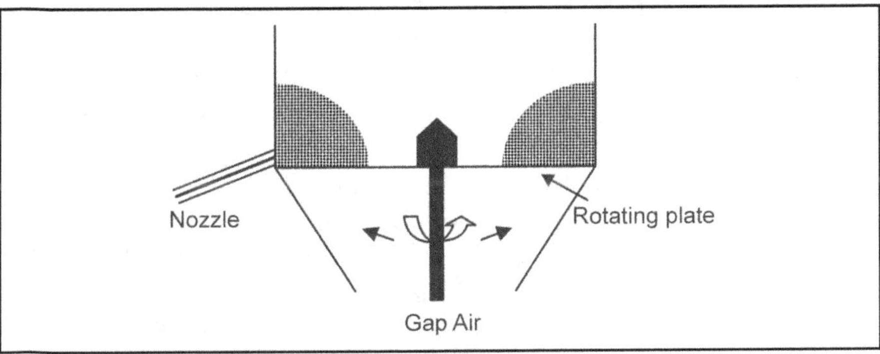

FIGURE 9.4 The schematic diagram of a Rota granulator.

9.2.3 Solution and Suspension Layering

Layering a suspension or a solution of a drug on a seed material (usually, a coarse crystal or nonpareil) can produce pellets that are uniform in size distribution and generally possess very good surface morphology (Villar-Lopez et al., 1999). These characteristics are especially desirable when pellets are to be coated for the purpose of achieving a controlled release. The equipment employed for this kind of processes consists of custom modified conventional coating pans (perforated pans) and various configurations of fluid-bed equipment (Vojnovic D., 1993).

There are many factors that determine the economic and performance feasibility of pellet coating. Besides the process variables mentioned before, there are other formulation variables, such as the drug solubility in the media used for solution layering, or the suspension concentration in solid particles for the suspension layering of the pellets, which need to be taken into account (Vojnovic D., 1993).

9.2.4 Dry Powder Layering

This process is similar to the solution or suspension layering. Instead of these dispersions, the layering is performed using a drug powder. Usually, the process is carried out in conventional coating pans. Initially, the nonpareils or starter seeds (neutral or inert pellets, beads, spheres) are charged into a rotating pan followed by wetting spraying an adhesive solution. As the wet seeds reach the front end of the pan, the powder added in the vortex adheres to them (Goodhart F., 1989). A baffle inserted into the rolling bed enhances the vortex action, which in turn intensifies the mixing and shear, improving the adhesion of the powder to the wet seeds. After the wet seeds pick up the powder, they are directed back into the upward moving bed and the entire process is repeated. In an intermittent powder layering process, the layering solution is added until the bed is wet and tacky. The drug powder is then added, until the bed is dry (Hirjau M., 2011).

Warm drying air may be used after each cycle. The process continues until the entire drug powder has been added. In a continuous process, the layering solution and the drug powder are added simultaneously. When using a centrifugal granulator, as the pellets rotate in a rope-like fashion, they are first wetted by the adhesive solution and the powder is added to the wet pellets immediately afterwards. This cycle continues until the desired pellet size is obtained (Goodhart F., 1989).

9.2.5 Cryopelletization

Cryopelletization is a process whereby droplets of a liquid formulation are converted into solid spherical particles or pellets by using liquid nitrogen as the fixing medium. These pellets are then freeze dried or lyophilized to remove water or organic solvents. Solid content and temperature of the liquid formulation determines the amount of liquid nitrogen used in the whole process. This technology was first developed to lyophilize bacterial suspension in the nutrition industry and now-a-days it is used in the pharmaceutical industry to produce drug loaded pellets for immediate as well as controlled release formulations (Hirjau M., 2011).

Immediate release formulation typically consists of drugs, fillers (lactose and mannitol) and binders (gelatin and PVP) while cross-linked polymers of collagen derivatives are used in the sustained release formulations (Rahman et al., 2009). The equipment consists of a perforated plate below which a reservoir of liquid nitrogen having conveyer belt of varying speed with transport baffle is dipped. The varying speed of the conveyer belt can be adjusted to provide the residence time required for freezing the pellets. The frozen pellets are transported into storage container at – 60°C before drying and are finally dried into the freeze dryer. Droplet formation is the most critical step in this technique and is influenced by formulation related variables, such as solid content, viscosity, surface tension, equipment design and process variables (Heng P., 1999).

9.2.6 Spray Drying and Spray Congealing

Spray drying and spray congealing, known as globulation processes, involve atomization of hot melts, solutions, or suspensions to generate spherical particles or pellets. Spray drying is a process in which, the drug entities in solution or suspension are sprayed, with or without excipients, into a hot air stream to generate dry and highly spherical particles (Hincal A., 1994). This process is commonly used for improving the dissolution rate and hence bioavailability of poorly soluble drugs. Spray congealing is the process in which a drug is allowed to melt, disperse or dissolve in hot melts of gums, waxes or fatty acids, and is sprayed into an air chamber where the temperature is kept below the melting point of the formulation components, to produce spherical congealed pellets under appropriate processing conditions (Eldem et al., 1991b; Helen L., 1993) (Fig. 9.5).

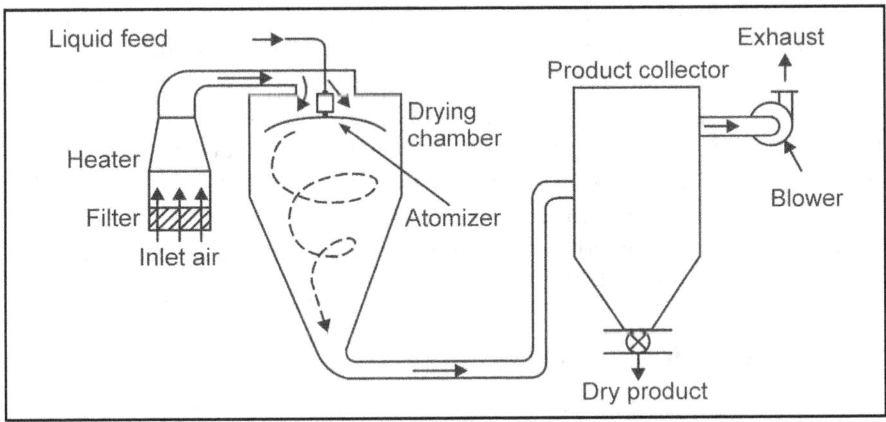

FIGURE 9.5 The schematic diagram of a spray-drier.

9.2.7 Freeze Pelletization

Freeze pelletization technique is a novel technique for producing spherical matrix pellets containing active ingredients. In this technique, a molten solid carrier along with a dispersed active ingredient is introduced as droplets into an inert and immiscible column of liquid. These droplets can move either in upward or downward directions, depending on their density with respect to the liquid in the column and solidify into spherical pellets. The technique involves less process variables and also offers several advantages over other pelletization methods, in terms of quality of pellets and process cost (Melia C.D., 1994). The pellets produced by this technique are spherical in shape with narrow size distribution. Since the pellets are solid at room temperature, they do not require drying (Vojnovic D., 1993).

9.2.8 Melt-Induced Agglomeration

Melt-induced agglomeration processes are similar to liquid-induced processes except that the binding material is a melt. Therefore, the pellets are formed with the help of congealed material without having to go through the formation of solvent-based liquid bridges (Wong T.W., 2005). If the surface moisture is not optimum, some particles may undergo nucleation and coalescence at different rates and form different sizes of nuclei admixed with the larger pellets. As a result, spherical agglomeration tends to produce pellets with a wide particle size distribution.

9.2.9 Melt Spheronization

Melt spheronization is a process whereby a drug substance and excipients are converted into a molten or semi molten state and subsequently shaped using appropriate equipment to provide solid spheres or pellets. The drug substance is first blended with the appropriate pharmaceutical excipients, such as polymers and waxes, and extruded at a predetermined temperature (Hincal A., 1994). The extrusion temperature must be high enough to melt at least one or more of the formulation components. The extrudate is cut into uniform cylindrical segments with a cutter. The segments are spheronized in a jacketed spheronizer to generate uniformly sized pellets (Heng et al., 1999).

9.2.10 Fluid-Bed Granulation

The process is carried out continuously in a fluid-bed granulator. It consists in the spraying of a granulation solution onto the suspended particles, which then are dried rapidly in the hot air stream. The following steps are involved in the fluid-bed granulation process (Hirjau M., 2011; Sövgren, 1992) (Fig. 9.6):

- The pre-blending of the formulation powder, including the active ingredients, fillers, disintegrants, in a flow of air.

- The granulation of the mixture by spraying a suitable liquid binder onto the fluidized (suspended) powder bed.

- The drying of the granulated product to the desired moisture content.

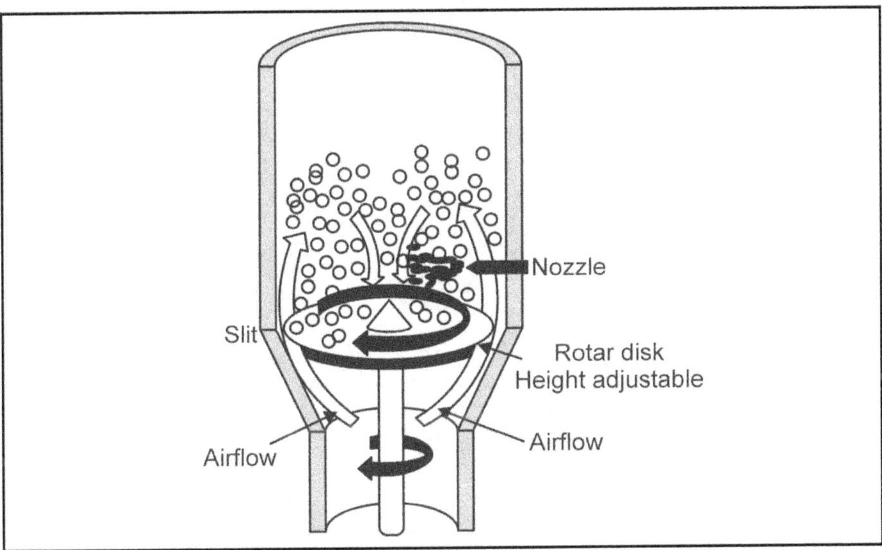

FIGURE 9.6 The schematic representation of a fluid-bed granulator.

9.2.11 Bottom Spray Coating Process

The most commonly known fluid-bed process for coating in the pharmaceutical industry is the bottom-spray (Wurster) process (Fig. 9.7). Developed by Dr. Dale Wurster in the late 1950s, the technique is well recognized for providing excellent coating uniformity and efficiency (Eldem et al., 1991b). The unique features of bottom-spraying are an air distribution plate and a partition that together organize fluidization of particles through the partition (coating zone). The nozzle is mounted at the bottom of the product container and is centred in the coating zone. The short distance between the coating materials and particles during the coating process minimizes spray-drying and contributes to high coating uniformity and coating efficiency (Eldem et al., 1991a).

9.2.12 Tangential Spray Fluid Bed Granulation

The second fluid-bed technique for wet granulation is the tangential-spray (rotary) process, available since the early 1980s. Fig. 9.7 depicts a tangential-spray processor. The nozzle is introduced at the side of a product container and is imbedded in the substrate during processing. The primary feature of a tangential-spray processor is a spinning, variable-speed disk. During processing, three mechanical forces cause particle movement, mixing, and granulation. First, the spinning of the disk generates a centrifugal force. Second, a lifting force is generated by the process air volume that passes through the adjustable disk gap. Third, gravity causes material to fall down onto the disk. These forces, resembling a spiralling helix, provide good mixing and result in granules with good content uniformity (Eldem et al., 1991a).

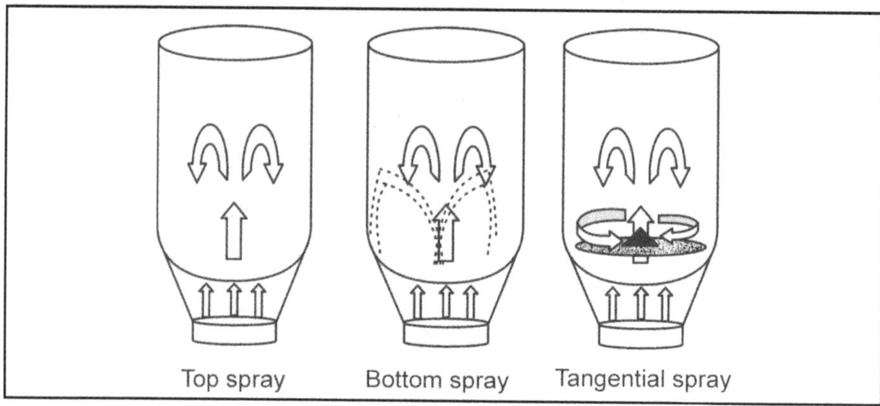

Figure 9.7 Different patterns of fluid bed processing.

9.2.13 Suspension/Solution Layering Technique

This technique involves deposition of successive layer of solution and/or suspension of drug substances and binders on starter seeds which may be inert material or crystals of granules of the same drug. In this technique drug particles and other components are dissolved or suspended in the application medium. The droplets impinge on the starter seeds or cores and spread evenly as the solution or suspension is sprayed on the cores. The drying process allows dissolved material to crystallize and form solid bridges between the cores and initial layer of the drug substances and among the successive layer of drug substances or polymer. This process is continued until the desired layer of drug or polymer is formed (Ghai, 2011).

9.2.14 Innovative Technologies

Nowadays pelletization technologies symbolize an efficient pathway for manufacture of drug delivery system. We have focused on commonly used pelletization techniques for producing pellets for oral drug delivery. Each technique has its own advantages and disadvantages. Layering processes have been used over the years for manufacturing of pellets. Most of the scientists have focused research on refining and optimizing existing pelletization techniques and also focused on the development of novel approaches and procedures of manufacturing pellets employing innovative formulation and processing equipment. These pelletization techniques have great impact on the development of different types of novel drug delivery systems. A number of pelletized products are being designed to maximize the *In vivo* performance of medications already in the market and to meet all regulatory requirements   .

The well explained multiparticulate pellet units can be formulated to prepare different drug application forms e.g., oral suspension, multiparticulate tablets etc.

In addition to existing and established pelletizing technologies, some recent advanced and innovative technologies have been explored such as CPS™ Technology (Controlled Release Pelletizing Technology); MicroPx™ Technology; ProCell™ Technology, allowing new formulation options and product qualities.

9.2.14.1 CPS™ Technology

CPS™ Technology is a direct pelletization process resulting in matrix type pellets. Release characteristics of API (active pharmaceutical ingredient) from CPS™ pellets depend both on the pellet formulation and on the pelletizing process. The CPS™ technology is an advanced fluid bed rotor technology allowing the preparation of matrix pellets with particular properties in a batch process. Extremely low dosed as well as high dosed APIs can be formulated as CPS™ matrix pellets (Srivastava S., 2010).

Some specific and outstanding product characteristics of CPS™ pellets are as follows:

- Dust free surfaces of the pellets having mean particle size range in between 100-1500 μm with narrow particle size distribution.

- Spherical and smooth pellet surfaces, best suited for coating applications

- High density/low porosity of pellets with low attrition and friability
- Broad potency range for APIs
- Controlled drug release from the CPS matrix

9.2.14.2 MicroPx™ Technology

The MicroPx™ Technology is a fluid bed agglomeration process resulting in matrix type pellets. Particle size could be rather small (<400 µm) together with a high drug loading of typically up to 95%. Functional pharmaceutical excipients, e.g., for bioavailability enhancement or controlled drug release can be integrated in the pellet matrix. The MicroPx™ Technology is a continuous fluid bed process: again, for the pelletization, no starting cores are required. Typically, all formulation components like the API, pharmaceutical binder(s) and other functional ingredients are contained in a liquid which is fed into the MicroPx™ process via spray guns; the spraying liquid can be a solution, suspension, emulsion or the like (Srivastava S., 2010). Here are some potential exceptional product characteristics of MicroPx™ pellets:

- Spherical and smooth pellet surfaces, ideal for coating applications like taste masking controlled release coating etc.

- High density/low porosity of pellets with high drug loading: typically up to 95%

- Low attrition and friability with dust free surfaces

- Mean particle size range: 100-500 µm with narrow particle size distribution

- Inclusion of bioavailability enhancers or controlled release polymers is feasible.

9.2.14.3 ProCell™ Technology

The ProCell™ Technology is a spouted-bed type pelletizing process for the preparation of very high concentrated pellet shaped particles. The ProCell™ Technology is a direct granulation and pelletizing process like CPS™ and the MicroPx™ technology. No inert starting beads are required and either, solutions, suspensions or emulsions containing the API, can be processed. With ProCell™ Technology formation of granules and pellets takes place by means of spray solidification and agglomeration (Srivastava S., 2010).

Specific product characteristics of ProCell™ granules and pellets are as follows:

- High density/low porosity of particles with very high drug load up to 100%
- Mean particle size range from 50-1500 µm with optimum narrow particle size distribution
- Low attrition and friability justifying its suitability for processing of particular products with inherent stickiness

9.3   Factors Affecting Pelletization Process

The shape size and characteristics of the pellets depends on various factors which in turn ensure the desired functions and applications. These factors are responsible for the effectiveness of the resulting product. Fig. 9.8 depicts some factors that need to be optimized to get better results.

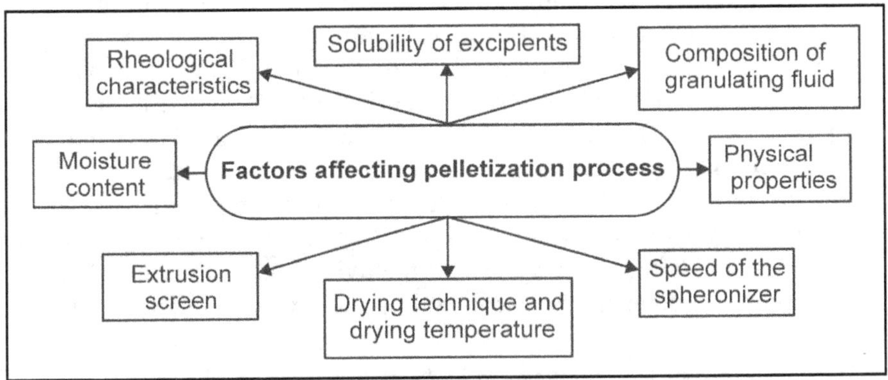

FIGURE 9.8 Factors affecting pelletization process.

9.3.1 Moisture Content

It is one of the critical parameters for pellet growth in pelletization technique. Moisture in the wet mass brings cohesiveness to the powder so that the wet mass can be extruded and spheronized resulting in spherical shape of the product. High moisture content leads to agglomeration of pellets during the process of spheronization which is one of the techniques of pelletization. This is due to the presence of excess of water in the surface of pellets while low moisture content leads to generation of fines with large variation in size distribution (Mehta K, 2005).

9.3.2 Rheological Characteristics

The rheological properties of wet powder masses used in the preparation of pharmaceutical pellets by extrusion/spheronization have been evaluated utilizing capillary and rotational rheometers. Rheological characters should be taken into account during pellet formation (Goodhart F., 1989; Hirjau M., 2011).

9.3.3 Solubility of Excipients and Drug in Granulating Fluid

A soluble drug gets dissolved in a granulating liquid. This increases the volume of liquid phase leading to over wetting of pellets. Increase in wetting liquid increases plasticity but also induces stickiness. Therefore, solubility of excipients and drug in granulating fluid must be considered and determined (Summers M., 2002).

9.3.4 Composition of Granulating Fluid

Besides water, alcohol, water/alcohol mixture, ethyl ether, dilute acetic acid, isopropyl alcohol is also used as a granulating liquid. According to Millili and Schwartz, a minimum 5% of granulation liquid has to be water in order to produce pellets containing Avicel pH (101) and theophylline (Vojnovic D., 1993). Some researchers using water and dilute acetic acid in different ratio (powder:liquid) concluded that mass fraction can be increased up to 100% by using dilute acetic acid for granulation step in place of demineralized water (Hirjau M., 2011). Aqueous polymer dispersion containing Hydroxy propyl methylcellulose, Eudragit, Gelatin, Poly vinyl pyrolidone can be use in conjugation with granulating fluid.

9.3.5 Physical Properties of Starting Material

Formulation variable such as type and content of starting material, type of filler and particle size of constituent have the effect on the pelletization process. Quality of pellets depends not only on composition but also on different grades of the same product (Eldem et al., 1991b). The swelling property of material used in pelletization technique decides the release behaviour of the drug in pellets.

9.3.6 Speed of the Spheronizer

The speed of the spheronizer affects the size, hardness, sphericity and density of pellets. High speed gives high sphericity, lower friability, smooth surface and higher crushing strength (Ghebre-Sellassie et al., 1985).

9.3.7 Drying Technique and Drying Temperature

It is important to get proper size, shape and flow of pellets and it must be reproducible and consistent in all the batches. Variation in pellet's size, shape and flow will lead to difference in physicochemical properties of final dosage form like weight variation, improper filling etc., which will further affect the therapeutic efficiency of the delivery system. Wider particle size distribution may lead to variation in the dose of the drug to be delivered. Variation in shape may lead to alteration in flow and compressibility (Fielden et al., 1992a; Ghebre-Sellassie et al., 1985).

9.3.8 Extrusion Screen

The characteristic of the orifice screen determines the quality of the extrudate/pellets to a significant extent. An increase in orifice dimension results in increased mean pellet size (Dietrich et al., 1988).

9.4　Characterization of Pellets

The pellets are characterized with reference to various parameters which are represented in Fig. 9.9.

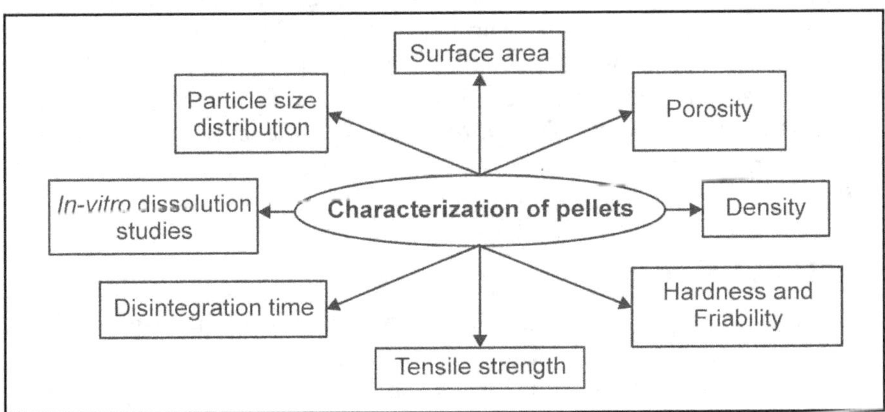

FIGURE 9.9 Characterization parameters for pellets.

9.4.1 Particle Size Distribution

The sizing of pellets is necessary because it has significant influence on the release kinetics (Mehta K, 2005). Mean ferret diameter, geometric mean diameter, mean particle width and length, are the parameters by which size of pellets can be determined. Particle size distribution should be as narrow as possible to ensure minimum variation in coating thickness and to facilitate blending process if blending of different types of pellets is required. Sieve analysis using sieve shaker is the most widely used method for measuring particle size distribution (Wan, 1989). Microscopy is direct method for determining distribution of particles based on size. Optical microscopy and scanning electron microscopy techniques are used to measure the diameter of pellets.

9.4.2 Surface Area

The characteristics of pellets, those controlling the surface area, are mainly size, shape, porosity and surface roughness. There are three methods of measuring the surface area of pellets. It can be calculated from the particle-size distribution by measuring/using the mean diameter. Two other techniques, i.e., gas adsorption and air permeability, permit direct calculation of surface area. Air permeability methods are widely used pharmaceutically for specific surface measurement, especially to control batch to batch variations. The principal resistance to the flow of a fluid such as air, through a plug of compacted material is the surface area of the material (Fielden et al., 1989). Gas adsorption is carried out by placing a powder sample in a chamber and evacuating the air within. Nitrogen is introduced in the chamber and the volume of nitrogen that is adsorbed by the substrate contained in an evacuated glass bulb is measured at different pressures. From the knowledge of pressure and temperature before and after introduction of the adsorbing gas, total sample surface area can be estimated (Dietrich et al., 1988; Summers M., 2002).

9.4.3 Porosity

The porosity of pellets influences the rate of release of drug from the pellets by affecting the capillary action of the dissolved drug. The porosity of the pellets can be measured quantitatively by mercury porosimetry (Hirjau M., 2011). The porosity of pellets can also be estimated qualitatively as well as quantitatively by using optical microscopy and scanning electron microscopy (Vojnovic D., 1993).

9.4.4 Density

The density of pellets can be affected by changes in the formulation and/ or process, which may influence other processing steps such as capsule filling, coating, and mixing. The bulk density of the pellets can be measured by an automated tapper. True density indicates the extent of densification or compactness of substances which can be determined by an air-comparison pycnometer, a helium pycnometer or by the solvent displacement method (Eldem et al., 1991b; Goodhart F., 1989).

9.4.5 Hardness and Friability

The quantitation of hardness and friability of the pellets is essential as the pellets have to encounter untoward pressure during handling and shipping and due to various other processing steps such as coating. The instrument such as the Kaul pellet hardness tester provides relative hardness value and friability of pellets is determined by using Erkewa type tablet friabilator. Friability can also be determined using fluidized bed with wurster insert by using stream of air (Fielden et al., 1992a; Ghebre-Sellassie et al., 1985).

9.4.6 Tensile Strength

The tensile strength of the pellets is determined by using tensile apparatus with a 5 kg load cell where the pellets are strained until failure occurs. The load is recorded and the tensile strength is calculated applying the value for the failure load and the radius of the pellets (Dietrich et al., 1988).

9.4.7 Disintegration Time

Disintegration of pellets is one of the foremost characteristics for immediate release pellets. (Huyghebaert *et al.,* 2005) reported disintegration test using the reciprocating cylinder method (USP Apparatus 3) (Huyghebaert et al., 2005). Thommes and Kleinbudde in 2006 performed it in a tablet disintegration tester specially designed by inserting special transparent tubes of certain diameter and length with sieve of 710 μm mesh size at the top and bottom of the tube (Thommes and Kleinebudde, 2006).

9.4.8 *In vitro* Dissolution Studies

In vitro dissolution has been recognized as an important element both in drug development as well as in quality assessment, especially in controlled released formulations. Drug release from pellets mainly depends on the composition, hardness and size of pellets and it is determined by using USP Apparatus I or by USP Apparatus II. The release behaviour of drug from pellets also depends on the nature of the excipient, aqueous solubility of the drug, physical state of the drug in the matrix, drug load and the presence of additives such as surfactants. In case of wax based freeze dried pellets, the release of the drug is decreased as the hydrophobicity of wax is increased whereas the drug release is increased on increment in the aqueous solubility of the drug (Hirjau M., 2011).

9.5 Applications

9.5.1 Taste Masking

Micropellets are ideal for products where perfect abatement of taste is required. Although various technique have been utilized to mask the bitter taste of a drug such as the addition of sweetners and flavours, filling in capsules, coating with water insoluble polymers or pH dependent soluble polymers, complexing with ion-exchange resins, microencapsulation with various polymers, compelxing with cyclodextrins and chemical modifications such as the use of insoluble prodrugs, few reports have described the masking of unpleasant taste without lowering of bioavailability (Singh et al., 2010). Micropelletization technique is a good alternative to resolve these problems. Furthermore, due to sophisticated manufacturing process, dust fractions that representing an uncoated fragments which could cause taste problems are absent in micropellets. Many products, such as antibiotics (clarithromycin, roxithromycin and cephelexin) and anti-inflammatory drugs with a prohibitively bitter taste, can now be formulated as products with high patient compliance leading to marked increase in the sales potential of the product (Hirjau M., 2011).

9.5.2 Immediate Release

Administering drugs in pellet form leads to an increased surface area as compared to traditional compressed tablets and capsules. This would considerably reduce the time required for disintegration and have the potential for use in rapidly dispersible tablets.

9.5.3 Sustained Release

The pellet form provides a smoother absorption profile from the gastrointestinal tract as the beads pass gradually through the stomach in to the small intestine at a steady rate. Pellets are being increasingly used in the manufacture of sustained release dosage form of drugs. The use of pellets with sustained release characteristics have following advantages:

- Extend day time and night time activity of the drugs
- Potential for reduced incidence of side effects
- Reduced administration frequency of dosage forms
- Increased patient compliance; patients who are required to take one or two doses of the formulation in a day are thought to be less likely to forget a dose then if they are required to take 3 or 4 times a day,
- Potential lower daily cost to patient due to fewer dosage units,

Different types of polymers e.g., carboxymethylcellulose, ethylcellulose, eudragit etc., are utilized for coating different drugs to enable the sustained/controlled release of drugs.

Pellets ensure improved flow properties and flexibility in formulation development and manufacture. If the pellet surface is smoother it allows thin or thick coat of the polymer on its surface. The thickness of the coat determines the rate at which the drug is released from the coated pellets. The coating material may be colored with a dye material so that the beads of different coating thickness will be darker in colour and distinguishable from those having fewer coating. It is widely used for frequently administered drugs having a half-life of 0.5-2 hr. The excellent reproducibility and homogeneity of the particle size and the round shape and smooth surface of the particles in micropellets with sizes smaller than 200 μm makes them suitable to fulfil the objective of powder for injections (Goodhart F., 1989).

Micropellets have thus, opens a new dimension in parenteral depot technologies. Drug substance particles can either be coated with biodegradable polymers or embedded in a polymer matrix. Using these approaches, release profiles ranging from days to months and even pulsed release can be obtained at wish (Fielden et al., 1992b).

9.5.4 Chemically Incompatible Products

Some situations can occur where chemically incompatible ingredients are required to be delivered in a single dose. In the compressed tablet dosage form separate tablets would have to be administered, but the pellets can be administered in a single capsule.

9.5.5 Varying Dosage without Reformulation

Pellets have excellent flow properties, due to this, they can be conveniently used for filling capsules and the manufacturer can vary the dosage by varying the capsule size without reformulating the product (Hirjau M., 2011).

9.6   Conclusion

Pelletization has gained an increased attention, principally due to the potential to use pellets in the formulation of modified-release solid oral dosage forms. Presently there are several pelletization methods, the most widely used being extrusion/spheronization. Due to the superior pharmacokinetic, technological and biopharmaceutics features of the pellets and the flexibility of the manufacturing processes implicated, pellets are expected to continue to play a major role in design and production of solid dosage forms.

The innovative fluid bed pelletizing technologies; CPS™, MicroPx™, ProCell™, potentially complement the actual capabilities of existing fluid bed technology as an added advantage. New possibilities for drug product development are demonstrated using advanced fluid bed technologies leading towards better therapeutic benefits and financial outcomes. The new era of innovative fluid bed technologies has potential not only for line-extensions of new chemical entity development but also for the by-pass of existing specific patent landscape in the generic business. Utilizing all the available fluid bed process technologies different product qualities related with different product throughputs and manufacturing cost are realizable. Now-a-days pelletization represents a proficient pathway for novel drug delivery in developing possibilities for different oral immediate or controlled delivery systems. Because of its simple design, high efficiency of producing spherical systems and fast processing, pelletization has found a special position in pharmaceutical industry and especially in case of production of multiparticulate oral controlled release dosage forms.

References

Chambliss, W. (1989). Conventional and specialized coating pans. In In Pharmaceutical Pelletization Technology, S. G, ed. (New York: Marcel Dekker), pp. 15-38.

Cimicata, L.E. (1951). How to manufacture and polish smallest pan goods-nonpareil seeds. *Confectioners J*, 41-43.

Crowley, M.M., Zhang, F., Repka, M.A., Thumma, S., Upadhye, S.B., Battu, S.K., McGinity, J.W., and Martin, C. (2007). Pharmaceutical applications of hot-melt extrusion: part I. *Drug Dev Ind Pharm* **33**, 909-926.

Dietrich, R., Brausse, R., Benedikt, G., and Steinijans, V.W. (1988). Feasibility of in-vitro/in-vivo correlation in the case of a new sustained-release theophylline pellet formulation. *Arzneimittel-Forschung* **38**, 1229-1237.

Eldem, T., Speiser, P., and Altorfer, H. (1991a). Polymorphic behavior of sprayed lipid micropellets and its evaluation by differential scanning calorimetry and scanning electron microscopy. *Pharmaceutical research* **8**, 178-184.

Eldem, T., Speiser, P., and Hincal, A. (1991b). Optimization of spray-dried and -congealed lipid micropellets and characterization of their surface morphology by scanning electron microscopy. *Pharmaceutical research* **8**, 47-54.

Fielden, K.E., Newton, J.M., and Rowe, R.C. (1989). The effect of lactose particle size on the extrusion properties of microcrystalline cellulose-lactose mixtures. *The Journal of pharmacy and pharmacology* **41**, 217-221.

Fielden, K.E., Newton, J.M., and Rowe, R.C. (1992a). A comparison of the extrusion and spheronization behaviour of wet powder masses processed by a ram extruder and a cylinder extruder. *International Journal of Pharmaceutics* **81**, 225-233.

Fielden, K.E., Newton, J.M., and Rowe, R.C. (1992b). The influence of lactose particle size on spheronization of extrudate processed by a ram extruder. *International Journal of Pharmaceutics* **81**, 205-224.

Ghai, D. (2011). Pelletization: An Alternate to Granulation. *Pharma Times* **43**, 13-15.

Ghebre-Sellassie, I., Gordon, R.H., Fawzi, M.B., and Nesbitt, R.U. (1985). Evaluation of A High-Speed Pelletization Process and Equipment. *Drug Development and Industrial Pharmacy* **11**, 1523-1541.

Goodhart F., J.S. (1989). Dry Powder Layering In Pharmaceutical Pelletization Technology, G.-S. I, ed. (New York: Marcel Dekker Inc), pp. 165 – 187.

Helen L., Y.J., Muttonen E (1993). Process Variables of the Radial Screen Extruder, II, Size and Size Distribution of Pellets. *Pharm Techn Int* **5**, 44–53.

Heng P., W.W., Shu J. and Wan L. (1999). A new method for the control of size of pellets in the melt pelletization process with a high shear mixer. *Chem Pharm Bull* **47**, 633-638.

Heng, P.W., Wan, L.S., and Wong, T.W. (1999). Effect of off-bottom clearance on properties of pellets produced by melt pelletization. *Pharmaceutical development and technology* **4**, 27-33.

Hicks D., F.H. (1989). Extrusion Spheronization Equipment. In Pharmaceutical Pelletization Technology, G.-S. .I, ed. (New York: Marcel Dekker, Inc), pp. 71-100.

Hincal A., K.H. (1994). Preparaton of micropellets by spray congealing. In Multiparticulate Oral Drug Delivery, Ghebre-Sellasie, ed. (New York: Marcel Dekker. Inc), pp. 17-34.

Hirjau M., N.A., Hirjau V., Lupuleasa D. (2011). Pelletization techniques used in pharmaceutical fields. *Practica Farmaceutica* **4**, 206-211.

Huyghebaert, N., Snoeck, V., Vermeire, A., Cox, E., Goddeeris, B.M., and Remon, J.P. (2005). Development of an enteric-coated pellet formulation of F4 fimbriae for oral vaccination of suckling piglets against enterotoxigenic Escherichia coli infections. European journal of pharmaceutics and biopharmaceutics: official journal of Arbeitsgemeinschaft fur Pharmazeutische Verfahrenstechnik eV 59, 273-281.

Jones, D. (1989). Solution and suspension layering. In Pharmaceutical Pelletization Technology, S. G, ed. (New York: Marcel Dekker Inc), pp. 158-159.

Kristensen H. G., S.T. (1993). Granulations. In Encyclopedia of Pharmaceutical Technology, B.J.C. Swabrick J., ed. (New York: Marcel Dekker Inc), pp. 121-160.

Mehta K, R.S., Parikh D. (2005). Extrusion/Spheronization as a Granulation Technique. In Handbook of Pharmaceutical Granulation Technology, P. D.M, ed. (Taylor & Francis Group), pp. 333- 360.

Melia C.D., W.N., Wilson C.G. (1994). Advantages and disadvantages of multiparticulate delivery systems. In Multiparticulate Oral Dosage Forms: Technology and Biopharmaceutics, W.N. Melia C.D., Wilson C.G., ed. (Edinburgh: Scottish Academic Press), pp. 135-140.

Nobuo Nakahara, N. (1964). Method and Apparatus for Making Spherical Granules. In US Patent Office (U.S.A).

O'connor, R.E., and Schwartz, J.B. (1985). Spheronization II: Drug Release from Drug-Diluent Mixtures. *Drug Development and Industrial Pharmacy* **11**, 1837-1857.

Palmieri, G.F., Grifantini, R., Di Martino, P., and Martelli, S. (2000). Emulsion/solvent evaporation as an alternative technique in pellet preparation. *Drug Dev Ind Pharm* **26**, 1151-1158.

Rahman, M.A., Ahuja, A., Baboota, S., Bhavna, Bali, V., Saigal, N., and Ali, J. (2009). Recent advances in pelletization technique for oral drug delivery: a review. *Current drug delivery* **6**, 122-129.

Rubinstein, M.H. (2000). Tablets. In Pharmaceutics: The Science of Dosage Form Design, A. M.E, ed. (New York Churchill Livingstone), p. 305.

Sellassie G., K.A. (2000). Pelletization Techniques. In Encyclopedia of Pharmaceutical Technology, S. J, ed. (Informa Healthcare), pp. 2651-2663.

Shettigar, R., and Damle, A. (1996). Controlled release pellets of nitrofurantoin. *Indian journal of pharmaceutical sciences* **58**, 179-183.

Singh, M.N., Hemant, K.S., Ram, M., and Shivakumar, H.G. (2010). Microencapsulation: A promising technique for controlled drug delivery. *Research in pharmaceutical sciences* **5**, 65-77.

Sövgren, K. (1992). Pellet Preparation. In Industrial Aspects of Pharmaceutics S. E, ed. (Stockholm: Swedish Pharmaceutical Press), pp. 200-212.

Srivastava S., M.G. (2010). Fluid Bed Technology: Overview and Parameters for Process Selection. *IJPSDR* **2**, 236-246.

Summers M., A.M. (2002). Granulation. In Pharmaceutics: The science of Dosage Form Design, A. M, ed. (Churchill-Livingstone), pp. 364-378.

Thommes, M., and Kleinebudde, P. (2006). Use of kappa-carrageenan as alternative pelletisation aid to microcrystalline cellulose in extrusion/ spheronisation. II. Influence of drug and filler type. European journal of pharmaceutics and biopharmaceutics : official journal of Arbeitsgemeinschaft fur Pharmazeutische Verfahrenstechnik eV 63, 68-75.

Villar-Lopez, M.E., Nieto-Reyes, L., Anguiano-Igea, S., Otero-Espinar, F.J., and Blanco-Mendez, J. (1999). Formulation of triamcinolone acetonide pellets suitable for coating and colon targeting. *Int J Pharm* **179**, 229-235.

Vojnovic D., R.P., Moneghini M., Rubessa F., Coslovich S., Phan-Tan-Luu R., Sergent M. (1993). Experimental research methodology applied to wet pelletization in a highshear mixer. Part 1. *STP Pharma Sci* **3**, 130-135.

Wan L.S.C. (1989). Manufacture of Core Pellet Formation and Growth. In Pharmaceutical Pelletization Technology, S. G, ed. (New York: Marcel Dekker, Inc.), pp. 123-143.

Wong T.W., C.W.S., Heng P.W (2005). Melt Granulation and Pelletization. In Handbook of Pharmaceutical Granulation Technology, P. D.M, ed. (Taylor & Francis Group), pp. 385-406.

10   Colloidal Drug Delivery Systems

Vinod K. Dhote[1], Kanika Dhote[1], Tripti Shukla[2], Sharad P. Pandey[1] and Piush Khare[3]

[1]Truba Institute of Pharmacy, Karond - Gandhi Nagar Bypass Road, Bhopal-462 038, India.

[2]School of Pharmacy, Peoples University, Bhanpur Bypass Road, Bhopal-462 037, India.

[3]Eiman Pharma Pvt Limited, 1/1 Palm Road, Shipra Sun City (Gaziabad), National Capital Region, 201 014, India.

10.1 Colloidal Nanocarriers: General Considerations

In the past many of the terms used to refer to therapeutic systems of controlled and sustained release have been used in an inconsistent and confusing manner. Although sustained release dosage form constitutes any dosage form that provides medication over specified period of time. Controlled release denotes that the system is able to provide some actual therapeutic control; this may be temporal or spatial nature or both. In other words, the system attempts to control drug concentrations in the target issue (Asiyanbola and Soboyejo, 2008).

In general, the goal of a sustained-release dosage form is to maintain therapeutic blood or tissue levels of the drug for an extended period and shows *zero order release* from the dosage form. Zero-order release constitutes drug release for the dosage from that is independent of the amount of drug in the delivery system. Sustained release systems generally do not attain this type of release by providing drug in a slow first-order fashion (Kingsley et al., 2006; Koo et al., 2005a).

Two basic types of controlled-delivery dosage forms have been designed in which diffusion is the rate-limiting step to generate temporal input profiles for drug delivery: matrix- and reservoir-type systems.

A *matrix type system* consists of a rate-controlling ingredient such as a polymer with drug uniformly dissolved or dispersed in it, and typically, a half order drug release corresponds to desorption from the preloaded matrix. A *reservoir-type system* separates a drug compartment from a polymer membrane that presents a diffusional barrier to yield drug flux of either zero order (with infinite dose) or first order (by dose depletion) (Muller et al., 2000). Broadly two methods are used to achieve site specific or targeted drug delivery. The first approach is synthesis of prodrug (new drug) by chemical modification in which the active moiety is released after metabolism *In vivo*. The second approach covers use of colloidal drug delivery systems (liposomes, niosomes, microemulsions, nanoparticles etc.) which provides targeting and controlled delivery for drugs.

During the last century, progress in medicine has been associated with the development of new drugs, which has led to improved therapeutics. However, in some instances such as cancer, the results are not proportionally linked to the amount of research that has been performed. This is often due to impaired pharmacokinetics or pharmacodynamics leading to elimination of the drug or severe side effects (Asiyanbola and Soboyejo, 2008; Kingsley et al., 2006; Koo et al., 2005b; Muller et al., 2000). To overcome this problem, several approaches have been tried aiming to protect the drug, to slow down its degradation, to optimize its targeting, to limit its accumulation in healthy organs, to reduce its potential toxicity, and/or to control its release either through natural processes or by external stimuli (Shrivastava, 2008).

Due to tremendous progress in field of drug discovery, organic synthesis and physical chemistry, it is now possible to design and elaborate colloidal systems made of lipids, polymers, or other similar materials. Their size, typically between 10 nm and 1 μm, renders their biodistribution completely different from that of small molecules (Shrivastava, 2008; zur Muhlen et al., 1998). Therefore, by encapsulating a drug within a colloidal system (that will act as nanovector or nanocarrier), the biodistribution of the drug will be determined by that of the nanocarrier leading to improvement in therapeutic effect (Fig. 10.1). Owing to the difficulties encountered in their administration, several generations of nanovectors have been developed (Kingsley et al., 2006). The early ones, called first generation, are constituted of simple colloids, such as simple liposomes or polymeric NPs which can be used to achieve passive delivery. According to another classification, this first generation can be divided into two classes: carriers without surface modification and another category includes 'stealth' carriers with surfaces modified exhibiting antifouling properties that enable longer blood circulation times (zur Muhlen et al., 1998). Actually the surfaces of such carriers are modified using some hydrophilic materials in order to avoid their recognition and clearance by the mononuclear phagocyte system. The second generation nanocarriers also allow active targeting using specific ligand–receptor interactions. Finally, the third generation group aims at passing all biological barriers before targeting (metabolic clearance, osmotic pressure gradients, hemodynamics, etc.) and at organizing time sequences of different functions on the vector. After 30 years of development of colloidal drug nanovectors (Asiyanbola and Soboyejo, 2008; Kingsley et al., 2006) a few systems are reaching the market and many are currently in preclinical or clinical trials, creating the new field of nanopharmaceutics that will complement nanomedicine. The number of scientific papers dealing with drug delivery by nanovectors and the number of reviews on this subject continues to grow, showing the importance of this new field.

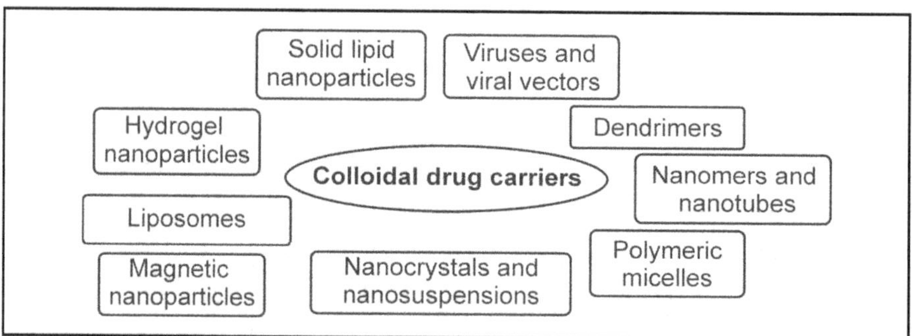

FIGURE 10.1 Classification of various colloidal drug carriers.

10.1.1 Colloidal Drug Delivery Systems

Colloidal drug delivery systems (CDDS) are particulate or vesicular dosage form in nanometer size range. They include liposomes, niosomes, nanoparticles, nanospheres, multiple emulsion and ceramics. CDDS are essentially required for effective transportation of loaded drug to the target site (Garcia-Garcia et al., 2005).

Colloidal drug carriers such as liposomes and nanoparticles are able to modify the distribution of an associated entity. They can therefore be used to improve the therapeutic index of drugs by increasing their efficacy and/or reducing their toxicity (Bromberg, 2008; Seow et al., 2007).

Colloidal drug carrier is one of the most important entities essentially required for successful transport of loaded drugs. They are drug vectors, which sequester, transport and retain the active drug en route, while they elute or deliver it within or in the vicinity of target area. Targeting the drug to the desired site of action would not only improve the therapeutic efficacy but also enable a reduction of the amount of drug, which must be administered to achieve a therapeutic response, thus minimizing unwanted toxic effects. The overall drug consumption and untoward effects can be lowered significantly by depositing the active agent in the morbid region only and in a concentration that does not exceed the desired limit. This highly selective approach reduces systemic side effects to a great degree (Cesur et al., 2009).

CDDS such as micellar solutions, vesicle and liquid crystal dispersions, as well as nanoparticle dispersions consisting of small particles of 10–400 nm diameter show great promise as drug delivery systems (Fig. 10.2). When developing these formulations, the goal is to obtain systems with optimized drug loading and release properties, long shelf-life and low toxicity. The incorporated drug participates in the microstructure of the system, and may even influence it due to molecular interactions, especially if the drug possesses amphiphilic and/or mesogenic properties.

A drug's therapeutic efficacy depends on four fundamental pathways of drug transport and modification within the body – absorption, distribution, metabolism, and elimination. Failure in therapy includes insufficient drug concentration due to poor absorption, rapid metabolism and elimination, poor drug solubility, and high fluctuation of plasma levels due to unpredictable bioavailability. A promising strategy to overcome these problems involves the development of a suitable drug colloidal carrier system (Khatri et al., 2008).

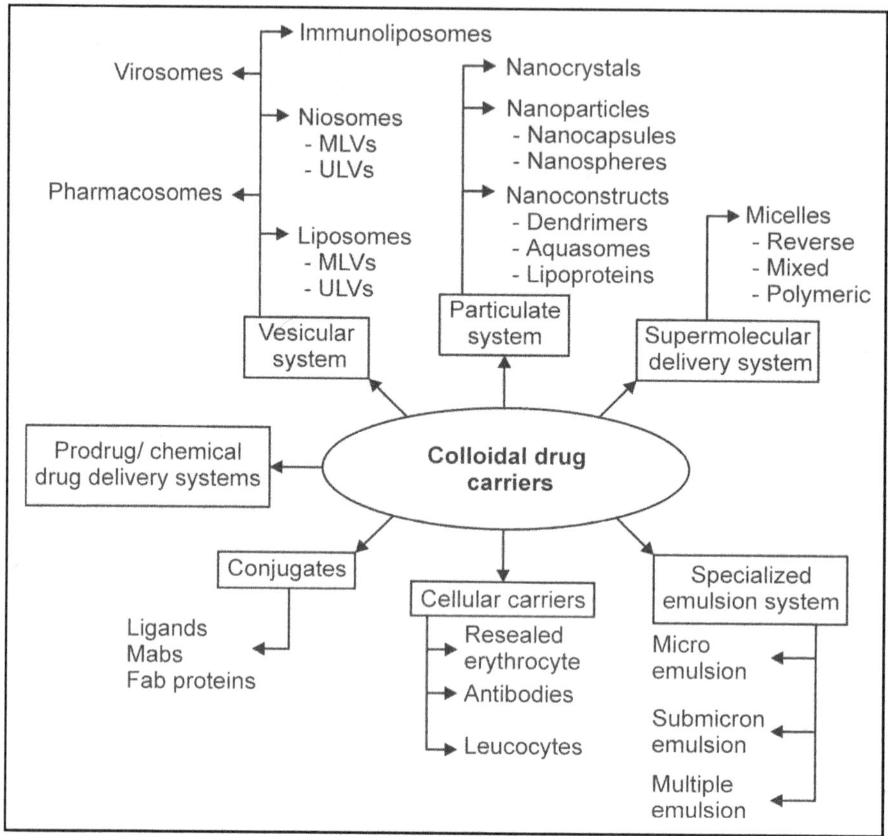

FIGURE 10.2 Classification of colloidal drug carriers.

10.1.2 Properties of an Ideal CDDS

An ideal colloidal drug carrier should be engineered to have the following features (Jung et al., 2008; Krauland and Bernkop-Schnurch, 2004; Sahoo and Labhasetwar, 2003):

- It must be able to cross anatomical barriers.

- It must be recognized specifically and selectively by the target cells and must maintain the avidity and specificity of the surface ligands.

- The linkage of the drug and the ligand should be stable in plasma, interstitial and other biofluids.

- Carrier should be non-toxic, non-immunogenic and biodegradable particulate or macromolecule and after internalization avoid recognition by the host's defence mechanisms.

- The carrier system should release the active moiety inside the target cells or organs tissues or else they may intersect to other sites, defeating the concept of targeting.

10.1.3 Applications of CDDS

- Nano-drug delivery systems that deliver large but highly localized quantities of drugs to specific areas to be released in controlled ways (Cesur et al., 2009)
- Controllable release profiles, especially for sensitive drugs
- CDDS are found applicability in development of materials for nanoparticles that are biocompatible and biodegradable (Khatri et al., 2008)
- CDDS offers virus-like systems for intracellular delivery
- Combined therapy and medical imaging, for example, nanoparticles for diagnosis and manipulation during surgery (e.g., thermotherapy with magnetic particles) (Carino et al., 2000)
- To improve devices such as implantable devices/nanochips for nanoparticle release, or multi reservoir drug delivery-chips
- Nanoparticles for tissue engineering e.g., for the delivery of cytokines to control cellular growth and differentiation, and stimulate regeneration; or for coating implants with nanoparticles in biodegradable polymer layers for sustained release
- For the delivery of therapeutic peptide/proteins (biopharmaceutics)
- Universal formulation schemes that serve as platform technology and can be used for preparation of formulations for IV, IM or peroral delivery (Cesur et al., 2009)
- Cell and gene targeting systems
- Devices for detecting changes in magnetic or physical properties after specific binding of ligands on paramagnetic nanoparticles that can correlate with the amount of ligand (Khatri et al., 2008)
- Better disease markers in terms of sensitivity and specificity

(Damge et al. 2007) reported oral delivery of insulin associated to polymeric nanoparticles (PNPs) in diabetic rats by multiple emulsions as colloidal nanocarriers which shows sustained release over 12 hr with 96% drug entrapment. A variety of therapeutic agents like anticancer drugs, protein and peptides, vaccine, and so forth, can be effectively delivered and targeted through. Insulin, a treatment of choice for type 1 and many type 2 diabetes, undergoes extensive enzymatic degradation when administered orally (Damge et al., 2007). Polymeric biodegradable and biocompatible nanoparticles of insulin have been developed to protect its degradation and facilitate the uptake across intestinal epithelium through paracellular or transcellular routes. U.S. patents on oral insulin delivery using the nanocarrier approach have been well proved in animal models and are being tested for human beings (Krauland and Bernkop-Schnurch, 2004).

Bioavailability of the other protein and peptide drugs can be improved using suitable mucoadhesive polymers, for example, those containing thiol groups attached to their backbone (thiomers). The mucoadhesive properties of five different poly(acrylic acid)-cysteine conjugates were compared; among which PAA450-Cys conjugate was proved to be the best (Leitner et al., 2003). Colloidal nanocarriers have a bright future in the delivery of therapeutics and diagnostic agents. Various novel ideas like oral delivery of proteins and peptides, targeted cancer therapy, *In vivo* tumor imaging, and so forth, can be crystallized into reality by a prudent use of this technology. It would result in a concomitant improvement in the quality, efficacy, and safety profile of drugs.

Pandey and co-workers reported successful oral delivery of therapeutics through solid lipid nanoparticle-based antitubercular chemotherapy displaying sustained release and maintenance of therapeutic plasma level for 8 days (Pandey et al., 2005). Zhang and his team reported Lectin-modified solid lipid nanoparticles as carriers for oral administration of insulin. The results showed 60% drug entrapment in colloidal nanocarriers (Zhang et al., 2006). Bromberg reported application of polymeric micelles in oral chemotherapy. Pluronic-PAA micelles were prepared by co-polymerization technique for successful treatment of solid tumor and the results showed increased solubility of hydrophobic drugs (Bromberg, 2008).

10.2 Colloidal Drug Carriers

10.2.1 Liposomes

An attractive option for the design of delivery systems is to mimic structures already present *In vivo*. Thus, a great deal of research has focused on the design of liposome-based systems (Bawarski et al., 2008). The structure of a liposome consists of a vesicle assembled from a lipid bilayer, with an aqueous interior and a hydrophobic membrane. Lipids are readily degradable *In vivo*, allowing the components of the delivery system to be removed easily from the body. In addition, the presence of a hydrophobic and hydrophilic domain within the structure allows flexibility in loading a variety of therapeutic cargos (Colas et al., 2007). Liposomes are commonly prepared using a number of approaches, including thin-film hydration, solvent injection or reverse-phase evaporation techniques. To engineer the vesicles to smaller or more uniform sizes both sonication and extrusion can be used. Liposomes have been one of the most successful delivery systems so far, with a number of therapies clinically available for treatment of cancer, including doxorubicin (Doxil®) and daunorubicin (DaunoXome®) (Bharali and Mousa, 2010).

Furthermore, the loading of liposomes is typically non-covalent and therefore cargo leakage can be an issue, especially in the case of hydrophobic drugs when the liposome is in contact with plasma proteins or cell membranes. Table 10.1 represents various types of liposomes used for drug delivery.

TABLE 10.1

Various types of liposomes used in drug delivery

Vesicle types	Abbreviation	Size	Number of lipid bilayers	Reference
Small unilamellar vesicles	SUV	20-100 nm	1	(Al-Jamal and Kostarelos, 2011)
Large unilamellar vesicles	LUV	> 100 nm	1	(Ariga et al., 2011)
Multilamellar vesicles	MLV	> 0.5 µm	5-20	(Mehnert and Mader, 2001)
Oligolamellar vesicles	OLV	0.1-1 µm	~5	(Matsumura and Kataoka, 2009)
Multivesicular vesicles	MVV	> 1 µm	Multicompartmental structure	(Kim and Dobson, 2009)

10.2.1.1 Advantages of Liposomes

- Controlled drug delivery systems.
- Liposomes can carry both hydrophilic and lipophilic drugs.
- Solubilize insoluble compounds.
- Selective passive targeting to tumor.
- Increase efficacy and therapeutic index.

- Reduce the toxicity of encapsulated drug.
- Improve pharmacokinetics (reduce elimination and increase circulation life time)
- Increase stability via encapsulation (protection against metabolic degradation).

Issues to consider when selecting lipids (Bertrand and Leroux, 2012) :

- *Phase transition temperature:* The temperature required to induce physical change in the lipid from the ordered gel state to disordered liquid crystalline state is known as phase transition temperature. The Phase transition temperature of a lipid depends on acyl chain length, degree of saturation and polar head group.
- *Stability:* Unsaturated lipids from biological source are less stable than saturated synthetic ones.
- *Charge:* It affects physical stability of formulation.
- *Cholesterol:* It can modulate membrane fluidity, elasticity, and permeability. It fills gaps created by imperfect packing of other lipid species and increases membrane rigidity. Fig. 10.3. Represents mechanism of vesicle formation and various steps involved.

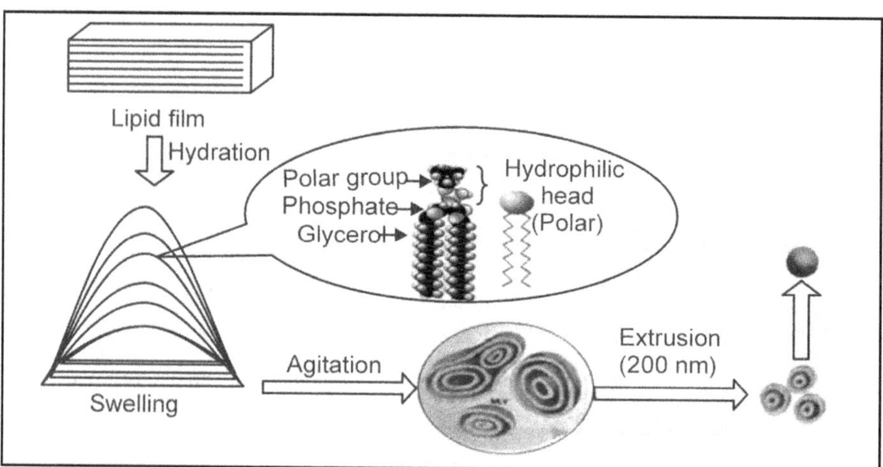

FIGURE 10.3 Lipid film preparation, hydration with agitation, sizing to produce homogenous distribution.

10.2.1.2 Pharmaceutical Applications of Liposomes

- *In vitro* enhancement of the antibacterial activity.
- *In vivo* enhancement of biological activity.

- Oral administration (Enhancing of buccal delivery of insulin) (Kim and Dobson, 2009)

- Topical and transdermal application (corticosteroids)

- Ophthalmic drug delivery system sustained release (Croy and Kwon, 2006)

- Prolonged retention of drugs

- Pulmonary administration (immunoglobulin's) (Garcia-Garcia et al., 2005)

10.2.2 Polymer Micelles and Polymersomes

In the last decade there has been significant research in the field of self-assembled polymer architectures (Maya et al., 2013). Polymers can self-assemble into a variety of different structures, with two of the most common structures being micelles and polymersomes. Polymer micelles are generally nanometre-sized spheres, 20–100 nm in size, with a hydrophobic core and a hydrophilic exterior, and are significantly more stable than their surfactant-based counterparts (Moretton et al., 2013). These structures spontaneously form above the critical micelle concentration of the polymers. Other shapes such as worm-like micelles can also be engineered and these structures have shown high promise for prolonging circulation times in the systemic circulation (Jung et al., 2008; Neekhra and Padh, 2004; Sahoo and Labhasetwar, 2003). In contrast to micelles, polymersomes have a hollow vesicle structure, similar to liposomes, with a hydrophobic membrane, hydrophilic surface and an aqueous interior (Krauland and Bernkop-Schnurch, 2004). As with liposomes, thin-film hydration, solvent injection or reverse-phase evaporation techniques are employed to form the polymersome structure. Sonication, extrusion and size exclusion chromatography can be used to lower the polydispersity of the dispersions. While there are a range of polymer structures that can be used to assemble micelles and polymersomes, they are typically formed from amphiphilic block copolymers. Many factors influence the architecture of the nanostructure formed, including the copolymer structure and composition, the copolymer concentration in solution, and the solvent properties. Both micelles and polymersomes have been successfully loaded with a range of therapeutics and active components (Sakhrani and Padh, 2013). Micelles are somewhat more limited for loading, as they only contain a hydrophobic interior, thus making them suited for loading hydrophobic cargo. In contrast, polymersomes have a similar structure to liposomes, lending them capable of accommodating both hydrophobic and hydrophilic drugs (Shrivastava et al., 2013). They also have a number of advantages over their lipid counterparts. For example, they are more stable and robust to a range of conditions. Also, as the copolymers that form the structure are synthetic, they can be readily modified to tune their fluidity and permeability.

10.2.3 Polymer Particles

While a significant amount of research has been focused on designing highly ordered self-assembled structures, bulk processes for particle synthesis are also of interest, as they offer the advantage of easier scale up for commercial application (Wirth et al., 1998). Polymer nanoparticles are commonly designed from polymers that can be readily degraded *In vivo*. These include poly(lactic acid), poly(glycolic acid) or poly(lacticco-glycolic acid), which degrade to form natural by-products of cellular metabolism (Zhang et al., 2013). Polymer nanoparticles can be synthesised through the polymerisation of monomers (emulsion or dispersion polymerisation) or by dispersion of polymers (nanoprecipitation or solvent evaporation) (Zhu et al., 2011). Loading these particles is generally achieved by incorporating the cargo during the synthesis process.

The size of spontaneously self-assembled systems is to a large extent governed by the intrinsic properties of the assembling molecules. Thus, there are limitations to controlling the size of the particles formed. Sonication and extrusion can be used to narrow the polydispersity of liposomes, micelles and polymersomes systems, and size exclusion chromatography can be used to fractionate the preparations.

10.2.4 Solid Lipid Nanoparticles

Among the colloidal carrier systems solid lipid nanoparticles (SLNs) have many advantages and limited disadvantages as compared to other colloidal carrier systems. SLNs have gained attention as carriers for the preparation of a wide variety of poorly water soluble drugs due to their biodegradable and biocompatible properties and low toxicity. They are typically spherical with an average diameter between 1 and 1000 nm (Khare et al., 2009a; Khare et al., 2009b; Zhu et al., 2011). It is an alternative carrier system to traditional colloidal carriers, such as, emulsions, liposomes, and polymeric micro and nanoparticles. The SLNs possess a lipid core matrix in the nanometer range stabilized by a layer of surfactants. They have been used as ideally suited drug delivery systems for the proteins, vaccines and other drugs for controlled release compared to other colloidal drug delivery systems. Their ability to penetrate through several anatomical barriers, sustained release of their contents, and their nanometre size range makes the implementation of SLN as successful drug delivery systems (Jing et al., 2013). SLNs combine the advantages of both polymeric nanoparticles and liposomes such as possibility of controlled drug release and drug targeting, increased drug stability and incorporation of lipophilic and hydrophilic drugs.

10.2.5 Microemulsion

The microemulsion concept was introduced as early as 1940s by *Hoar and Schulman* who generated a clear single-phase solution by titrating a milky emulsion with hexanol (Gabizon, 1992). However, the microemulsion definition provided by Danielson and Lindman in 1981 will be used as the point of reference. Microemulsion is thus defined as 'a system of water, oil and amphiphile which is single optically isotropic and thermodynamically stable liquid solution' Or microemulsions can be defined as: Transparent thermodynamically stable dispersion of water and oil stabilized by surfactant and co-surfactant having particle size smaller than 0.1 um (Gupta et al., 2014).

Advantages of the use of microemulsion as drug carrier systems including following: Thermodynamic stability allows self-emulsification.

1. Technology is very simple, no significant energy required.
2. Super solvents of drugs due to SAA and cosurfactant.
3. W/O or O/W types microemulsions can serve as potential reservoirs to drugs.
4. Droplet size is below 100 nm allowing higher interfacial area from which the drug is quickly absorbed *In vivo* or *In vitro*.
5. Sterilized by filtration as mean diameter below 0.22 um.
6. Auto-oxidation of lipids in O/W is slower than in case of emulsions or micellar solution.
7. Both hydrophilic and lipophilic drugs can be carried in the same microemulsion.
8. They are of low viscosity.
9. They can improve the efficacy of drugs; allow the total dose to be reduced.

10. May become unstable at high or low temperature however this is reversible as they return back to stable forms at room temperature.

10.3 *In-vivo* Fate of Colloidal Drug Carriers

The *In vivo* fate of the CDDS will depend mainly on the administration route and distribution process (adsorption of biological material on the particle surface and desorption of carrier components into the biological surrounding). The administration of colloidal particles to the blood stream has been considered for many years for a variety of reasons. The development of artificial blood has been a long-term research interest and has not been diminished by the risks associated with HIV infection in donor blood. In the field of drug targeting, many different types of delivery systems have been considered ranging from numerous synthetic carriers like emulsions, lipoprotein, erythrocytes and viruses. These approaches have had varying degrees of success in laboratory experiments (Bromberg, 2008). Therefore, pathways for transportation and metabolism are present in the body which may contribute to a large extent to the *In vivo* fate of the carrier.

Various colloidal systems either drug loaded vesicular systems (liposomes, niosomes etc.) or particulate systems such as micropatrticles, nanoparticles, nanocapsule etc., have the ability to taken up by the macrophages of RES system and this ability makes them special for passive targeting to RES organs specially liver and spleen (Chourasia and Jain, 2004). Biological particles are usually negatively charged, while the administered particles can be positively or negatively charged, and the charge can be changed as a consequence of change in the fluid. Charged particles are surrounded by associated charged species of the opposite charge, creating an electrical double layer. When a charged carrier and a bio-molecule are in close proximity, their associated charged layers will overlap. If the two materials have the same charge this will cause repulsion but if they have opposite charges, this will result in attraction (Gupta and Vyas, 2007).

The DLVO theory describes the net interaction between two particles of the same charge as they approach each other. In plasma, the ionic strength is such that a secondary minimum is probable, and thus the materials of the same charge will exhibit net attraction in this region. At short distances of separation different forces dominate, and in this region it is the surface nature which becomes important. It might reasonably be asserted that, as bio-molecules are generally negatively charged, administered carriers might best be designed to be also negatively charged (or at least not positively charged) (Maulding et al., 1986; Zhou and Po, 1991). In most cases, however, this is not adequate to prevent opsonisation.

Fate of colloidal drug carriers in biological environment after oral delivery is a contentious issue, as a wide spectrum of reports exists in this regard. Some researchers have claimed contribution of specialized transports for colloidal drug carriers whereas; others advocate solubilisation followed by absorption of hydrophobic drugs. The oral route presents formidable challenge to carrier integrity due to presence of acidic environment of stomach, digestive enzymes and secretions like bile salts etc. The majority of liposomal formulations are destroyed under these circumstances; however nanoparticles seem to be more stable (Gupta and Vyas, 2007). Some studies show that intact nanoparticles can be absorbed from the gut, possibly by transcytosis across M cells of Peyer's patches, but the extent of uptake is not clear.

Following oral administration, colloidal drug carriers can be inured to protect a labile drug from degradation or to protect the gut from the redundant effects of the drug, e.g., non steroidal anti-inflammatory agents (Maulding et al., 1986). Peptides and proteins remain poorly bioavailable upon oral administration. Association of these agents with colloidal carriers offer protection in terms of stability in gastrointestinal tract and competence to modulate physicochemical properties, release behaviour and biological activity.

10.4 Advantage and Successes

Colloidal drug carriers offer a number of potential advantages as delivery systems for, for example, poorly soluble compounds. The first generation of colloidal carriers, in particular liposomes and submicron-sized lipid emulsions are, however, associated with several drawbacks which so far have prevented the extensive use of these carriers in drug delivery. As an alternative colloidal delivery system melt-emulsified nanoparticles based on solid lipids have been proposed. Careful physicochemical characterization has demonstrated that these lipid-based nanosuspensions (solid lipid nanoparticles) are not just emulsions with solidified droplets (Gupta et al., 2014; Gupta and Vyas, 2007).

Colloidal drug carriers such as liposomes and nanoparticles can be used to improve the therapeutic index of both established and new drugs by modifying their distribution, and thus increasing their efficacy and/or reducing their toxicity. This is because the drug distribution then follows that of the carrier, rather than depending on the physicochemical properties of the drug itself. If these delivery systems are carefully designed with respect to the target and the route of administration, they may provide one solution to some of the delivery problems posed by new classes of active molecules, such as peptides and proteins, genes and oligonucleotides. They may also offer alternative modes for more conventional drugs, such as highly hydrophobic small molecules (Mathiowitz et al., 1990).

Nanoparticle-based drug delivery systems have considerable potential for treatment of tuberculosis (TB). Colloids from an aqueous suspension can cross the skin barrier only through hydrophilic pathways. Various colloids have a different ability to do this by penetrating narrow pores of fixed size in the skin, or the relevant nano-pores in barriers modelling the skin (Maulding et al., 1986).

Engineering drug itself in nanoparticulate form has emerged as a new strategy for the delivery of hydrophobic drugs due to their unique advantages over colloidal drug carriers. Nanoparticles and nano formulations have already been applied as drug delivery systems with great success; and nanoparticulate drug delivery systems have still greater potential for many applications, including anti-tumour therapy, gene therapy, and AIDS therapy, radiotherapy, in the delivery of proteins, antibiotics, virostatics, vaccines and as vesicles to pass the blood - brain barrier (Gupta et al., 2014; Gupta and Vyas, 2007; Mathiowitz et al., 1990; Maulding et al., 1986).

Polymeric micelles have recently emerged as a novel promising colloidal carrier for the targeting of poorly water soluble and amphiphilic drugs. Polymeric micelles are considerably more stable than surfactant micelles and can solubilize substantial amounts of hydrophobic compounds in their inner core. Due to their hydrophilic shell and small size they sometimes exhibit prolonged circulation times *In vivo* and can accumulate in tumoral tissues (Zhou and Po, 1991).

Nanoparticles provide advantages regarding drug targeting, delivery and release and, with their additional potential to combine diagnosis and therapy, emerge as one of the major tools in nanomedicine. The main goals are to improve their stability in the biological environment, to mediate the bio-distribution of active compounds, improve drug loading, targeting, transport, release, and interaction with biological barriers (Gupta and Vyas, 2007; Mathiowitz et al., 1990). The cytotoxicity of nanoparticles or their degradation products remains a major problem, and improvements in biocompatibility obviously are a main concern of future research (Willard et al., 1988). Carrier systems like SLN and NLC were developed with a perspective to meet industrial needs like scale up, qualification and validation, simple technology, low cost etc. The ability to incorporate drugs into nanocarriers offers a new prototype in drug delivery that could be used for secondary and tertiary levels of drug targeting (Sahoo and Labhasetwar, 2003). Table 10.2 illustrates comparison between various drug carrier systems.

TABLE 10.2

Comparison of available novel drug carrier systems

S. No.	Properties	SLN	Polymeric nanoparticles	Liposomes	Lipid emulsion
1.	Definition	Submicron colloidal carriers (50-1000 nm) which are composed of phospholipids.	Sub nano-sized colloidal structure composed of synth. /semi synthetic polymers.	Outer bilayer of Amphipatic molecules (phospholipids) with an aqueous component inside.	Neutral lipophilic oil core surrounded by mono- layer of amphilic lipid (phospholipids).
2.	Systemic Toxicity	Low	> or = SLN	Low	Low
3.	Cytotoxicity	Low	> or = SLN	Low	Low
4.	Residue from organic solvent	No	Yes	May/may not	No
5.	Large scale Production	Yes	No	Yes	Yes
6.	Sterilization by autoclave	Yes	No	No	Yes
7.	Sustained release	Yes	Yes	< or = SLN	No
8.	Avoidance of Reticuendothelial system	Yes	No	Yes	Yes

10.5 Conclusion

In the case of orally administered therapeutics, low bioavailability and low half-life presents major challenge in the therapy, especially with drugs having high dose and dosing frequency. These issues could be greatly minimized by designing the appropriate colloidal delivery systems. At the similar time the therapeutic index of the drug could also be improved by enhancing the safety and efficacy of the drug. The colloidal systems can be engineered in a way that can increase the absorption with consequent increase in bioavailability of the drug. Predicted release pattern of the delivery system and higher surface area because of their size can be used to modulate the dissolution pattern, solubility properties and other related properties to result in an efficient oral delivery. Enormous research is being carried out on colloidal drug delivery systems with special reference to delivery of proteins/peptides, vaccines and therapeutics via oral route. Emphasis is also being laid out on the design and development of the targeted oral colloidal delivery systems which could serve delivery of an active agents to site of action, increase uptake through receptor mediated transport and transport to the cells through endocytosis. By careful selection of excipients and sound design, the colloidal carriers can be used as a better tool for delivery of peptides, proteins, genes and oligonucleotides.

References

Al-Jamal, W.T., and Kostarelos, K. (2011). Liposomes: from a clinically established drug delivery system to a nanoparticle platform for the ranostic nanomedicine. *Accounts of chemical research* **44,** 1094-1104.

Ariga, K., McShane, M., Lvov, Y.M., Ji, Q., and Hill, J.P. (2011). Layer-by-layer assembly for drug delivery and related applications. *Expert opinion on drug delivery* **8,** 633-644.

Asiyanbola, B., and Soboyejo, W. (2008). For the surgeon: an introduction to nanotechnology. *Journal of surgical education* **65,** 155-161.

Bawarski, W.E., Chidlowsky, E., Bharali, D.J., and Mousa, S.A. (2008). Emerging nanopharmaceuticals. *Nanomedicine: nanotechnology, biology, and medicine* **4,** 273-282.

Bertrand, N., and Leroux, J.C. (2012). The journey of a drug-carrier in the body: an anatomo-physiological perspective. *Journal of controlled release: official journal of the Controlled Release Society* **161,** 152-163.

Bharali, D.J., and Mousa, S.A. (2010). Emerging nanomedicines for early cancer detection and improved treatment: current perspective and future promise. *Pharmacology & therapeutics* **128,** 324-335.

Bromberg, L. (2008). Polymeric micelles in oral chemotherapy. *Journal of controlled release: official journal of the Controlled Release Society* **128,** 99-112.

Carino, G.P., Jacob, J.S., and Mathiowitz, E. (2000). Nanosphere based oral insulin delivery. *Journal of controlled release: official journal of the Controlled Release Society* **65,** 261-269.

Cesur, H., Rubinstein, I., Pai, A., and Onyuksel, H. (2009). Self-associated indisulam in phospholipid-based nanomicelles: a potential nanomedicine for cancer. *Nanomedicine : nanotechnology, biology, and medicine* **5,** 178-183.

Chourasia, M.K., and Jain, S.K. (2004). Design and development of multiparticulate system for targeted drug delivery to colon. *Drug Deliv* **11,** 201-207.

Colas, J.C., Shi, W., Rao, V.S., Omri, A., Mozafari, M.R., and Singh, H. (2007). Microscopical investigations of nisin-loaded nanoliposomes prepared by Mozafari method and their bacterial targeting. *Micron* (Oxford, England: 1993) **38,** 841-847.

Croy, S.R., and Kwon, G.S. (2006). Polymeric micelles for drug delivery. *Current pharmaceutical design* **12,** 4669-4684.

Damge, C., Maincent, P., and Ubrich, N. (2007). Oral delivery of insulin associated to polymeric nanoparticles in diabetic rats. *Journal of controlled release : official journal of the Controlled Release Society* **117,** 163-170.

Gabizon, A.A. (1992). Selective tumor localization and improved therapeutic index of anthracyclines encapsulated in long-circulating liposomes. *Cancer research* **52,** 891-896.

Garcia-Garcia, E., Andrieux, K., Gil, S., and Couvreur, P. (2005). Colloidal carriers and blood-brain barrier (BBB) translocation: a way to deliver drugs to the brain? *International journal of pharmaceutics* **298,** 274-292.

Gupta, R., Mehra, N.K., and Jain, N.K. (2014). Fucosylated multiwalled carbon nanotubes for Kupffer cells targeting for the treatment of cytokine-induced liver damage. *Pharm Res* **31,** 322-334.

Gupta, S., and Vyas, S.P. (2007). Development and characterization of amphotericin B bearing emulsomes for passive and active macrophage targeting. *J Drug Target* **15,** 206-217.

Jing, F., Li, J., Liu, D., Wang, C., and Sui, Z. (2013). Dual ligands modified double targeted nano-system for liver targeted gene delivery. *Pharmaceutical biology* **51,** 643-649.

Jung, J., Matsuzaki, T., Tatematsu, K., Okajima, T., Tanizawa, K., and Kuroda, S. (2008). Bio-nanocapsule conjugated with liposomes for *In vivo* pinpoint delivery of various materials. *Journal of controlled release : official journal of the Controlled Release Society* **126,** 255-264.

Khare, P., Jain, A., Gulbake, A., Soni, V., Jain, N.K., and Jain, S.K. (2009a). Bioconjugates: harnessing potential for effective therapeutics. *Critical reviews in therapeutic drug carrier systems* **26,** 119-155.

Khare, P., Jain, A., Jain, N.K., Soni, V., and Jain, S.K. (2009b). Glutamate-conjugated liposomes of dopamine hydrochloride for effective management of parkinsonism's. *PDA journal of pharmaceutical science and technology / PDA* **63,** 372-379.

Khatri, K., Goyal, A.K., Gupta, P.N., Mishra, N., Mehta, A., and Vyas, S.P. (2008). Surface modified liposomes for nasal delivery of DNA vaccine. *Vaccine* **26,** 2225-2233.

Kim, D.K., and Dobson, J. (2009). Nanomedicine for targeted drug delivery. *Journal of Materials Chemistry* **19,** 6294-6307.

Kingsley, J.D., Dou, H., Morehead, J., Rabinow, B., Gendelman, H.E., and Destache, C.J. (2006). Nanotechnology: a focus on nanoparticles as a drug delivery system. *Journal of neuroimmune pharmacology: the official journal of the Society on NeuroImmune Pharmacology* **1,** 340-350.

Koo, O.M., Rubinstein, I., and Onyuksel, H. (2005a). Camptothecin in sterically stabilized phospholipid micelles: a novel nanomedicine. *Nanomedicine : nanotechnology, biology, and medicine* **1,** 77-84.

Koo, O.M., Rubinstein, I., and Onyuksel, H. (2005b). Role of nanotechnology in targeted drug delivery and imaging: a concise review. Nanomedicine: nanotechnology, biology, and medicine 1, 193-212.

Krauland, A.H., and Bernkop-Schnurch, A. (2004). Thiomers: development and *In vitro* evaluation of a peroral microparticulate peptide delivery system. European journal of pharmaceutics and biopharmaceutics: official journal of *Arbeitsgemeinschaft fur Pharmazeutische Verfahrenstechnik eV* **57,** 181-187.

Leitner, V.M., Marschutz, M.K., and Bernkop-Schnurch, A. (2003). Mucoadhesive and cohesive properties of poly(acrylic acid)-cysteine conjugates with regard to their molecular mass. European journal of pharmaceutical sciences: official journal of the European Federation for *Pharmaceutical Sciences* **18,** 89-96.

Mathiowitz, E., Kline, D., and Langer, R. (1990). Morphology of polyanhydride microsphere delivery systems. *Scanning microscopy* **4,** 329-340.

Matsumura, Y., and Kataoka, K. (2009). Preclinical and clinical studies of anticancer agent-incorporating polymer micelles. *Cancer science* **100,** 572-579.

Maulding, H.V., Tice, T.R., Cowsar, D.R., Fong, J.W., Pearson, J.E., and Nazareno, J.P. (1986). Biodegradable microcapsules: Acceleration of polymeric excipient hydrolytic rate by incorporation of a basic medicament. *Journal of Controlled Release* **3,** 103-117.

Maya, S., Kumar, L.G., Sarmento, B., Sanoj Rejinold, N., Menon, D., Nair, S.V., and Jayakumar, R. (2013). Cetuximab conjugated O-carboxymethyl chitosan nanoparticles for targeting EGFR overexpressing cancer cells. *Carbohydrate polymers* **93,** 661-669.

Mehnert, W., and Mader, K. (2001). Solid lipid nanoparticles: production, characterization and applications. *Adv Drug Deliv Rev* **47**, 165-196.

Moretton, M.A., Chiappetta, D.A., Andrade, F., das Neves, J., Ferreira, D., Sarmento, B., and Sosnik, A. (2013). Hydrolyzed galactomannan-modified nanoparticles and flower-like polymeric micelles for the active targeting of rifampicin to macrophages. *Journal of biomedical nanotechnology* **9**, 1076-1087.

Muller, R.H., Mader, K., and Gohla, S. (2000). Solid lipid nanoparticles (SLN) for controlled drug delivery - a review of the state of the art. *European journal of pharmaceutics and biopharmaceutics:* official journal of Arbeitsgemeinschaft fur Pharmazeutische Verfahrenstechnik eV **50**, 161-177.

Neekhra, N., and Padh, H. (2004). An insight into molecular mechanism of endocytosis. Indian journal of biochemistry & biophysics 41, 69-80.

Pandey, R., Sharma, S., and Khuller, G.K. (2005). Oral solid lipid nanoparticle-based antitubercular chemotherapy. *Tuberculosis (Edinburgh, Scotland)* **85**, 415-420.

Sahoo, S.K., and Labhasetwar, V. (2003). Nanotech approaches to drug delivery and imaging. *Drug discovery today* **8**, 1112-1120.

Sakhrani, N.M., and Padh, H. (2013). Organelle targeting: third level of drug targeting. *Drug design, development and therapy* **7**, 585-599.

Seow, W.Y., Xue, J.M., and Yang, Y.Y. (2007). Targeted and intracellular delivery of paclitaxel using multi-functional polymeric micelles. *Biomaterials* **28**, 1730-1740.

Shrivastava, P.K., Shrivastava, A., Sinha, S.K., and Shrivastava, S.K. (2013). Dextran Carrier Macromolecules for Colon-specific Delivery of 5-Aminosalicylic Acid. *Indian J Pharm Sci* **75**, 277-283.

Shrivastava, S. (2008). Nanofabrication for drug delivery and tissue engineering. *DJNB* **3**, 257-263.

Willard, H.H., Merritt, L.L., Dean, J.A., and Settle, P.A. (1988). Instrumental Methods of Analysis, 7 edn (Belmont, CA: Wadsworth).

Wirth, M., Fuchs, A., Wolf, M., Ertl, B., and Gabor, F. (1998). Lectin-mediated drug targeting: preparation, binding characteristics, and antiproliferative activity of wheat germ agglutinin conjugated doxorubicin on Caco-2 cells. *Pharm Res* **15**, 1031-1037.

Zhang, N., Ping, Q., Huang, G., Xu, W., Cheng, Y., and Han, X. (2006). Lectin-modified solid lipid nanoparticles as carriers for oral administration of insulin. *International journal of pharmaceutics* **327**, 153-159.

Zhang, X., Liu, L., Chai, G., Zhang, X., and Li, F. (2013). Brain pharmacokinetics of neurotoxin-loaded PLA nanoparticles modified with chitosan after intranasal administration in awake rats. *Drug development and industrial pharmacy* **39**, 1618-1624.

Zhou, X.H., and Po, A.L.W. (1991). Peptide and protein drugs: II. Non-parenteral routes of delivery. *International journal of pharmaceutics* **75**, 117-130.

Zhu, L., Chen, L., Cao, Q.R., Chen, D., and Cui, J. (2011). Preparation and evaluation of mannose receptor mediated macrophage targeting delivery system. *Journal of controlled release:* official journal of the Controlled Release Society **152** Suppl 1, e190-191.

zur Muhlen, A., Schwarz, C., and Mehnert, W. (1998). Solid lipid nanoparticles (SLN) for controlled drug delivery-drug release and release mechanism. *European journal of pharmaceutics and biopharmaceutics:* official journal of Arbeitsgemeinschaft fur Pharmazeutische Verfahrenstechnik eV **45**, 149-155.

11 *In-situ* Gel and Liquid Crystals as Potential Drug Delivery Systems

Ashish Parashar[1], Ankit Jain[2], Kamlendra Bhadoriya[3], Piush Khare[4] and Punit Bhatnagar[5]

[1]School of Pharmacy & Technology Management, NMIMS, SHIRPUR Campus, Dhule-425 405 Maharashtra, India.

[2]Sri Aurobindo Institute of Pharmacy SAIMS Campus, Indore-Ujjain Highway, Indore-453 111, India.

[3]School of Pharmacy, ITM University, AH-43, Bypass, Jhansi Road, Gwalior-475 001, India.

[4]Eiman Pharma Pvt Limited, 1/1 Palm Road, Shipra Sun City (Gaziabad), National Capital Region, 201 014, India.

[5]Rishiraj College of Pharmacy, Behind SAIMS Campus, Indore-Ujjain Highway, Indore-453 331, India.

11.1 Introduction

Drug discovery and development process is tedious and cumbersome job, hence pharmaceutical companies face a constant pressure for improvising the drug delivery system which is able to meet the two basic requirements i.e., desired drug release and improved bioavailability. Hence, researchers and academicians are looking for novel innovations which are able to improve patient compliance and provide maximum therapeutic benefits over a prolong period of time. The idealized conception can be fulfilled by sustained release drug delivery systems (SRDDS) and controlled release drug delivery systems (CRDDS). SRDDS are those which are able to maintain the rate of drug release over a prolonged period of time; while CRDDS are those which are somewhat similar to SRDDS but there is a predictability of plasma drug concentration.

But these days, we have ameliorated the SRDDS and CRDDS by conjugating it with targeted release drug delivery systems (TRDDS). This TRDDS are able to release the drug at controlled rate but appreciably in the vicinity of target organ. This system distributes the drug in body in a selective manner that it will interact only with target cells and tissue, thus minimize the systemic toxicity issues.

In the current scenario of drug delivery, *in-situ* gelling systems (ISGS) have emerged as potential candidates imparting drug delivery with desirable features. This *in-situ* gelling system remains liquid at room temperature but transform to gel when it is exposed to body fluid or change in temperature or change in pH etc. In analogy to conventional CRDDS, *in-situ* gels outfitted with admirable merits like ease of manufacturing and administration, reduction in dose frequency, improved patient compliance, reproducible drug-plasma profile, greater stability, and biocompatibility. Polymers which act as backbone of ISGS may be of natural, semi-synthetic and synthetic origin like Alginic acid, gellan gum, carboxymethyl chitin, pectin, chitosan, polyglycolic acid, polylactic acid, poly ε-caprolactone etc. *In-situ* gelling system (ISGS) has gained considerable cognizance and it can be capitalized as effective dosage form for treatment of multifarious diseases (Rathod et al., 2010). Advantages of ISGS include ease to administration with good patient compliance, higher gastric retention with slower drug release, reduced dosing frequency and can be utilized for both local action as well as site specific targeting (Sangeetha et al., 2010). The disadvantages associated with ISGS include, occasional instability due to higher chemical degradation inside the body, large volume of fluid is required and issues of stability during storage (Singh and Kim, 2000).

This chapter delineates basic principles of ISGS, polymer used, methods of preparation, evaluations and its pharmaceutical applications.

11.2 *In-Situ* Gelling System

In-Situ Gelling System (ISGS) is basically a hydrogel which undergoes *'Sol-to-Gel transformation'* under the influence of some vital factors like alteration in pH, temperature, crosslinking etc. It is basically a viscous, biocompatible, possibly biodegradable (natural polymer), mucoadhesive, polymer-based liquid system which transmogrify into a polymeric gel with tailored drug release profile. ISGS commits two basic advantages; prolonged residence time and homogenization of drug in dosage form prior to gelation. Various mechanism involved in preparation of *in-situ* gels are outlined in Fig. 11.1.

11.2.1 Physiological Stimuli Approach

Physiological parameters like temperature and pH of body fluid always play a vital role in modifying the drug release from dosage forms. These factors also influence the performance of ISGS, where by slight variation in temperature and body pH triggers the ISGS to release the drug.

11.2.1.1 Temperature Induced

It is one of the most common and popular mechanism used to produce an ISGS. Temperature sensitive ISGS can be broadly classified into 2 basic types:

(i) Positively thermosensetive;
(ii) Negatively thermosensetive.

Positively thermosensetive polymers has an upper critical solution temperature (UCST), which simply means that such polymers when get exposed to a cool temperature front they get consolidated themselves and form an ISGS for example poly acrylic acid (PAA) and poly-acrylamide (PAAm). Negatively thermosensetive polymers are those which has a lower critical solution temperature (LCST), which means they get solidify in presence of hot weather conditions. They usually remain liquid at room temperature but get solidified when exposed to body temperature e.g. poly-N-isopropylacrylamide (PNIPAAm) (Nirmal et al., 2010).

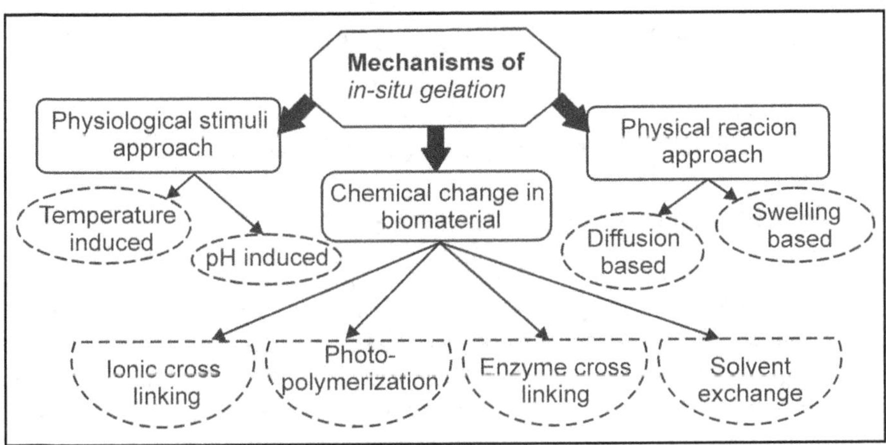

FIGURE 11.1 Mechanisms of *in-situ* gelation.

11.2.1.2 pH Induced

Among various types of *in-situ* gel systems, pH-sensitive gels have a potential use in site-specific delivery of drugs to specific regions of the gastrointestinal tract. The pH prone polymers contain either acidic or basic groups which are ionizable in nature and hence by performing an exchange of protons with the body fluids they will lead to the formation of an ISGS. pH sensitive polymers are polyvinylacetal diethylamino-acetate and carbopol. The above mentioned polymers are liquid at lower pH approx 4 but get solidified at neutral pH 7.4 and act as drug delivery system. In some cases some researchers have also used hydroxyl propyl methyl cellulose (HPMC) as viscosity enhancers for ISGS. In some cases the optimization of gelation has also been tried using combinations of polymers like combinations of poly-ethyleneglycols and poly-methacrylic acid (Soppimath et al., 2002). The effect of pH can be visualized through Fig. 11.2 where the gel is solidified upon change of pH.

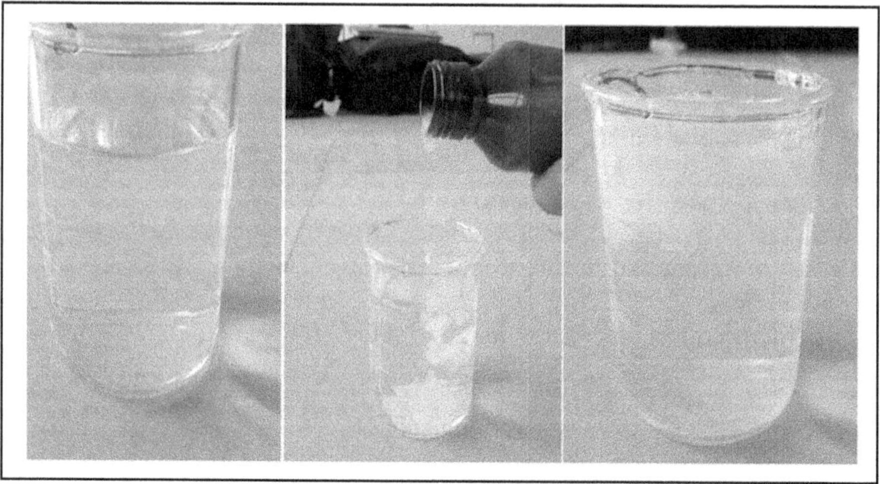

FIGURE 11.2 Sequence of formation of pH based floating *in-situ* gel.

11.2.2 Physical Reaction Approach

It is usually operated on two basic principles; diffusion and swelling. Diffusion is a physical approach in which solvent gets diffused out from the polymer solution into surrounding tissues, resulting in precipitation and solidification of polymer matrix. N-methyl pyrrolidone is one of the most commonly used polymers for development of ISGS by diffusion approach. Swelling is the second type of physical approach which acts on the principle of endosmosis. The polymers imbibe the surrounding fluid from the external environment and swells from inside to outside thus retard the drug release. ISGS formed by glycerol mono-oleate represents this approach (Mottu et al., 2000).

11.2.3 Chemical Changes in Biomaterial

Chemical changes may include ionic crosslinking, enzymatic crosslinking, photo-polymerization and solvent exchange. These mechanisms are summarized as follows:

11.2.3.1 Ionic Crosslinking

Polymers based on this approach undergoes gelation in the presence of monovalent or divalent ions e.g., alginic acid when exposed to an environment flourished with Ca^{2+} ions undergoes gelation. It actually happened due to active interaction of Ca^{2+} with gluronic acid of alginic acid. Similarly gellan gum undergoes gelation in the presence of Ca^{2+}, Mg^{2+}, Na^+, and K^+ (Podual et al., 2000).

11.2.3.2 Photo-Polymerization

These types of polymers are transformed to ISGS by using electro-magnetic radiations (EMR). The process involves the administration of initiator, monomer and reactive macromer to the site of application in the solution form. When this solution gets exposed to EMR, it leads to photo-polymerization of the system. EMR are delivered by using fiber optics concept at the site of application and basically long wavelength UV or visible light is used as source of EMR (Burkoth and Anseth, 2000).

11.2.3.3 Enzymatic Cross Linking

Enzymatic cross linking has emerged as the most convenient approach to produce in-situ gelling system. In this approach, gel is formed by cross linking with the enzymes that are present in the body fluids avoiding the use of potentially harmful chemicals such as monomers and initiators. Another advantage of the enzymatic crosslinking is presence of mild gelation conditions (e.g., physiological conditions) which is favourable for tissue regeneration. Horseradish peroxidase (HRP) a single-chain b-type hemoprotein has recently been employed in the preparation of ISGS that catalyzes the coupling of phenols or aniline derivatives in the presence of hydrogen peroxide. Crosslinking reaction takes place at ortho position via a carbon-carbon bond and/or between the carbon atom at the ortho position and the phenoxy oxygen in the phenol moieties via a carbon-oxygen bond. However use of hydrogen peroxide at higher concentration (>0.2 mM) may prove to be disadvantageous and lead to cell apoptosis (Kobayashi, 2001). Thus a controlled fraction of hydrogen peroxide should be utilized. HRP-mediated enzymatic crosslinking is well seen in formation of dextran-tyramine hydrogels for cartilage tissue engineering (Jin et al., 2007).

11.3 Methods of Preparation of *In-Situ* Gel Systems

In-situ gel systems can be developed by several methods based on copolymerization or crosslinking of monomer units. Polymerization may be done in solution or suspension phase. Cross linking is the second method of *in-situ* gel formation and done by either irradiation or chemical reaction.

11.3.1 Solution Polymerization/Crosslinking

This method involves mixing of ionic or neutral monomers with the multifunctional crosslinking agent. Here the polymerization can be initiated either thermally, or by UV light or by redox initiator system. Reaction solvent sinks heat and thus helps to control problems associated with irregular temperature rise. The prepared gel system is washed with distilled water to remove excess of unreacted monomers, crosslinking agent, and the initiator. Poly (2-hydroxyethyl methacrylate) gel system is prepared by this method using hydroxyl ethyl methacrylate as monomer unit and ethylene glycol dimethacrylate as crosslinking agent (Vyas et al., 2011).

11.3.2 Suspension Polymerization

To develop a spherical hydrogel micro particulate system with a size range of 1μm to 1mm, suspension polymerization is the method of choice. In this method, solution of monomer units is dispersed in a non solvent system resulting in the formation of fine droplets, which are further stabilized by addition of stabilizer. Here the polymerization is stimulated by thermal decomposition of free radicals. Microparticles obtained in this method are then washed with distilled water to remove excessive and unreacted monomers and initiator molecules (Langer and Peppas, 1981). Hydrogel micro particles of poly (vinyl alcohol) and hydroxyl ethyl methacrylate have been prepared by this method.

11.3.3 Polymerization by Irradiation

In-situ gel system for unsaturated compounds can be prepared by using radiation energy of gamma rays and electron beam. In this method aqueous polymer solution is exposed to irradiation energy which develops microradicals on the polymer chains. These microradicals, rejoins with each other on different polymeric chains forming covalent bonds and finally a cross linked structure. To prevent the interaction of oxygen with microradicals during polymerization an inert environment of nitrogen or argon gas is preferred (Peppas and Mikos, 1986). Example of polymers crosslinked by radiation method includes poly (vinyl alcohol), poly (ethylene glycol), and poly (acrylic acid).

11.3.4 Chemically Crosslinked Hydrogels

Many water soluble polymers containing functional groups like –OH, -COOH, -NH$_2$, can be used to prepare *in-situ* gels by forming covalent linkages between the polymer chains and complementary groups such as amine-carboxylic acid, isocyanate-OH/NH$_2$ etc. Gluteraldehyde is well established as a crosslinking agent in the formation of hydrogels of polymers containing –OH groups like poly (vinyl alcohol). Cross linking agents exhibit addition reaction with the functional groups present on the polymer, however they are highly toxic, and hence unreacted agents should be well removed. Cross linker may react with water and hence full polymerization reaction is carried out in organic solvents instead of water (Berger et al., 2004).

11.3.5 Physically Crosslinked Hydrogels

Hydrogels can be prepared by reversible ionic crosslinking in order to avoid the toxicity related issues of croslinking agents and to eliminate the purification step. Chitosan a polycationic polymer forms a network of polymers through ionic bridges by reacting with positively charged ions or molecules. Ionic crosslinking is a simple and mild procedure that requires no auxiliary molecules such as catalysts to prepare the gel system (Plourde et al., 2005).

11.4 *In-Situ* Gelling Polymers

There are a number of polymers which can be utilized for the formulation of *in-situ* gel system. Some of these polymers are discussed below:

11.4.1 Pectin

Pectin belongs to polysaccharides family with α-(1-4)-Dgalacturonic acid residues as polymer backbone. Galacturonic acid chains of this backbone readily form gel in presence of free calcium ions in aqueous solution creating a suitable vehicle for sustained drug delivery. Pectin being water soluble, also avoid the use of organic solvents in development of formulations and thus contribute additional advantages (Dumitriu et al., 1996). To maintain the fluid state of pectin during storage sodium citrate may be added to the pectin solution containing calcium ions. Sodium citrate forms a complex with free calcium ions in pectin solution and restricts them to form gel state. However this complex is broken in acidic environment of the stomach and free calcium ions present in the stomach; carry out the transition of pectin to gel state when administered orally. To develop a successful oral formulation it is necessary to optimize the quantities of calcium and citrate ions to maintain the fluidity of the formulation at storage condition and gelation when administered orally. Such *in-situ* gelling pectin formulation is already reported for the sustained delivery of paracetamol for oral administration (Kubo et al., 2004).

11.4.2 Gellan Gum

Gellan gum is another type of polysaccharide anionic in nature and secreted by *Pseudomonas elodea*, which is comprised of one α-L-rhamnose, one β-D-glucuronic acid and two β-D-glucuronic acid residues. It shows gelation property either on temperature variation or cationic induction. This gelation involves the formation of three-dimensional network by complexation of cations and hydrogen bonding with water. Similar to pectin formulation, gellan solution is also prepared with calcium chloride and sodium citrate complex and forms *in-situ* gel with the calcium ions released in acidic environment of stomach, when administered orally. Theophylline is reported to be delivered as *in-situ* gelling gellan formulation (Miyazaki et al., 1999).

11.4.3 Xyloglucan

Xyloglucan, a derived polysaccharide from tamarind seeds contains a (1-4)-β-D-glucan backbone chain, with (1-6)-α-D xylose as branches. Xyloglucan can be partially degraded by β- galactosidase to form a thermally reversible product. Aforesaid product exhibits a sol-gel transition temperature which varies with the degree of galactose elimination and forms thermally reversible gels when warm to the body temperature. However its slow gelation time property restricts its use as *in-situ* gelling vehicle in oral drug delivery and make it suitable for the use in intraperitoneal, ocular and rectal drug delivery. Xyloglucan *in-situ* gel has been reported for intraperitoneal sustained release formulation of mitomycin C (Suisha et al., 1998).

11.4.4　Guar Gum

Guar gum is a water soluble naturally occurring gum which is obtained from the endosperm of the seed. It forms a high viscous gelling solution at low concentrations in water. However alteration in temperature causes reversible change in gelling property of gaur gum and plays an important role in transition of its sol-gel status. Guar gum is also available as its semi synthetic form, carboxy methyl guar which shows a better release rate profile, safety and stability properties and used extensively for transdermal drug delivery (Prabaharan, 2011).

11.4.5　Xanthum Gum

Xanthan gum is a water soluble high molecular weight polysaccharide obtained from bacteria *Xanthomonas campestris*. It exhibits anionic nature due to the presence of both glucuronic acid and pyruvic acid groups that are present in the side chain. It is extensively used to stabilize emulsions or suspensions formulations either alone or in combination of hydrocolloids. It is also used as a polymer in formulation of in-situ gelling systems due to its property to form gel in aqueous solution. Water molecules bind with xanthan gum molecules and form lumps that rearrange at moderate temperature and on cooling forms firm and stiff gel (Fujiwara et al., 2000).

11.4.6　Carbopol

Carbopol express its sol gel properties on alteration of pH. It remains in solution form at acidic pH and forms a low viscosity gel at alkaline pH. However to reduce the acidity and to increase the gelling property, HPMC is added to the carbopol solution. The water soluble polymers such as carbopol-hydroxypropylmethylcellulose system, and poly (methacrylic acid)-poly (ethylene glycol) come under the category of pH-induced in-situ precipitating polymeric systems. This concept is well seen in sustained delivery of indomethacin ocular drug delivery.

11.4.7 Synthetic Polymers

Biodegradable synthetic polymers are extensively investigated for parenteral *in-situ* gel preparations. Advantages of biodegradable polymers include no need of surgical follow up and removal of polymer after the drug is completely released from the ISGS. Majority of these polymers act on sol-gel transition temperature principle and remain liquid outside the body with capability to be injected by a syringe and needle, however once inside the body, they form gel. Poly (lactic acid), poly (glycolic acid), poly (lactide- coglycolide), poly (decalactone), poly ε-caprolactone are the names among most extensively investigated and applied synthetic polymers for *in-situ* gel system.

11.5 Evaluation and Characterizations of *In-Situ* Gel System

11.5.1 Clarity

It is important to remove all the visible impurities from the formulation as clarity is an important factor. The clarity of formulated solutions may be determined by visual inspection under black and white background.

11.5.2 Texture Analysis

In case of parenteral administration, formulation is evaluated for the firmness, consistency and cohesiveness using texture analyzer to assess the syringeability of sol. However greater values of adhesiveness of gels are needed to maintain an intimate contact with surfaces like tissues.

11.5.3 pH of Gel

pH of the gel can be determined using digital pH meter.

11.5.4 Sol-Gel Transition Temperature and Gelling Time

In case of temperature regulated *in-situ* gel system it is necessary to determine the sol-gel transition temperature, which is actually the temperature at which the phase transition of sol to gel is first noted when heated at a specified rate. Gelling time is the time for first detection of gelation as defined above (Kashyap et al., 2007).

11.5.5 Gel-Strength

Gel strength is determined using a rheometer. The gel is placed in a beaker which is then raised at a certain rate, pushing a probe slowly through the gel. Gel strength is measured by the changes in the load on the probe, as a function of depth of immersion of the probe below the gel surface (Kashyap et al., 2007).

11.5.6 Viscosity and Rheology

This is an important parameter for evaluation of *in-situ* gel system. The viscosity and rheological properties of the polymeric formulations can be determined using Brookfield viscometer in both sol and gel phase. The viscosity of these formulations should be such that no difficulties should be encountered during their administration by the patient, especially during parenteral and ocular administration (Kashyap et al., 2007).

11.5.7 Fourier Transform Infrared Spectroscopy and Thermal Analysis

At the time of transition of sol to gel, alteration in bonding arrangement and interacting forces can be determined using FTIR and potassium bromide pellet method. To determine the percentage of water in gel structure thermogravimetric analysis can be conducted. Differential scanning calorimetry can also be utilized to determine the drug interactions in comparison to pure ingredients used (Kashyap et al., 2007).

11.5.8 *In-vitro* Drug Release Studies

For the *in-situ* gel formulations to be administered by oral, ocular or rectal routes, the drug release studies are carried out by using the Franz diffusion cell .The cell is composed of two half, a donor compartment and a receptor compartment, separated by the cellulose membrane. The sol form of the formulation is placed in the donor compartment and receptor compartment is filled with simulated fluid. The whole assembly is kept on constant temperature of 37 ± 0.5 °C.

Certain volume of receptor solution is withdrawn at pre decided time intervals and the volume is replaced with the fresh media. Sample withdrawn is analyzed for the drug release either by UV spectroscopy or HPLC technique.

11.6 Applications of *In-Situ* Polymeric Drug Delivery System

In-situ gel systems may be applied to a wide variety of drug delivery through different routes of administration.

11.6.1 *In-Situ* Gel based Oral Drug Delivery

The oral delivery of drugs with a narrow absorption window in the gastrointestinal tract is often limited by poor bioavailability with conventional dosage forms due to incomplete drug release and short residence time at the site of absorption and hence novel *in-situ* based drug delivery systems have been developed. Liquid orals exhibit low bioavailability profile for stomach specific drug deliveries due to faster transit from the stomach and thus liquid *in-situ* floating gel system may be used which produces sustained release effect of same formulation. Among various types of *in-situ* gel systems, pH-sensitive gels have a potential use in site-specific delivery of drugs to specific regions of the gastrointestinal tract.

Many polysaccharide based *in-situ* gel systems are popular for oral drug delivery. Cross-linked dextran hydrogels with a faster swelling under high pH conditions is one of them. Pectin, guar gum and inulin are the other examples of polysaccharides investigated to develop a potential colon-specific drug delivery system. The gelation of pectin occurs in the presence of H^+ ions, a source of divalent ions, generally calcium ions is required to produce the gels that are suitable as vehicles for drug delivery. Sodium citrate may be added to the pectin solution to form a complex with most of the Ca^{+2} ions added in the formulation. By this means, the formulation may be maintained in a fluid state (sol), until the breakdown of the complex in the acidic environment of the stomach, where release of calcium ions causes gelation to occur. The quantities of calcium and citrate ions may be optimized to maintain the fluidity of the formulation before administration and resulting in gelation, when the formulation is administered in the stomach. Oral delivery of theophylline through *in-situ* gelling gellan formulation consisting calcium chloride and sodium citrate complex is an example of increased bioavailability and sustained drug release profile. When taken orally, the calcium ions released in acidic environment of stomach leading to gelation of gellan thus forming a gel *in-situ*. Oral delivery of paracetamol through pectin *in-situ* gel is reported showing advantages of replacing organic solvents with water (Kubo et al., 2004; Miyazaki et al., 1999).

Wu and co-workers in 2008, designed and prepared *in-situ* gel systems for the oral delivery of ibuprofen (IBU-ISG) and studied its pharmacokinetics in beagle dogs. They also optimized the binary IBU-ISG formulation by monitoring the complex viscosity before gelling *In vitro* release property (Wu et al., 2008).

Liquid formulations of xyloglucan and sodium alginate in appropriate proportions were prepared for oral administration of paracetamol to dysphagic patients which forms gel *in-situ* in the stomach. This formulation was capable of sustaining the release of paracetamol over a 6-hour period (Itoh et al., 2010). (El Maghraby et al., 2012) developed a modified *in-situ* gelling system for sustained dextromethorphan release in the stomach and intestine. However, this formulation failed to sustain the release in the intestinal conditions.

11.6.2 Ocular Delivery

Gellan gum, alginic acid and xyloglucan are the most commonly used polymers for development of *in-situ* gels based ocular delivery. These *in-situ* gel based systems are most suitable for local ophthalmic delivery of antimicrobial, antiinflammatory and autonomic drugs. Poor bioavailability and therapeutic response of conventional delivery systems can be improved using ISGS because of their high residential time in eye. Gellan gum based *in-situ* gel system is extensively utilized for this purpose. Slower drug release profile and long residential time of these systems also help in prolonging drug action at ocular site compared with the conventional eye drops. Miyazaki and co-workers developed an *in-situ* gel formulation of xyloglucan for ocular delivery which showed an overwhelming mitotic response for a period of 4 h (Miyazaki et al., 2001). *In-situ* gel based sustained release indomethacin ophthalmic formulation has been developed for the treatment of uveitis which was found to be responsive for a period of more than 8 h *in-vitro* and proved to be superior over the conventional systems.

11.6.3 Nasal Delivery

Gallan gum and xanthan gum are polymers of choice for in-situ gel system based nasal drug delivery. *In-situ* gel based system for mometasone furoate has been developed and evaluated for the treatment of allergic rhinitis (Miyazaki et al., 2001; Sarasija and Shyamala, 2005). A sustained and more effective result obtained when *in-situ* gel of mometasone was applied to antigen induced allergic rhinitis rats. A comparative study of this formulation with marketed preparation nosonex (mometasone furoate suspension 0.05%) proved that *in-situ* gel is safe and more effectively inhibit the increase in nasal symptoms (Cao et al., 2009).

11.6.4 Rectal and Vaginal Drug Delivery Systems

In-situ gel possesses potential applications for rectal and vaginal delivery. Rectal and vaginal route may be considered as a route of drug administration for different types of dosage forms including solution, suspension, ointments, creams, foams and suppositories, when the oral route either lacks feasibility (in comatose patients) or is not suitable for the delivery of certain drugs (drugs having low bioavailability or degrade in gastric juice). However conventional dosage forms like suppositories often cause discomfort during insertion and sometimes they can migrate upward to the colon causing first-pass metabolism of the drug. Problems associated with conventional suppositories may be rectified using novel *in-situ* gelling liquid suppositories with gelation temperature at 30-36°C. A combination of poloxamer 407 and poloxamer 188 may be used to prepare the temperature-sensitive gelation suppositories. Similarly xyloglucan has been utilized to prepare thermo reversible gel of indomethacin for rectal drug delivery (Miyazaki et al., 1998). In comparison to marketed suppository, a better drug absorption and prolonged drug action was observed when Indomethacin loaded xyloglucan based system was inserted into rectal cavity of rabbit. A mucoadhesive, thermosensitive and prolonged release vaginal gel containing clotrimazole-β-cyclodextrin complex is also developed and evaluated for better therapeutic efficacy and patient compliance for treatment of vaginitis (Bilensoy et al., 2006).

11.6.5 Injectable Drug Delivery Systems

In-situ gel forming formulations are also evaluated for their application as injectable drug delivery systems. An anticancer drug loaded chitosan based hydrogel is developed for the treatment of tumor that is based on injectable thermosensitive *in-situ* system. For local delivery of paclitaxel at tumor site *in-situ* based system was developed and investigated using EMT-6 tumors implanted subcutaneously on albino mice. Ito et al. developed an *in-situ* based injectable hydrogel using hydrazide modified hyaluronic acid cross-linked with aldehyde modified carboxymethylcellulose, hydroxypropylmethylcellulose and methylcellulose. These *in-situ* forming gels were used for preventing postoperative peritoneal adhesions thus avoiding pelvic pain, bowel obstructions and infertility (Ito et al., 2007). A marketed formulation of *in-situ* gel based injectable system ReGel ® (triblock copolymer PLGAPEG- PLGA) has been developed for the continuous release of human insulin up to day 15 when injected subcutaneously. Such types of the formulations release the drug in a sustained manner by formation of a depot. The gel system is injected into the body upon application of the pressure and once the pressure is released the liquid system turns into gel leading to formation of a depot (sol-gel theory). This mechanism is depicted in Fig. 11.3.

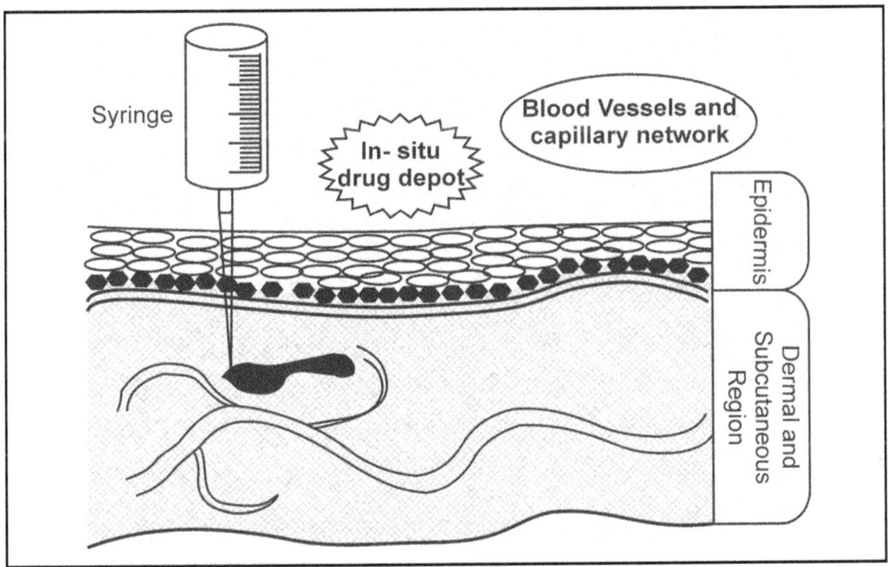

FIGURE 11.3 Subcutaneous drug delivery through *in-situ* gel system.

11.7 Liquid Crystals as Drug Delivery Systems

Liquid crystals (LCs) is the emerging technology for sustained drug delivery that exists between the liquid and the crystalline solid state. The liquid state is related with their ability to flow, whereas the solid state is characterized by an ordered, crystalline structure (Kelker and Hatz, 1980). Thus LCs may show mechanical stability like solids as well as flow like liquids. Solid crystal exhibits both short as well as long range order with regard to the position and orientation of the molecules (Fig. 11.4A). However liquids are amorphous and show short-range order with regard to position and orientation (Fig. 11.4B). But in case of liquid crystals at least orientational long-range order and short-range order may be appeared, whereas positional long-range order disappears (Mueller-Goymann and Hamann, 1993). This intermediate state of LCs is also called as mesophases. LCs elicit general properties like birefringence, response to magnetic and electric fields, optical activity in twisted nematic phases and sensitivity to temperature resulting in color changes (Larsson, 2009).

It is necessary to have an anisometric molecular shape with a marked anisotropy of the polarizability for the development of liquid crystalline phase. Molecules that are able to form mesophases are known as mesogens that are either rod like or disc like in shape. Rod like mesogens form calamitic mesophases and disc like mesogens form discotic mesophases. Rod-shaped molecules are often excipients of drugs (e.g., surfactants). Even drug compounds themselves (e.g., the salts of organic acids or bases with anisometric molecular shape) fulfill the requirements for the formation of calamitic mesophases (Fig. 11.5).

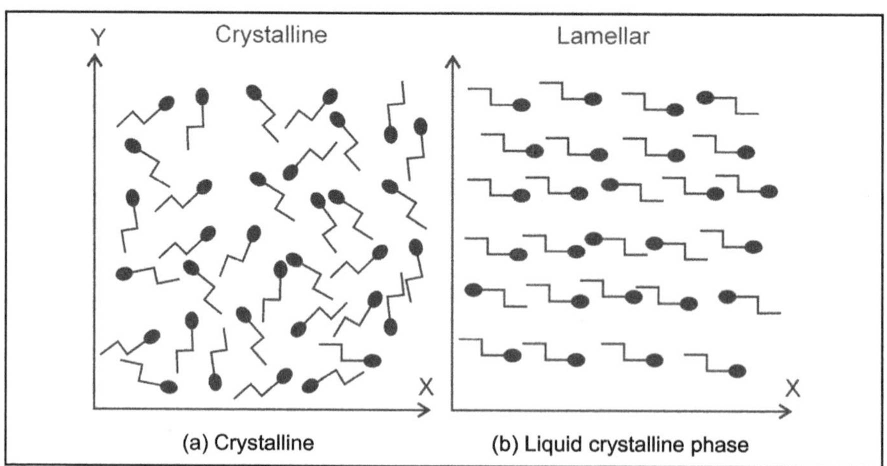

FIGURE 11.4 Difference in position and orientation of the molecules in (a) Crystalline and (b) Liquid crystalline phase.

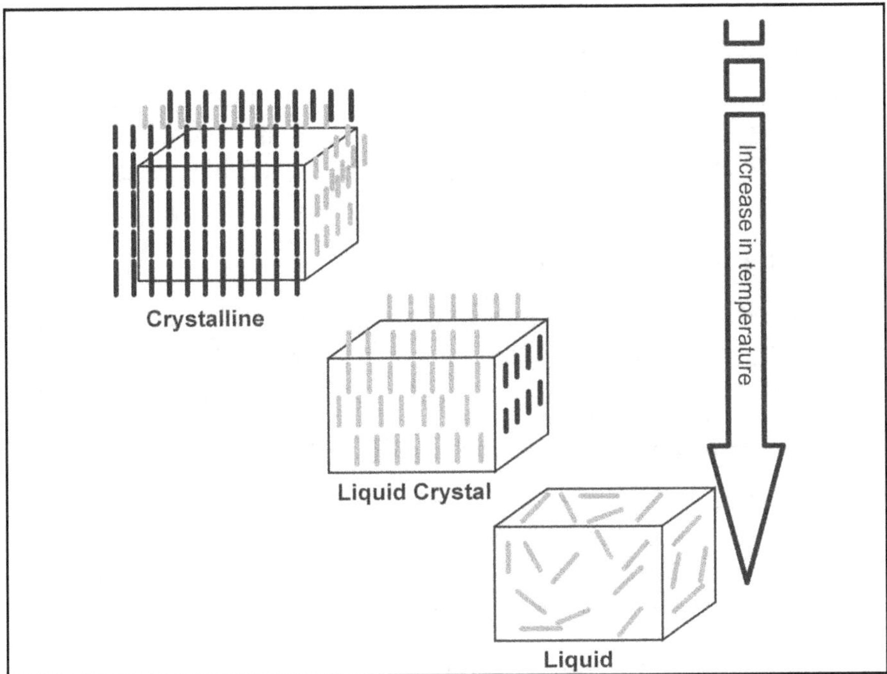

FIGURE 11.5 Appearance of mesophases on temperature change.

11.7.1 Classification of Liquid Crystals

LCs are broadly classified on the basis of method of preparation into lyotropic and thermotropic. They are further subdivided into different groups on the basis of positional and orientational order of the molecules.

11.7.1.1 Lyotropic Liquid Crystals

Lyotropic liquid crystalline systems are composed of rod like micelles, which show a long-range orientational order with respect to symmetry axis of the micelle, but no long-range positional order. They are formed by mesogens that are not the molecules themselves but their hydrates or solvates as well as by associates of hydrated or solvated molecules. The three main types of LLCs are characterized as being lamellar, hexagonal and cubic (Bennett et al., 1999).

11.7.1.1.1 Lamellar Liquid Crystals

Lamellar LCs are bilayered structures of repeating units, showing long-range positional order in one dimension and long-range orientational order within the layer (Makai et al., 2003).

11.7.1.1.2 Hexagonal Liquid Crystals

If the molecules are arranged in long-range positional order in two dimensions, they form hexagonal LCs, which can be identified using polarized light microscopy. These types of liquid crystals are also known as middle phase.

11.7.1.1.3 Cubic Liquid Crystals

Liquid crystals showing long-range positional order in three dimensions are known as cubic LCs. They have a high viscosity and poor flow property comparison to lamellar and hexagonal LCs (Shah et al., 2001).

11.7.1.2 Thermotropic Liquid Crystals

Thermotropic mesophases are developed by heating the crystalline substance alone and they may be regarded as special polymorphic form (Patterson et al., 2002). The three types of thermotropic liquid crystalline phases are characterized as being nematic, smectic, and cholesteric.

11.7.1.2.1 Smectic Liquid Crystals

Smectic liquid crystal consists of parallel molecules to one another and perpendicular to the plane in given layers. These liquid crystals are viscous, however fluid enough due to free slip and travel of layers over each other.

11.7.1.2.2 Nematic Liquid Crystals

Nematic liquid crystals look like a thread under a polarized light microscope. In the nematic state, the molecules are not as extremely ordered as in the smectic state, but they maintain their parallel order.

11.7.1.2.3 Cholesteric Liquid Crystals

Cholesteric arrangement may be described as the combination of the nematic and smectic states. In cholesteric liquid crystals molecules are arranged parallel in layers. However, the molecular layers in cholesteric liquid crystals are very thin (Kawamoto, 2002).

11.7.2 Characterization of Liquid Crystals

The liquid crystals can be characterized with respect to variety of parameters which are mentioned below.

11.7.2.1 Polarized Light Microscopy

Liquid crystals can be characterized using polarized light microscope except cubical mesophases. They show birefringence in presence of polarized light just like real crystals. Each liquid crystal shows typical black and white texture.

11.7.2.2 Transmission Electron Microscopy

Microstructure of liquid crystals can be visualized and measured under the electron microscope with high magnification power. However, aqueous samples do not survive the high vacuum of an electron microscope and hence freeze fracture technique is utilized for the sample preparation before electron microscopy.

11.7.2.3 X-Ray Scattering Pattern

X-ray scattering technique can be utilized to determine the characteristic interferences that are generated from an ordered microstructure (Fontell, 1974). Interferences may be detected either by film detection or X-ray scintillation counters. X-ray diffraction technique detects not only the interferences from which the interlayer spacings can be calculated, but also the type of liquid crystal.

11.7.2.4 Differential Scanning Calorimetry

Differential Scanning Calorimetry (DSC) determines the total energy required for the transition of crystalline to liquid crystalline or amorphous form. The transition from crystalline to liquid crystalline and from liquid crystalline to amorphous and particularly the transition between different liquid crystals consume low amounts of energy. Hence instrument with high level of sensitivity should be deployed.

11.7.2.5 Rheology

With the alteration in microstructural organization of the liquid crystal, a large variation in rheological properties of different types of liquid crystals is observed. A more viscous and consistent behavior of liquid crystals is seen with an in increase in its microstructural organization. A mechanical oscillation measurement is the method of choice for determining the elasticity and rheology of the liquid crystalline gels.

11.7.2.6 Determination of Vesicle Size

Determination of vesicle size of liquid crystals is an important parameter with reference to quality assurance and in process control and thus ensuring the maximum physical stability of the vesicular dispersion. Most appropriate and quick method to determine the vesicle size and size distribution is laser light scattering and diffraction technique (Jain et al., 2007).

11.7.3 Applications of Liquid Crystals

A huge amount of research is being levied on liquid crystals in order to explore their properties for use in pharmaceutical and other related fields. Some of the applications are being focused below.

11.7.3.1 Liquid Crystalline Drug Substances

Some drugs are able to form liquid crystals while retaining their pharmacological property. Arsphenamin is the very first example of antibacterial drug that exists as thermotropic nematic mesomorph and used widely under the name of Salvarsan (Freundlich et al., 1923). Diethylammonium flufenamate, fenoprofen, ketoprofen, ibuprofen and diclofenac are some other examples of drugs that exhibit lamellar type of liquid crystalline state.

11.7.3.2 Liquid Crystalline Formulations for Dermal Application

Amphiphilic drug molecules and surfactants are able to form lyotropic liquid crystals and may be utilized as excipients in the development of drug formulations. Ringing gels with cubic liquid crystalline microstructure are used for topical NSAIDs formulations.

11.7.3.3 Liquid Crystalline Formulations for Sustained Release Drug Delivery

Sustained release from disperse systems such as emulsions and suspensions can be achieved by the adsorption of appropriate mesogenic molecules especially multilamellar liquid crystals at the interface. Drug present in the dispersed phase cannot pass the liquid crystals easily and thus diffuses slowly into the continuous phase, providing a sustained drug release profile (Mueller-Goymann and Hamann, 1993).

11.7.3.4 Liquid Crystals in Cosmetics

Liquid crystals may be utilized for decorative purposes in cosmetics. Cholesteric liquid crystals having iridescent color effects are exclusively applied as coloring for nail varnishes, eye shadows, and lipsticks. The structure of these thermotropic liquid crystals undergo change with body temperature, resulting in the required color effect.

11.8 Conclusion

In-situ gel systems and liquid crystals have been explored recently in the field of drug delivery. It is evident from the previous work and data available that these systems can be efficiently utilized for development of newer strategies in the dynamic field of drug delivery and drug formulation. A great deal of work has been done and lot of research has contributed towards the development of these newer systems. However, much more remains to be explored in this regard to harness the properties and qualities of these systems to a greater extent for the cause of design and development of safe and efficacious drug delivery systems.

References

Bennett, D.B., Cabot, K.M., Foster, L.C., Lechuga-Ballesteros, D., Patton, J.S., and Tan, T.K. (1999). Liquid crystal forms of cyclosporin, U. Patent, ed. (U.S.A: Google Patents).

Berger, J., Reist, M., Mayer, J.M., Felt, O., Peppas, N.A., and Gurny, R. (2004). Structure and interactions in covalently and ionically crosslinked chitosan hydrogels for biomedical applications. *European Journal of Pharmaceutics and Biopharmaceutics* **57**, 19-34.

Bilensoy, E., Rouf, M.A., Vural, I., Sen, M., and Hincal, A.A. (2006). Mucoadhesive, thermosensitive, prolonged-release vaginal gel for clotrimazole:beta-cyclodextrin complex. *AAPS Pharm Sci Tech* **7**, E38.

Burkoth, A.K., and Anseth, K.S. (2000). A review of photocrosslinked polyanhydrides: in-situ forming degradable networks. *Biomaterials* **21**, 2395-2404.

Cao, S.L., Ren, X.W., Zhang, Q.Z., Chen, E., Xu, F., Chen, J., Liu, L.C., and Jiang, X.G. (2009). In-situ gel based on gellan gum as new carrier for nasal administration of mometasone furoate. *International journal of pharmaceutics* **365**, 109-115.

Dumitriu, S., Vidal, P.F., and Chornet, E. (1996). Hydrogels based on polysaccharides. In Polysaccharides in medical applications, S. Dumitriu, ed. (New York: Marcel Dekker Inc), pp. 125-242.

El Maghraby, G.M., Elzayat, E.M., and Alanazi, F.K. (2012). Development of modified in-situ gelling oral liquid sustained release formulation of dextromethorphan. *Drug development and industrial pharmacy* **38**, 971-978.

Fontell, K. (1974). X-ray Diffraction by Liquid Crystals- Amphiphilic Systems. In Liquid Crystals and Plastic Crystals, G. Gray, and P. Winsor, eds. (Chichester: Ellis Horwood).

Freundlich, H., Stern, R., and Zocher, H. (1923). The colloidal chemistry of arsphenamine and neoarsphenamine. *Biochem Zeit* **138**, 307-317.

Fujiwara, J., Iwanami, T., Takahashi, M., Tanaka, R., Hatakeyama, T., and Hatakeyama, H. (2000). Structural change of xanthan gum association in aqueous solutions. *Thermochimica Acta* **352-353**, 241-246.

Ito, T., Yeo, Y., Highley, C.B., Bellas, E., Benitez, C.A., and Kohane, D.S. (2007). The prevention of peritoneal adhesions by in-situ cross-linking hydrogels of hyaluronic acid and cellulose derivatives. *Biomaterials* **28**, 975-983.

Itoh, K., Tsuruya, R., Shimoyama, T., Watanabe, H., Miyazaki, S., D'Emanuele, A., and Attwood, D. (2010). In-situ gelling xyloglucan/alginate liquid formulation for oral sustained drug delivery to dysphagic patients. *Drug development and industrial pharmacy* **36**, 449-455.

Jain, S., Tiwary, A.K., Sapra, B., and Jain, N.K. (2007). Formulation and evaluation of ethosomes for transdermal delivery of lamivudine. *AAPS Pharm Sci Tech* **8**, E111.

Jin, R., Hiemstra, C., Zhong, Z., and Feijen, J. (2007). Enzyme-mediated fast in-situ formation of hydrogels from dextran-tyramine conjugates. *Biomaterials* **28**, 2791-2800.

Kashyap, N., Viswanad, B., Sharma, G., Bhardwaj, V., Ramarao, P., and Ravi Kumar, M.N. (2007). Design and evaluation of biodegradable, biosensitive in-situ gelling system for pulsatile delivery of insulin. *Biomaterials* **28**, 2051-2060.

Kawamoto, H. (2002). The history of liquid crystal display. *Proceedings of the IEEE* **90**, 460-500.

Kelker, H., and Hatz, R. (1980). Handbook of liquid crystals (Weinheim: Verlag Chemie).

Kobayashi, S. (2001). Enzymatic polymerization. *Chem Review* **101**, 3793-3818.

Kubo, W., Konno, Y., Miyazaki, S., and Attwood, D. (2004). *In-situ* gelling pectin formulations for oral sustained delivery of paracetamol. *Drug development and industrial pharmacy* **30**, 593-599.

Langer, R.S., and Peppas, N.A. (1981). Present and future applications of biomaterials in controlled drug delivery systems. *Biomaterials* **2**, 201-214.

Larsson, K. (2009). Lyotropic liquid crystals and their dispersions relevant in foods. *Current Opinion in Colloid & Interface Science* **14**, 16-20.

Makai, M., Csányi, E., Németh, Z., Pálinkás, J., and Erős, I. (2003). Structure and drug release of lamellar liquid crystals containing glycerol. *International journal of pharmaceutics* **256**, 95-107.

Miyazaki, S., Aoyama, H., Kawasaki, N., Kubo, W., and Attwood, D. (1999). *In-situ* -gelling gellan formulations as vehicles for oral drug delivery. *Journal of controlled release: official journal of the Controlled Release Society* **60**, 287-295.

Miyazaki, S., Suisha, F., Kawasaki, N., Shirakawa, M., Yamatoya, K., and Attwood, D. (1998). Thermally reversible xyloglucan gels as vehicles for rectal drug delivery. *Journal of controlled release: official journal of the Controlled Release Society* **56**, 75-83.

Miyazaki, S., Suzuki, S., Kawasaki, N., Endo, K., Takahashi, A., and Attwood, D. (2001). *In-situ* gelling xyloglucan formulations for sustained release ocular delivery of pilocarpine hydrochloride. *International journal of pharmaceutics* **229**, 29-36.

Mottu, F., Gailloud, P., Massuelle, D., Rufenacht, D.A., and Doelker, E. (2000). *In vitro* assessment of new embolic liquids prepared from preformed polymers and water-miscible solvents for aneurysm treatment. *Biomaterials* **21**, 803-811.

Mueller-Goymann, C.C., and Hamann, H.J. (1993). Sustained release from reverse micellar solutions by phase transformations into lamellar liquid crystals. *Journal of Controlled Release* **23**, 165-174.

Nirmal, H.B., Bakliwal, S.R., and Pawar, S.P. (2010). *In-Situ* gel: New trends in Controlled and Sustained Drug Delivery System. *Int J PharmTech Research* **2**, 1398-1408.

Patterson, J., Bary, A., and Rades, T. (2002). Physical stability and solubility of the thermotropic mesophase of fenoprofen calcium as pure drug and in a tablet formulation. *International journal of pharmaceutics* **247**, 147-157.

Peppas, N.A., and Mikos, A.G. (1986). Preparation Methods and Structure of Hydrogels. In Hydrogels in Medicine and Pharmacy Vol 1 Fundamental, N.A. Peppas, ed. (Boca Raton: CRC Press), pp. 1-25.

Plourde, F., Motulsky, A., Couffin-Hoarau, A.C., Hoarau, D., Ong, H., and Leroux, J.C. (2005). First report on the efficacy of l-alanine-based *in-situ* -forming implants for the long-term parenteral delivery of drugs. *Journal of controlled release: official journal of the Controlled Release Society* **108**, 433-441.

Podual, K., Doyle, F.J., 3rd, and Peppas, N.A. (2000). Dynamic behavior of glucose oxidase-containing microparticles of poly(ethylene glycol)-grafted cationic hydrogels in an environment of changing pH. *Biomaterials* **21**, 1439-1450.

Prabaharan, M. (2011). Prospective of guar gum and its derivatives as controlled drug delivery systems. *International journal of biological macromolecules* **49**, 117-124.

Rathod, H., Patel. V, and Modasia. M. (2010). In-situ gel as a novel approach of gastro retentive drug delivery. *Int J. Pharmacy and Life Sci* **1,** 440-447.

Sangeetha, S., Harish, G., Medapati, R., Gantasala, P., Raju, B., and Damodharan, N. (2010). Oral sustained delivery of salbutamol using *in-situ* gelation of sodium alginate. *Int J Current Pharma Research* **2,** 61-64.

Sarasija, S., and Shyamala, B. (2005). Nasal Drug Delivery: An Overview. *Indian J Pharm Sci* **67,** 19- 25.

Shah, J.C., Sadhale, Y., and Chilukuri, D.M. (2001). Cubic phase gels as drug delivery systems. *Adv Drug Deliv Rev* **47,** 229-250.

Singh, B.N., and Kim, K.H. (2000). Floating drug delivery systems: an approach to oral controlled drug delivery via gastric retention. *Journal of controlled release : official journal of the Controlled Release Society* **63,** 235-259.

Soppimath, K.S., Aminabhavi, T.M., Dave, A.M., Kumbar, S.G., and Rudzinski, W.E. (2002). Stimulus-responsive "smart" hydrogels as novel drug delivery systems. *Drug development and industrial pharmacy* **28,** 957-974.

Suisha, F., Kawasaki, N., Miyazaki, S., Shirakawa, M., Yamatoya, K., Sasaki, M., and Attwood, D. (1998). Xyloglucan gels as sustained release vehicles for the intraperitoneal administration of mitomycin C. *International journal of pharmaceutics* **172,** 27-32.

Vyas, J., Ghedia, T., and Gajjar, V. (2011). Review on novel *in-situ* polymeric drug delivery system. *Int J Pharm Res Dev* **3,** 53-59.

Wu, R.L., Zhao, C.S., Xie, J.W., Yi, S.L., Song, H.T., and He, Z.G. (2008). Preparation of *in-situ* gel systems for the oral delivery of ibuprofen and its pharmacokinetics study in beagle dogs. *Yao xue xue bao Acta pharmaceutica Sinica* **43,** 956-962.

INDEX

A

Adsorption theory 163, 248

Agglomerates 228-232, 292, 293

Agglomeration 55, 203, 230, 231, 234, 239, 243, 292, 302, 306, 307

Amorphous 193, 214, 239, 354, 357

Amphiphilic 321, 327, 332, 358

Amphoteric surfactants 43

Angina pectoris 159, 169, 271

Anionic surfactants 43, 236

Antibodies 102, 112, 126

Antibody 126, 127 , 190

Aptivus 72

Asthma 271

Autoclaving 141

B

Backing membrane 164, 167, 168

Bile salt micelles 40, 62

Binding agent 278

Bioavailability 18, 24, 38-40, 42, 43, 53, 56-58, 60, 65, 67, 85, 101, 109, 158, 167, 168, 200, 218, 227, 239, 246, 270, 274, 301, 306, 312, 321, 324, 333, 334, 339, 350-352

Biodegradable 22, 28, 95, 99-101, 117, 120, 122, 139, 140, 168, 210, 313, 322-324, 328, 340, 348, 360

Biodegradable microspheres 100, 139

Biodistribution 319

Biopharmaceutical 54, 60, 86, 138, 215, 263, 272

Birefringence 354, 357

Brownian flocculation 145

Brownian motion 4, 5, 228, 234

Brownian movement 234

Buccal patches 160, 161, 167, 171-173

Buccal tablets 160, 161, 164, 165, 167-170, 173, 174, 208

Butylated hydroxyanisole 141, 202

Butylated hydroxytoluene 141, 202

C

Capmul 42, 66, 69

Capryol 44, 54, 66, 68

Caramel base medicated tablets 196, 197

Centrifugal 225, 299, 300, 304

Ceramics nanoparticle 320

Cetomacrogol 43

Cholesteric liquid crystals 356, 358

Chrono pharmaceutical delivery 283

Chronotherapeutic 159, 277, 288

Coagulation 230, 232, 239, 243

Coalescence 45, 59, 138, 142, 145, 146, 246, 247, 250-252, 255, 262, 263, 302

Colloidal drug delivery systems 318-320, 329, 334

Colloidal nanocarriers 318, 323, 324

Colloidal suspensions 227

Colloids 45, 141, 225, 226, 233, 237, 246-248, 255, 277, 319, 332, 347

Colon 78-104 , 158-160, 188, 191, 251, 271, 297, 350, 352

Colon specific drug delivery systems 78, 82, 84, 86, 103

Colon targeted drug delivery 78, 83, 84, 93, 95

Colonic microflora 80, 83, 84, 93, 99, 103

Commercial SEDDS 69

Compressed lozenge 197, 198

Compressibility 56, 309

Confocal laser scanning microscopy 125, 128

Congealed material 302

Controlled delivery 7, 11, 158, 184, 314, 318, 319

Controlled release 1-2, 11, 12, 15, 18, 39, 68, 78, 180, 183, 209, 214, 274, 277, 286-288, 292, 294, 295, 299, 300, 305, 306, 312-314, 318, 328, 339

Controlled release drug delivery system 1, 18, 78, 339

Co-solvents 39, 43, 45, 46, 58, 61

Co-surfactants 39, 45, 54, 58

Creaming 145, 146, 148, 149, 250, 251, 262

Crohn's disease 78, 84, 85, 159

Crosslinking 96, 340, 343-345

Crushing strength 170, 309

Cryopelletization 300

Cyclosporine 65, 69, 71, 72

D

Degradation 11, 42, 45, 46, 53, 54, 60, 61, 79, 83, 92, 94, 97-101, 103, 122, 140, 160, 165, 195, 196, 218, 239, 250, 256, 262, 277, 319, 324, 326, 331, 333, 340

Dermatological 141, 226

Differential scanning calorimetry 30, 349, 357

Diffusion controlled systems 2, 3, 10

Diffusion theory 163

Direct compression 4, 68, 168, 169, 198, 281

Direct milling 171

Disintegrating agent 278

Disintegrating tablets 25, 271, 293

Disproportionation 145

Distal colon 80, 81, 84

Dosing frequency 1, 108, 159, 188, 270, 271, 280, 333, 340

Drug release kinetics 6, 14, 55

E

Egalet® delayed release 212, 213

Egalet® prolonged release Tablets 212

Egalet® technology 160, 209

Electron microscopy 58, 116, 128, 310, 357

Electronic theory 163

Emulsifiers 39, 138, 140, 141, 147, 201, 247, 252, 253, 255, 256, 258

Emulsion 39, 41-43, 45-46, 52, 54, 55, 57-59, 62, 63, 70, 137-153, 225, 226, 245, 246-267, 306, 320, 323, 328, 329-331, 333, 347, 358

Endocytosis 111, 112, 115, 334

Enteric coating 13, 83, 87, 89-91, 189, 190

Enterion capsule technology 215

Enterion technology 160, 218

Erodible matrix 29, 273, 288

Erythrocytes 66, 330

Extrusion 4, 47, 55, 65, 68, 115, 293, 295-298, 302, 308, 309, 314, 325, 327, 328

F

Fate of SEDDS 61, 62, 63

Fatty acid 20, 27, 41, 42, 53, 62-64, 140, 147, 167, 253, 256, 262, 273, 301

Floating drug delivery systems 24

Flocculation 138, 145, 146, 230-234, 237, 239, 241, 250, 251

Flow properties 198, 293, 313, 314

Fluid bed granulation 302-304

Fluorescent activated cell sorter 129

Flux regulators 180, 183

Follicle associated epithelium 111, 112, 116, 119, 122, 126

Fortavase 72

Fracture theory 163

Freeze-thaw cycle 243

G

GALT 111

Gastric retention 18, 20, 21, 22, 26, 29, 33, 82, 340

Gel microbeads 139

Gelucire 42, 67

Gengraf 72

GMS 44

Goblet cells 110, 112

GRAS 41, 69, 99

Gravitational separation 138

H

Hemodynamics 320

Heterogeneous 58, 141, 213, 214, 224, 225

Heteropolysachharide 274

Hirchsprung's disorder 85

HLB 39, 40, 42-45, 53, 54, 70, 147, 160, 236, 252-255

Hydrocolloids 141, 237, 255, 277, 347

Hydrodynamic pressure 279, 285

Hydrogel 21, 22, 23, 27, 86, 87, 96-98 , 188-190, 192, 284, 285, 340, 344, 345, 350, 352, 353

Hydrophilic and hydrophobic Polymers 182, 183

Hydrophilic polymer 180, 181, 183, 188, 190, 218, 284-286

Hydrophilic sandwich 218, 219

I

IBD 84, 87, 93, 100, 101, 159

In situ gel 25, 27, 267, 339, 340, 341, 343-353, 359

In vitro dissolution 16, 59, 311

Incompatibility 252, 287

Injectable drug delivery 352

Inorganic particles 139

Interfacial complexation 139

Interfacial tension 45, 52, 54, 229, 230, 236, 246, 247, 253, 255, 260

Isotropic mixture 39, 43, 45-47, 54

K

Kinetic property 230

L

Labrafil 42-44, 54, 71

Labrasol 44, 68

Large intestine 79, 80, 82, 84, 90, 109, 110, 159

Lauroglycol 43, 54

Lectins 102, 112, 124, 125, 126

Lipid nanoparticles 125, 139, 266, 324, 328, 331

Liposomes 109, 116, 117, 122, 123, 125, 127, 266, 319, 320, 321, 324, 325-333

Liquid crystals 339, 353-358, 359

Liquid membrane system 138

Lozenges 160, 161, 192-199

Lymphatic uptake 40, 70

Lymphoid tissue 84, 110-112, 114, 121, 122

Lyotropic liquid crystals 355, 358

M

Macroemulsions 138

Maisine 42, 67

Matrix type system 319

M-cell 109, 111-117, 119-127, 130, 131

M-Cell mediated transport 114, 122, 130

Medicated chewing gum 160, 199-201, 206, 207

Melt spheronization 302

Mesogenic properties 321

Mesophases 354-357

Metabolic clearance 320

Microemulsions 138, 319, 329

Micro-heterogeneous 225

Microparticle 31, 100, 116-118, 120, 121, 123, 125, 126, 129, 143, 266, 344

Molecular dispersion 224, 225

Monoclonal antibodies 112

Mononuclear phagocyte system 320

Morning arthritic pain 271

Mucoadhesion 22, 162

Mucoadhesive polymers 22, 164, 165, 324

Multilayered tablet 4, 168, 280

Multiple emulsions 137-139, 142-153, 246, 320, 323

Multiple-unit doses 293

N

Nanocapsules 266

Nanomedicine 320, 332

Nanoparticles 59, 101-103, 109, 112, 114, 116-118, 120-122, 124, 125, 127, 129, 139, 263, 266, 319-321, 323, 324, 328-333

Nanovectors 319, 320

Nasal delivery 351

Natural polymer 4, 233, 234, 340

Nematic liquid crystals 356

Neoral 65, 69, 71

Niosomes 319, 320, 330

Non-ionic surfactants 42, 43, 236

Norvir 73

Noyes–Whitney equation 12

Nutritive 226

O

Ocular delivery 351

Oils 24, 39, 41-43, 46, 53, 54, 56, 61, 64, 139, 140, 147, 196, 201, 202, 226, 250, 258-261

Optical microscopy and scanning electron microscopy techniques 310

Oral delivery 109, 130, 157, 159, 160, 179, 188, 323, 324, 331, 334, 350, 351

Osmosis 22, 176, 177, 188, 189

Osmotic controlled drug delivery 86, 87

Osmotic pressure gradients 11, 320

Osmotic pump 177, 179, 180, 182, 184-186, 271

Osmotic tablets 160, 176, 179-181, 184, 186

Ostwald ripening 138, 234, 235, 240

Oxidative 141, 250, 258, 262

P

Paracellular pathway 114

Parenteral 41, 109, 121, 140, 141, 157, 227, 228, 236, 265, 313, 348, 349

Patient compliance 1, 9, 23, 109, 122, 159, 167, 168, 188, 270, 271, 280, 287, 312, 313, 339, 340, 352

Peceol 43

Pellet 59, 65, 68, 82, 91, 100, 215, 216, 273, 292-302, 305-314, 349

Pelletization 292-295, 302, 305-308, 314

Permeation enhancers 164, 166, 167
Peyer's patches 108-115, 117-123, 125, 127, 129, 130, 331
p-glycoprotein 40, 70
pH Induced 188, 190
Pharmacodynamic 236, 272, 319
Pharmacokinetic 66, 164, 217, 236, 272, 314
Pharmacokinetics 1, 33, 62, 319, 326, 351
Phase inversion 138, 144, 250-253
Phospholipids 42, 140, 333
Photomicroscopic examination 240
Plasticizers 182
Plurololeique 43
Polarized light microscopy 356, 357
Polymeric microspheres 139
Polymeric nanoparticle 101-103, 323, 329, 333
Polymeric nanoparticles 101, 102, 103, 323, 329, 333
Polymerization 96, 97, 139, 324, 343-345
Polymerosomes 139
Polysaccharides 27, 93-95, 99, 110, 183, 233, 274, 276, 277, 279, 346, 350
Pre-blending 303
Pressure-based systems 86
Prodrug 82, 84, 86, 93, 99, 312, 319
Prolonged release 85, 151, 164, 208, 212, 287, 288, 352
Proximal colon 80
Pulsincap 87, 160, 187-192, 283-286

R

Rancidity 140, 250, 256, 258
Rectal and vaginal drug delivery 352
Redox-sensitive polymers 98
Reservoir-type system 318, 319
Resuspendability 241
Reverse micellar 361

Rotary processor 299
Roto granulation 299

S

Sandimmune 71
Sandwich osmotic tablets 184, 186
SEDDS 39-72
Sedimentation 55, 145, 225, 227-230, 233-235, 239, 241, 242, 251
Self-emulsifying drug delivery system 38, 54
Semipermeable membrane 28, 88, 177-181, 184, 185, 189, 192
SLS 45, 236
Smectic liquid crystals 356
SMEDDS 39
SNEDDS 39
Sol-Gel transition 346, 348
Solvent casting 171
Spans 43, 254
Spectroscopy 30, 58, 244, 349
Spheronization 4, 65, 68, 293, 295, 296-298, 302, 307, 308, 314
S-SEDDS 47, 51
Stability 39, 41, 42, 45-47, 53, 55-58, 60, 61, 64-66, 82, 85, 86, 95, 140, 146-149, 151, 170, 226-229, 235, 238-243, 246, 247, 250, 253, 255, 261, 263, 265, 267, 296, 326, 329, 331, 332, 340, 347, 354, 358
Steric stabilization 139
Submicron emulsion 331
Surface free energy 229, 230, 240, 247
Surfactants 39, 40, 42-46, 52-56, 58, 60, 61, 63, 64, 69, 70, 140, 141, 167, 236, 312, 328, 354, 358
Sustained release 100, 122, 151, 246, 265, 266, 277-279, 287, 301, 313, 318, 323, 324, 327, 329, 333, 339, 347, 350, 351, 358

Sustained release drug delivery 339, 358

Synthetic polymers 101, 233, 333, 348

T

Targeted release drug delivery systems 340

Targeting 26, 89, 93, 96, 98, 102, 103, 108, 109, 113, 117, 118, 121-127, 130, 152, 153, 158, 179, 188, 319-321, 323, 325, 329, 330, 332, 333

Targeting delivery 332

Tensile strength 4, 56, 216, 311

Therapeutic plasma concentration 271

Thermodynamically 45, 138, 227, 230, 245, 251, 329

Thermotropic liquid crystals 356, 358

Timed release/delayed release dosage forms 86

Tocopherol 65, 71, 258

Transient time 293

Transmission electron microscopy 58, 128, 357

Triglycerides 41, 42

Tweens 43

V

Vaccines 109, 112, 118, 121, 122, 124, 130, 328, 332, 334

W

Wetting theory 163

Wicking agents 183

Wurster process 303

X

X-ray scattering 357

Z

Zero order release 177, 209, 276, 280, 288, 318

Zeta potential 57, 58, 234, 236, 237, 242, 243, 263

www.ingramcontent.com/pod-product-compliance
Lightning Source LLC
Chambersburg PA
CBHW050744150726
48196CB00003B/352